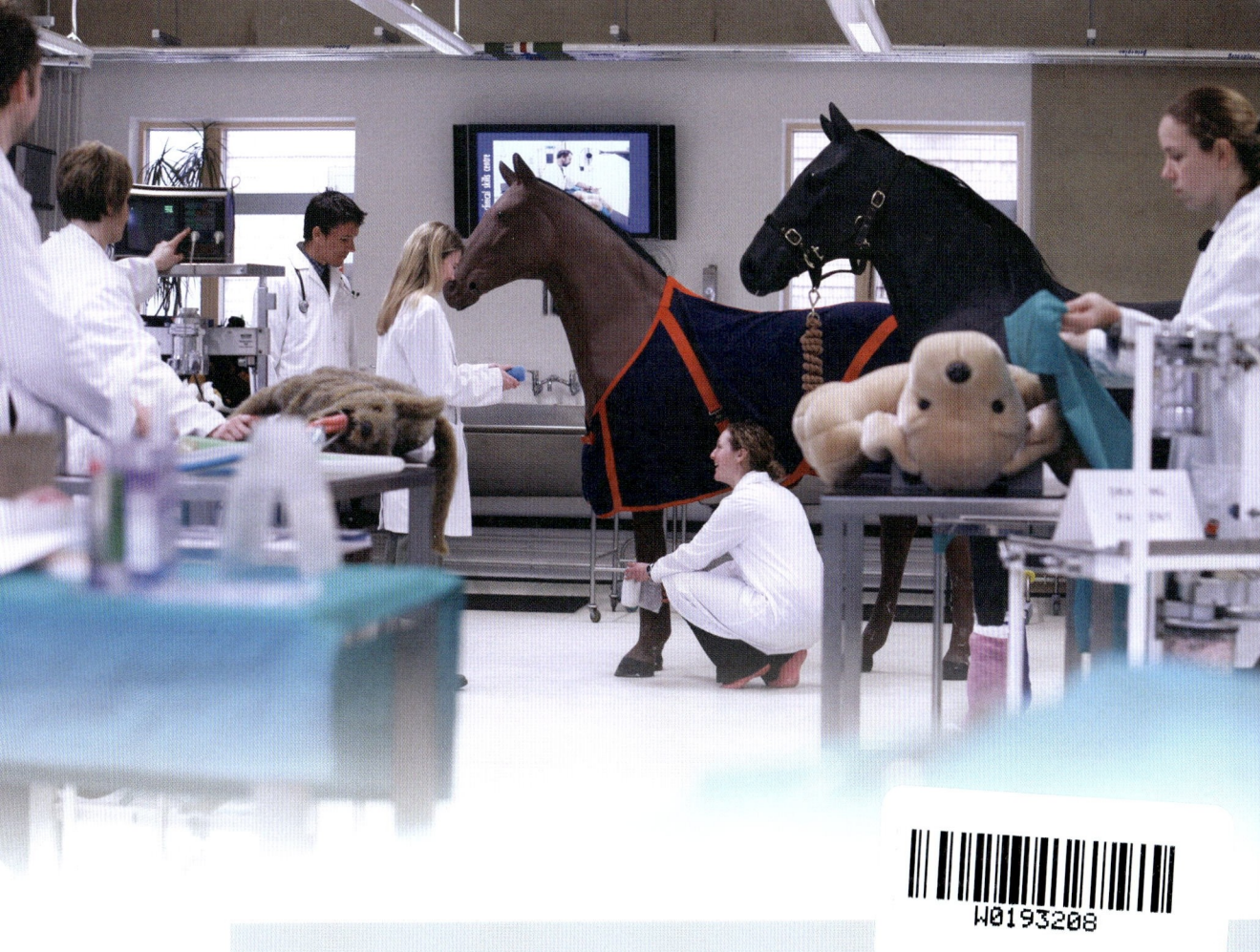

Veterinary Clinical
Skills Manual

W0193208

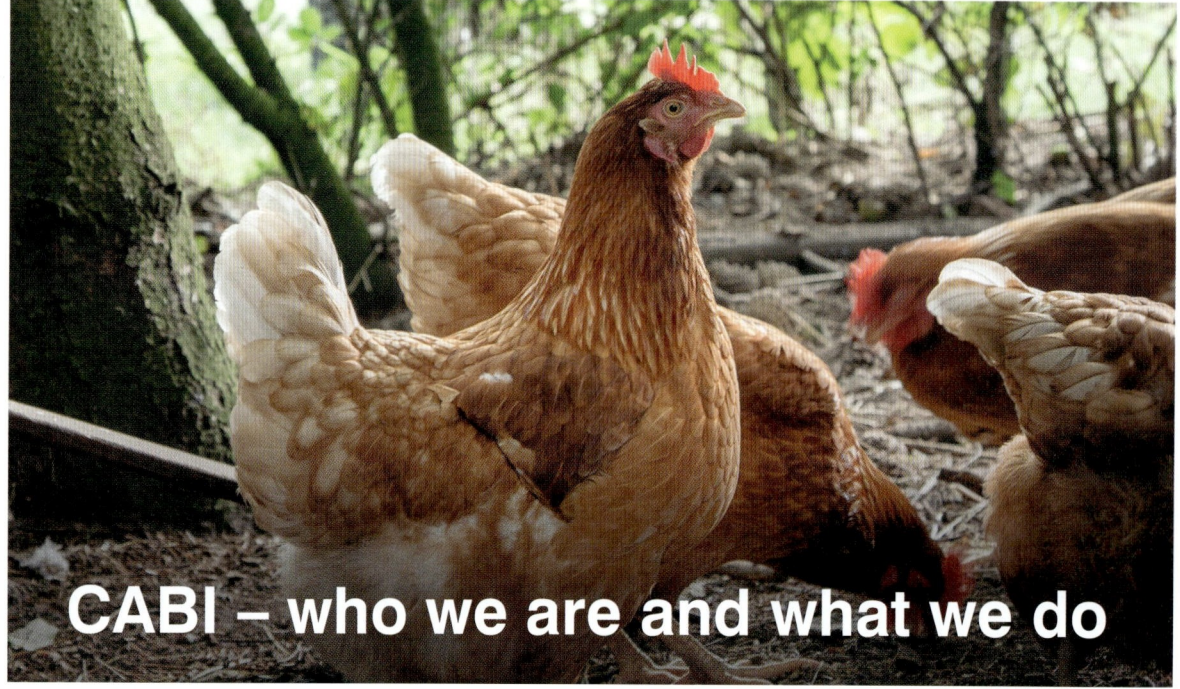

CABI – who we are and what we do

This book is published by **CABI**, an international not-for-profit organisation that improves people's lives worldwide by providing information and applying scientific expertise to solve problems in agriculture and the environment.

CABI is also a global publisher producing key scientific publications, including world renowned databases, as well as compendia, books, ebooks and full text electronic resources. We publish content in a wide range of subject areas including: agriculture and crop science / animal and veterinary sciences / ecology and conservation / environmental science / horticulture and plant sciences / human health, food science and nutrition / international development / leisure and tourism.

The profits from CABI's publishing activities enable us to work with farming communities around the world, supporting them as they battle with poor soil, invasive species and pests and diseases, to improve their livelihoods and help provide food for an ever growing population.

CABI is an international intergovernmental organisation, and we gratefully acknowledge the core financial support from our member countries (and lead agencies) including:

  Ministry of Agriculture People's Republic of China

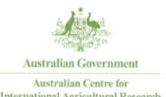 Australian Government
Australian Centre for International Agricultural Research

 Agriculture and Agri-Food Canada

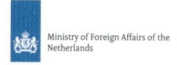 Ministry of Foreign Affairs of the Netherlands

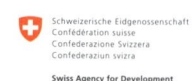 Schweizerische Eidgenossenschaft
Confédération suisse
Confederazione Svizzera
Confederaziun svizra

Swiss Agency for Development and Cooperation SDC

Discover more

To read more about CABI's work, please visit: **www.cabi.org**

Browse our books at: **www.cabi.org/bookshop**,
or explore our online products at: **www.cabi.org/publishing-products**

Interested in writing for CABI? Find our author guidelines here:
www.cabi.org/publishing-products/information-for-authors/

Veterinary Clinical Skills Manual

Edited by

Nichola Coombes and Ayona Silva-Fletcher

The Royal Veterinary College, London

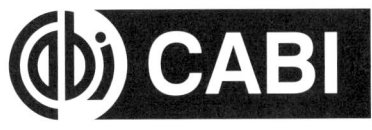

CABI is a trading name of CAB International

CABI
Nosworthy Way
Wallingford
Oxfordshire OX10 8DE
UK

Tel: +44 (0)1491 832111
Fax: +44 (0)1491 833508
E-mail: info@cabi.org
Website: www.cabi.org

CABI
745 Atlantic Avenue
8th Floor
Boston, MA 02111
USA

Tel: +1 (617)682-9015
E-mail: cabi-nao@cabi.org

© CAB International 2018. All rights reserved. No part of this publication may be reproduced in any form or by any means, electronically, mechanically, by photocopying, recording or otherwise, without the prior permission of the copyright owners.

A catalogue record for this book is available from the British Library, London, UK.

Library of Congress Cataloging-in-Publication Data

Names: Coombes, Nichola, editor. | Silva-Fletcher, Ayona, editor.
Title: Veterinary clinical skills manual / edited by Nichola Coombes and Ayona Silva-Fletcher.
Description: Wallingford, Oxfordshire ; Boston, MA : CABI, [2018] | Includes bibliographical references and index.
Identifiers: LCCN 2017054582 (print) | LCCN 2017056628 (ebook) | ISBN 9781786391636 (pdf) | ISBN 9781786391643 (ePub) |
    ISBN 9781786391629 (pbk. : alk. paper)
Subjects: | MESH: Education, Veterinary--methods | Animal Diseases--diagnosis | Animal Diseases--therapy
Classification: LCC SF756.3 (ebook) | LCC SF756.3 (print) | NLM SF 756.3 | DDC 636.089/069--dc23
LC record available at https://lccn.loc.gov/2017054582

ISBN-13: 978 1 78639 162 9 (pbk)
          978 1 78639 163 6 (PDF)
          978 1 78639 164 3 (ePub)

Commissioning editor: Caroline Makepeace
Associate editor: Alexandra Lainsbury
Production editor: Tim Kapp

Typeset by SPi, Pondicherry, India
Printed and bound in the UK by Bell & Bain Ltd, Glasgow, G46 7UQ

Contents

List of Contributors ix

List of Skill Sheets xiii

List of Videos xv

Acknowledgements xvii

Foreword xix
Holger Andreas Volk

Editors' Note xxi
Nichola Coombes and Ayona Silva-Fletcher

How to Use this Book xxiii

Section 1: Introduction 1
    Section Editor – Ayona Silva-Fletcher
    Background 2

1. **Developing Veterinary Clinical Skills: The Pedagogy** 3
    Stephen A. May

2. **The Modern Outcome-based Curriculum and the Role of the Clinical Skills Laboratory** 9
    Ayona Silva-Fletcher

3. **The Clinical Skills Centre Models Relevant to Location** 16
    Nichola Coombes, Ayona Silva-Fletcher, Julie Williamson, Stacy Anderson, B. Otgontugs,
    N. Odontsetseg, Aruna Amarasinghe, M.L.A.N.R Deepani, Catherine. J. Wager, Britt Coles,
    Desiree Karlsson, Pia Haubro Andersen, Zuhair Bani Ismail and Ehab Abu-Basha

Section 2: Surgical Theatre Skills 29
    Section Editor – Fiona Brown
    Introduction 30

4. **Theatre Practice** 31
    Fiona Brown

5. **Surgical Instruments** 49
    Alison Young

6. **The Fundamentals of Suturing** 60
    Nicola Jayne Kulendra

Section 3: Anaesthesia   93
Section Editor – Fiona Brown
Introduction   94

7. **The Anaesthetic Machine**   95
Fiona Brown and Chris Seymour

8. **Breathing Systems, Intubation and Monitoring**   105
Fiona Brown, Chris Seymour and Caroline Hoy

Section 4: Principles of Good Practice in the Laboratory   127
Section Editor – Alison Langridge
Introduction   128

9. **Laboratory Skills and Sample Collection**   129
Kate English and Alison Langridge

10. **Using a Microscope and Preparing Samples**   145
Kate English and Alison Langridge

11. **Urine and Faecal Analysis**   159
Alison Langridge and Kate English

Section 5: General Clinical Skills   169
Section Editor – Alison Langridge
Introduction   170

12. **Physical Examination, Fluid Therapy, Tube and Drain Management**   171
Karen Humm

13. **Principles of Small Animal Bandaging**   190
Alison Langridge

14. **Pharmacy**   203
Hilary Orpet

Section 6: Patient Handling and Diagnostics   213
Section Editor – Isobel Vincent
Introduction   214

15. **General Principles of Animal Handling**   217
Isobel Vincent

16. **Diagnostic Imaging**   249
Panagiotis Mantis and Victoria Watts

17. **Equine Radiography – Example Tarsus**   272
Renate Weller and Alana Cyman

Section 7: Large Animal Skills   291
Section Editor – Isobel Vincent
Introduction   292

18. **Udder Health**   293
John Fishwick and Isobel Vincent

19. **Equine Procedures**   298
    Imogen Johns

20. **Equine Foot Related Skills: Example Shoe Removal**   318
    Renate Weller and Peter Day

Section 8: Assessment of Clinical Skills   329
    Section Editor – Nichola Coombes
    Introduction   330

21. **Practical Assessments – Assessments in a Simulated Environment**   331
    Stephen A. May and Ayona Silva-Fletcher

22. **Objectively Structured Clinical Examinations – the Practicalities**   346
    Nichola Coombes

Section 9: Moving Forward   357
    Section Editor – Ayona Silva-Fletcher
    Introduction   358

23. **'Mind the Gap' – the Development, Validation and Evaluation of a Veterinary
    Clinical Skills Model**   359
    Rachel Lumbis

24. **Simulators in Veterinary Clinical Skills Education: Background and Examples** 368
    Tierney Kinnison

25. **The Transition between the Clinical Skills Lab and the Real World – Perspectives from a New
    Graduate 2 Years After Qualifying**   376
    Desiree Janine Herrick

Glossary   383

Index   387

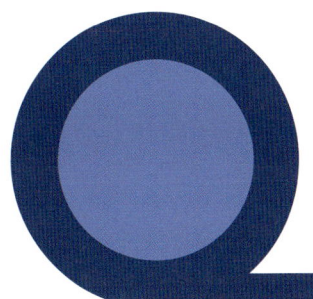

List of Contributors

Ehab Abu-Basha DVM MSc PhD, Professor of Pharmacology and Toxicology, Faculty of Veterinary Medicine, Jordan University of Science and Technology, PO Box 3030, Irbid 22110, Jordan. Email: Eabubasha@just.edu.jo

Aruna Amarasinghe BVSc MSc Mphil, Lecturer in Large Animal Reproduction, Faculty of Veterinary Medicine and Animal Science, University of Peradeniya, Sri Lanka. Email: arunavetlk@gmail.com

Pia Haubro Andersen DVM PhD DVSci, Professor of Large Animal Surgery, Department of Clinical Sciences: Equine Medicine Unit, Swedish University of Agricultural Sciences, Box 7054, 75007 Uppsala, Sweden. Email: pia.haubro.andersen@slu.se

Stacy Anderson DVM MVSc PhD DACVS-LA, Director of Large Animal Clinical Skills, Lincoln Memorial University – College of Veterinary Medicine, 6965 Cumberland Gap Parkway, Harrogate, TN 37752, USA. Email: stacy.anderson@lmunet.edu

Fiona Handyside Brown PGDipVetEd BSc(Hons) RVN FHEA, Assistant Lecturer in Veterinary Clinical Skills, Clinical Science and Services (CSS), Clinical Skills Centre, The Royal Veterinary College, Hawkshead Lane, North Mymms, Hatfield, Hertfordshire, AL9 7TA, UK. Email: fbrown@rvc.ac.uk

Britt Coles DVM PhD(Ecology), Research Assistant, Department of Clinical Sciences, Equine Medicine Unit, Swedish University of Agricultural Sciences, Box 7054, 75007 Uppsala, Sweden. Email: britt.coles@slu.se

Nichola A. Coombes RVN PGCert(MedEd) MScVetEd FHEA, Manager of the Clinical Skills Centre and Clinical Educator, Clinical Skills Centre, Clinical Science and Services (CSS), The Royal Veterinary College, Hawkshead Lane, North Mymms, Hatfield, Hertfordshire, AL9 7TA, UK. Email: ncoombes@rvc.ac.uk

Alana Cyman Equine Diagnostic Imaging, Clinical Science and Services (CSS), The Royal Veterinary College, Hawkshead Lane, North Mymms, Hatfield, Hertfordshire, AL9 7TA, UK. Email: acyman@rvc.ac.uk

Peter Day DipWCF, Farriery Services, Equine Referral Hospital, The Royal Veterinary College, Hawkshead Lane, North Mymms, Hatfield, Hertfordshire, AL9 7TA, UK. Email: pday@rvc.ac.uk

M.L.A.N.R. Deepani BVS MSc PGcert Vet Ed PhD, Senior Lecturer in Genetics and Animal Breeding, Statistics; Educator of Vet Surgery Clinical Skills, Department of Farm Animal Production and Health, Faculty of Veterinary Medicine and Animal Science, University of Peradeniya, Sri Lanka. Email: nirupa_deepani@yahoo.com

Kate English BSc BVetMed FRCPath MRCVS, Lecturer in Veterinary Clinical Pathology, Pathobiology and Population Sciences (PPS), The Royal Veterinary College, Hawkshead Lane, North Mymms, Hatfield, Hertfordshire, AL9 7TA, UK. Email: kenglish@rvc.ac.uk

John Fishwick MA VetMB DCHP DipECBHM MRCVS, Senior Lecturer in Dairy Herd Medicine, Pathobiology and Population Sciences (PPS), Farm Animal Health and Production Group, The Royal Veterinary College, Hawkshead Lane, North Mymms, Hatfield, Hertfordshire, AL9 7TA, UK. Email: jfishwick@rvc.ac.uk

Desiree Herrick BS BVetMed MRCVS, Veterinary Surgeon at Vets4Pets Basildon, Unit 1A Old Market Retail Park, High Street, Pitsea, Basildon, SS13 3BY, UK. Email: dherrick@rvc.ac.uk

Caroline Hoy RVN VTS (Anes/Analgesia) NCert (A&CC), Veterinary Nurse, Clinical Science and Services (CSS), Queen Mother Hospital for Animals (QMHA), The Royal Veterinary College, Hawkshead Lane, North Mymms, Hatfield, Hertfordshire, AL9 7TA, UK. Email: choy@rvc.ac.uk

Karen Humm MA VetMB MSc CertVA DACVECC DipECVECC FHEA MRCVS, Senior Lecturer in Emergency and Critical Care, Clinical Science and Services (CSS), Queen Mother Hospital for Animals (QMHA), The

Royal Veterinary College, Hawkshead Lane, North Mymms, Hatfield, Hertfordshire, AL9 7TA, UK. Email: khumm@rvc.ac.uk

Zuhair Bani Ismail DVM Diplomate ABVP, Professor, Veterinary Surgery, Faculty of Veterinary Medicine, Jordan University of Science & Technology, PO Box 3030, Irbid 22110, Jordan. Email: zuhair72@just.edu.jo

Imogen Johns BVSc PGCAP Dip ACVIM FHEA Dip ACVIM MRCVS, B and W Equine Vets, Breadstone Equine Hospital, Breadstone, Berkeley, Gloucestershire, GL13 9HG, UK. Email: imogen.johns@bwequinevets.co.uk

Desiree Karlsson RVN, Manager and Educator at the Clinical Teaching Centre (Kliniskt Träningscentrum), Department of Clinical Sciences at the Swedish University of Agricultural Sciences, Box 7054, 75007 Uppsala, Sweden. Email: desiree.karlsson@slu.se

Tierney Kinnison PGCertVetEd BSc MSc PhD FHEA, Postdoctoral Research Assistant, Pathobiology and Population Sciences (PPS), Veterinary Epidemiology, Economics and Public Health, The Royal Veterinary College, Hawkshead Lane, North Mymms, Hatfield, Hertfordshire, AL9 7TA, UK. Email: tkinnison@rvc.ac.uk

Nicola Jayne Kulendra BVetMed (Hons) MVetMed CertVDI DipECVS MRCVS, Lecturer in Small Animal Surgery, Clinical Science and Services (CSS), Queen Mother Hospital for Animals (QMHA), The Royal Veterinary College, Hawkshead Lane, North Mymms, Hatfield, Hertfordshire, AL9 7TA, UK. Email: nkulendra@rvc.ac.uk

Alison J. Langridge MScVetEd RVN BA(Hons) FHEA, Assistant Lecturer in Veterinary Clinical Skills, Clinical Skills Centre, Clinical Science and Services (CSS), The Royal Veterinary College, Hawkshead Lane, North Mymms, Hatfield, Hertfordshire, AL9 7TA, UK. Email: alangridge@rvc.ac.uk

Rachel H. Lumbis MSc(VetEd) BSc(Hons) PGCert(MedEd) RVN CertSAN FHEA, Lecturer in Veterinary Nursing & Course Director FdSc VN & BSc VN, Clinical Science and Services (CSS), Veterinary Nursing School, The Royal Veterinary College, Hawkshead Lane, North Mymms, Hatfield, Hertfordshire, AL9 7TA, UK. Email: rlumbis@rvc.ac.uk

Panagiotis Mantis DVM DipECVDI FHEA MRCVS, Consultant Radiologist, Hon. Assoc. Professor of Veterinary Diagnostic Imaging, University of Nottingham, Dick White Referrals, Station Farm, London Road, Six Mile Bottom, Newmarket, Cambridgeshire, CB8 0UH, UK. Email: pete.mantis@dwr.co.uk

Stephen A. May MA VetMB PhD DVR DEO FRCVS DipECVS FHEA NTF, Senior Vice Principal, Director, Lifelong Independent Veterinary Education (LIVE), Clinical Science and Services (CSS), The Royal Veterinary College, Hawkshead Lane, North Mymms, Hatfield, Hertfordshire, AL9 7TA, UK. Email: smay@rvc.ac.uk

N. Odontsetseg BVM PhD, Veterinarian, Animal Health Project, Swiss Agency for Development and Cooperation SDC, Ulaanbaatar, Mongolia. Email: odontsetseg@livestock.mn

Hilary A. Orpet MScVetEd BSc DipAVN(Surgical) FHEA CertEdDipCABT(COAPE) RVN, Senior Lecturer in Veterinary Nursing, Veterinary Nursing School, Clinical Science and Services (CSS), The Royal Veterinary College, Hawkshead Lane, North Mymms, Hatfield, Hertfordshire, AL9 7TA, UK. Email: horpet@rvc.ac.uk

Bat Otgontugs BVM, Lecturer, Department of Veterinary Basic Sciences, School of Veterinary Medicine, Mongolian University of Life Sciences, Zaisan-17024, Ulaanbaatar, Mongolia. Email: bat.otgontugs@yahoo.com

Chris Seymour MA VetMB DVA DipECVAA FHEA MRCVS, Veterinary Anaesthetist, Davies Veterinary Specialists, Manor Farm Business Park, Higham Gobion, Hitchin, Hertfordshire, SG5 3HR, UK. Email: chris.seymour@vetspecialists.co.uk

Ayona Silva-Fletcher BVSc PhD MA(Med Ed) FHEA FSLCVS NTF, Professor and Course Director in Veterinary Education, Lifelong Independent Veterinary Education (LIVE), Clinical Science and Services (CSS), The Royal Veterinary College, Hawkshead Lane, North Mymms, Hatfield, Hertfordshire, AL9 7TA, UK. Email: asilvafletcher@rvc.ac.uk

Isobel Vincent BSc PhD PgCertMedEd FHEA, Lecturer in Animal Husbandry and Veterinary Skills, Pathobiology and Population Sciences (PPS), Clinical Skills Centre, The Royal Veterinary College, Hawkshead Lane, North Mymms, Hatfield, Hertfordshire, AL9 7TA, UK. Email: ivincent@rvc.ac.uk

Holger Andreas Volk DVM PGCAP PhD DipECVN FHEA MRCVS, Head of Department, Clinical Science and Services (CSS), Professor of Veterinary Neurology and Neurosurgery, The Royal Veterinary College, Hawkshead Lane, North Mymms, Hatfield, Hertfordshire, AL9 7TA, UK. Email: hvolk@rvc.ac.uk

Catherine Wager GradDipVN RVN, Clinical Skills Centre Facilitator, University of Cambridge, Department of Veterinary Medicine, Madingley Road, Cambridge, CB3 0ES, UK. Email: cw619@cam.ac.uk

Victoria Watts BSc(Hons), Radiographer, Clinical Science and Services (CSS), Queen Mother Hospital for Animals (QMHA), The Royal Veterinary College, Hawkshead Lane, North Mymms, Hatfield, Hertfordshire, AL9 7TA, UK. Email: vwatts@rvc.ac.uk

Renate Weller Dr Med.Vet PhD MRCVS FHEA NTF, Professor in Comparative Imaging and Biomechanics, Clinical Science and Services (CSS), The Royal Veterinary College, Hawkshead Lane, North Mymms, Hatfield, Hertfordshire, AL9 7TA, UK. Email: rweller@rvc.ac.uk

Julie Williamson DVM MSc AFAMEE, Director of Small Animal Clinical Skills, Assistant Professor of Veterinary Clinical Skills, Lincoln Memorial University – College of Veterinary Medicine, 6965 Cumberland Gap Parkway, Harrogate, TN 37752, USA. Email: Julie.Williamson@lmunet.edu

Alison Young DipAVN (Surgery), VTS (Surgery), RVN, Head Theatre Nurse, Clinical Science and Services (CSS), Queen Mother Hospital for Animals (QMHA), The Royal Veterinary College, Hawkshead Lane, North Mymms, Hatfield, Hertfordshire, AL9 7TA, UK. Email: ayoung@rvc.ac.uk

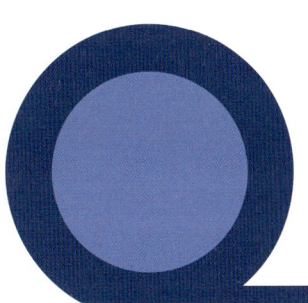

List of Skill Sheets (SS)

Section	Chapter	Sheet No.	Title
2	4	4.1	Surgical scrub
		4.2	Hand drying
		4.3	Gowning
		4.4	Closed gloving
		4.5	Open gloving
		4.6	Draping using the four-quadrant technique
	5	5.7	Opening a sterile instrument pouch
		5.8	Instrument handling and selection
	6	6.9	One-handed tie, right-hand method
		6.10	Two-handed tie (the 'bird's beak' version)
		6.11	Instrument suture – square knot or surgeon's knot
3	7	7.12	Anaesthetic machine set-up
	8	8.13	Parallel Lack breathing system
		8.14	Circle breathing system
		8.15	Bain breathing system
		8.16	Modified Ayres T-piece breathing system
		8.17	Anaesthesia help sheet: calculating fresh gas flow
4	9	9.18	Venepuncture techniques: blood collection by Vacutainer
		9.19	Venepuncture techniques: blood collection by syringe + needle
		9.20	Fine-needle aspirate biopsy (FNAB) and smear
		9.21	Packing a laboratory sample
	10	10.22	Microscope set-up
		10.23	Preparing and examining blood smear and stain
		10.24	Packed cell volume (PCV)
	11	11.25	Obtaining a urine specific gravity reading and a dipstick reading
		11.26	Preparing a urine sample for microscope analysis
		11.27	McMaster faecal egg count technique

Section	Chapter	Sheet No.	Title
5	12	12.28	Cranial nerve examination
		12.29	Ophthalmology practical: eye examination
		12.30	Assessing urinary output in a catheterized patient
		12.31	Catheterizing a limb
		12.32	Setting up intravenous fluids
	13	13.33	Applying a canine forelimb bandage
		13.34	Applying a canine chest drain bandage
		13.35	Applying an ear bandage
6	15	15.36	Rugging up a horse
		15.37	Tying up a horse using a quick-release knot
		15.38	Putting a tail bandage on a horse
		15.39	Putting a stable bandage on a horse
		15.40	Applying a lower-limb protective bandage on a horse
		15.41	How to halter a cow
	16	16.42	Imaging BVA/KC hips
		16.43	Imaging caudo-cranial stifle
		16.44	Ultrasound (U/S) set-up
	17	17.45	Radiography help sheet: understanding radiographic projections
		17.46	Radiographic projections of the foot
		17.47	Radiographic projections of the tarsus
7	18	18.48	Bovine sterile milk sampling method
		18.49	California Milk Test (CMT) sampling method
	19	19.50	Equine fluid therapy set-up
		19.51	Common sites for intramuscular injections
		19.52	Passing a nasogastric tube in a horse
	20	20.53	Shoe removal
		20.54	Paring the sole and trimming the hoof wall

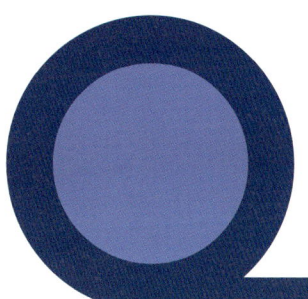

List of Videos (V)

4.1   WHO hand wash
4.2   Surgical gowning (fabric gown)
4.3   Surgical gowning (paper gown)
4.4   Closed gloving
4.5   Open gloving
4.6   Draping (4 drape)

6.1   One-handed tie
6.2   Two-handed tie
6.3   Modified Miller's knot
6.4   Slip knot
6.5   Aberdeen knot
6.6   Simple interrupted suture
6.7   Simple continuous suture

7.1   How to set up the anaesthetic machine

10.1   Microscope set-up (shorter video)
10.2   Blood smear and stain
10.3   Packed cell volume (PCV)

11.1   Urine SG

12.1   Ophthalmic examination.
12.2   Place an intravenous catheter in a dog.
12.3   Prepare and set up fluid admin (small animal).

13.1   Ear bandage

15.1   Restraint of a cat (out of a basket, jugular/cephalic blood sampling & wrapping cat in a towel)
15.2   Crush cage
15.3   Handling a cat
15.4   Check chain – dog
15.5   Restraint of a large dog for injection
15.6   Restraint techniques for a small to medium dog
15.7   Restraint of a large dog for jugular and cephalic sampling
15.8   Hamster handling
15.9   Rat handling
15.10 Rabbit lifting and carrying

15.11   Chicken Handling
15.12   Rugging up a horse
15.13   Quick-release knot
15.14   Lead rope over neck & put on head collar
15.15   Tying up a cow
15.16   Sheep handling including 1 & 2 person method
15.17   Lambing

19.1   Equine jugular placement in a horse
19.2   Equine fluid therapy

20.1   Removing a horse shoe

Acknowledgements

This book has been put together by many different contributors, as has the Clinical Skills Centre (CSC). Our sincere thanks to all the authors and specifically to the section editors, Fiona Brown, Alison Langridge and Isobel Vincent, who tirelessly worked with their author teams to develop coherent themes within individual sections.

A special word of thanks to Melanie Cappello, Brian Cox, Nina Davies (née Turnbull), Stan Head, Stephen May, Peter Nunn, Matthew Pead, Paul Probyn, Perdi Welsh and Belinda Yamagishi, without whose help the CSC and the book would not have flourished!

We are also indebted to many unnamed staff and students who over the years have and are continuously supporting us to make the CSC the best environment for skills learning at the RVC.

Foreword

Every modern veterinary curriculum will attempt to further close the educational gap to ensure that recently graduated veterinary professionals will have all the skills and competences required to hit the road running with confidence. Developing clinical skills needs repetitive practice in a safe learning environment. A game shifter has been the development of Clinical Skills Centres in veterinary teaching institutes worldwide to support skills development in students. Today at the Royal Veterinary College (RVC) it is hard for new students and some younger faculty and staff to imagine a time when these centres did not exist. The RVC set up its first Clinical Skills Centre in 2004 and it was greeted with such enthusiasm by students that the RVC quickly conceived a facility on a greater scale. This was created, in 2006, in purpose-designed spaces in the College's Lifelong and Independent Veterinary Education Centre (Centre of Excellence in Teaching and Learning), with funding from the Higher Education Funding Council for England. The centre started small, with a few stations, but today there are more than 50 stations for practice and assessments.

This centre, acting as a bridge from classroom to clinic, deals with the development of fluency in practical tasks that are a source of concern to new graduates, as they become independent practitioners. However, the past 11 years has been a period of iterative learning on how to convert the concept of the classroom to clinic, a bridge into a practical programme of sequential skills development across the 5-year veterinary programme.

This book represents another marker of our progress in clinical skills development. It captures the content and techniques of the modern veterinary clinical skills centre within a pedagogical framework spanning the last 3 years of a veterinary programme. Like the authors, I hope the lessons learned at the RVC will transfer to other clinical programmes nationally and internationally, so that students are helped in their personal skills development and curriculum designers are inspired to find ways to better develop veterinary Day One skills within the confines of the often overcrowded first clinical degree programme.

It gives me great pleasure to endorse this book and I hope it will inspire and support you all.

Holger Andreas Volk DVM PGCAP PhD DipECVN FHEA MRCVS
Head of Department, Clinical Science and Services (CSS)
Professor of Veterinary Neurology and Neurosurgery
The Royal Veterinary College, UK

Editors' Note

This book has come about as the culmination of a 14-year journey by the Royal Veterinary College (RVC) to enhance the teaching of practical skills in its Clinical Skills Centre (CSC). Since the establishment of the RVC, as the first Veterinary School in the UK in 1791, the teaching of clinical skills has progressed from direct practise by students on live animals to the use of a CSC as the starting point for training in practical techniques. This transition has been facilitated by the recognition that the first steps in development of practical skills, such as surgical instrument and anaesthetic machine usage as well as sample taking, is best practised on manikins and models rather than on live animals. When the original CSC concept was put forward there was no blueprint to follow in the world of veterinary education. In the absence of a veterinary model, the RVC turned to the experience gained in medical education, with visits from 2002 to Dundee, Sheffield and King's Medical Schools to collect ideas for models and learning materials and to understand how such centres are best managed and run. This pioneering endeavour by the RVC has proved to be the cornerstone of success of CSCs in the veterinary sector. Today many veterinary teaching institutions have reaped the rewards of RVC's initial model, developing and expanding their own CSCs to enhance the learning of skills by their students.

There have been successes as well as failures in this journey of CSC development at the RVC. Many staff members and students have contributed, from providing ideas to developing models, skills sheets, videos and assessments. Today many are still contributing by refining the CSC stations and assessment item checklists. The rich pool of experience gained by the CSC is reflected in the many ways that this book can be used, not least helping students to learn and enhance their clinical skills. In addition, this book may help educators to improve the teaching of complex skills and procedures that require multiple steps and repetition in the safe environment of a CSC. To be told that 'I've shown you how to do that before' is not enough for the learner to become proficient. An important premise behind the concept of a CSC is to take away the fear of making mistakes on a live animal, so that initial learning can be facilitated and then consolidated. Educators should also be aware of the importance within a CSC class of providing additional information and the context for the skill.

We hope that this book will illustrate better how a group of dedicated and diligent educators are working together to ensure that students have a safe learning environment with the necessary support to learn and practise clinical skills that they will need to practise veterinary medicine successfully. A CSC is an effective place to learn and is also an enjoyable experience for both students and trainers, leading to competent graduates who will go forth and practise with care and confidence.

Nichola Coombes and Ayona Silva-Fletcher

How to Use this Book

This book is firstly a practical guide to veterinary clinical skills, how they are practised in a simulated environment and how they transfer into the 'real' clinical environment. Over many years we have developed the Skills Sheets we routinely use for teaching students. These are included in the book within the relevant chapters, but are cross-referenced to other chapters where they may be useful. In many cases you will also be able to access online relevant videos demonstrating the skill, or additional skills relevant to that chapter.

This book is divided into nine sections, of which six are practical sections. The six practical sections are Sections 2–7.

Section 1 – Introduction

Section 2 – Surgical Theatre Skills

Section 3 – Anaesthesia

Section 4 – Principles and Good Practice in the Laboratory

Section 5 – General Clinical Skills

Section 6 – Patient Handling and Diagnostics

Section 7 – Large Animal Skills

Section 8 – Assessment of Clinical Skills

Section 9 – Moving Forward

Within each practical section there are two or more chapters. The chapter offers detailed guidance on how to perform a skill. This is done using skills sheets and videos to support your development. Some skills are fundamental 'Day One' skills, i.e. skills in which you would expect to be competent on the day you graduate from university. There are also 'Year One' skills, i.e. skills you should have knowledge of and maybe have performed, but are not competent in as yet because you need more experience in the skill, or the ability to perform the skill in real clinical situations.

Icons

Within each chapter you will find the following icons.

	Clinical point to consider
	Hint to make life easier

	Think about this before going further
	Watch this video
	Skills sheet
	Definitely do not do this
	Moving forwards – Year One skill competence
	Calculations

The icons within the chapters of the six practical sections are used to emphasize points to consider in practising the skill. You can follow the guidance offered by the skills sheets and watch the videos as you practise. Also pay attention to 'definitely do not do this' sections.

Section 1

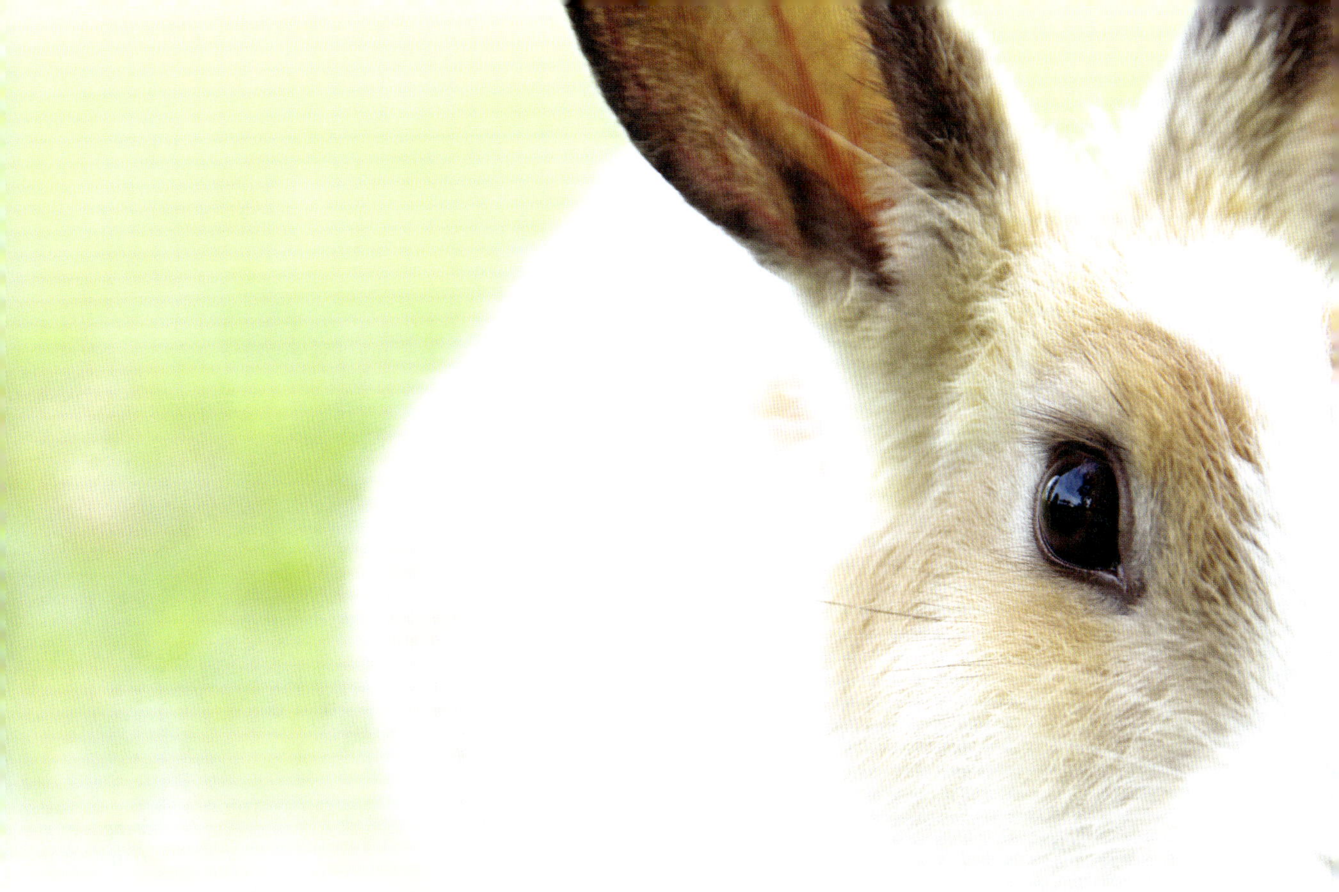

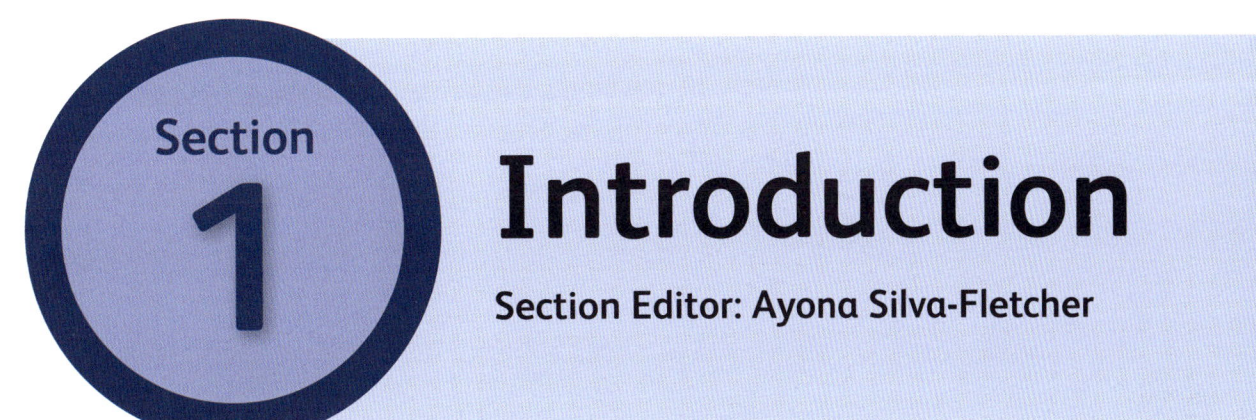

Introduction

Section Editor: Ayona Silva-Fletcher

Background

A busy veterinary clinic is probably not the best starting point to learn and practise clinical skills. Although the student can experience, observe and learn from the busy clinic it is not a safe and calm environment to learn a new skill; the presence of large or small animal patients, anxious clients, a veterinary team stressed and pressed for time and a multitude of clinical procedures may all hinder efficient learning. The starting point of a new skill should ideally happen elsewhere, away from onlookers and without risk to the patient.

The simulated environment created in a clinical skills centre (CSC), though far removed from the messy and complex clinical situation, is quiet and safe: the student can make mistakes, repeat procedures and learn from these to practise a skill until they are competent and confident. How does learning happen in a CSC? Can the skills be taught and learnt in an effective manner? Is there a correct way to guide the student? These are some of the questions that we answer in this introductory section of the book.

There is a growing body of evidence-based knowledge on learning theories and principles that contribute to effective learning. As more and more veterinary teaching institutions are moving towards competence/outcome-based curricula, it is necessary to understand how to guide our students and trainee tutors to develop these skills. A body of underlying knowledge is essential to perform an effective clinical skill and both educators and students should be fully aware of this before starting to teach and learn a clinical skill. The introductory section of this book explores the underlying theories that support student learning and how the trainers/educators can effectively use these theories and concepts to support student learning in a CSC environment. The aim is to provide an evidence-based approach, using examples from well-established and developing CSCs from around the world.

Within this section there are three chapters as outlined below.

Chapter 1: Developing Veterinary Clinical Skills: The Pedagogy

Chapter 2: The Modern Outcome-based Curriculum and the Role of the Clinical Skills Laboratory

Chapter 3: The Clinical Skills Centre Models Relevant to Location

Chapter 1 explores learning theories that underpin and enhance skills teaching, such as active learning, emotions that impact learning and how to overcome barriers such as fear, anxiety and lack of confidence. Chapter 1 provides essential knowledge for tutors to help them to utilize the principles of skills teaching and best practice guidelines on how to provide students with formative feedback. For students, Chapter 1 explains why CSCs provide an opportunity to move from a novice level of skill to competence and the advantages of participating in structured simulations and practicse within a supported and safe learning environment.

Chapter 2 explores the modern veterinary curriculum and the competences to be expected as an outcome of following an accredited veterinary degree. The growing demands exerted by national, regional and global veterinary curricula are to produce competent graduates who can perform immediately in the clinical workplace, rather than just having theoretical knowledge about a skill. The CSC can create opportunities to practise skills that are identified as outcomes by the curriculum. In Chapter 2 an attempt is made to answer how and what to teach as essential skills for veterinary and para-veterinary undergraduates. These experiential learning opportunities are designed to closely mimic (or to resemble) the clinical workplace.

Chapter 3 describes the successful practices of the growing number of CSC labs from different parts of the world. It shows how CSCs have adapted the core veterinary curricula to provide appropriate learning outcomes for local students and local community needs. In addition, Chapter 3 describes how successful CSCs promote self-directed learning through the provision of drop-in or appointment-based access.

Developing Veterinary Clinical Skills: The Pedagogy

Professor Stephen A. May
The Royal Veterinary College, London

The clinical professions are science based. This is part of the 'social contract' that in the case of the veterinary profession has led, in countries such as the UK, to monopoly powers for qualified individuals when it comes to the diagnosis and treatment of disease in animals (May, 2013). Society grants to veterinarians the privilege of caring for its animals provided that the profession regulates itself in a way that recognizes the need for its members to remain evidence based and up-to-date, and to look after the interests of animal owners and keepers by recognizing their needs and charging reasonably for the services provided (Rollin, 2006). In the century since Flexner's influential report on the quality of US medical education (Flexner, 1910), this has led to a considerable focus on scientific knowledge and the content of clinical curricula (Finnerty *et al.*, 2010), at times to the detriment of the balanced knowledge and skill set required by the practitioner (Christakis, 1995).

In the UK, the state of medical education was addressed by the General Medical Council in its first edition of *Tomorrow's Doctors* (GMC, 1993), when it called a halt to the overburdening focus on the passive acquisition of knowledge by students in a way that 'taxed the memory but not the intellect'. Medical schools were exhorted to define core knowledge so that their updated curricula enabled students to understand the principles of their discipline and have time to develop basic technical skills, as well as enhancing the attitudes and behaviours of the students as professional practitioners. Similar recognition of the mismatch between the attributes of new graduates and the requirements of society have led, in both the USA (Pritchard, 1988) and the UK (RCVS, 1991), to calls for a greater focus on the application of knowledge and problem solving, rather than the accumulation of facts, as well as the acquisition of basic technical and professional skills (RCVS, 2001; NAVMEC, 2011).

The Flexnerian curriculum, with its preclinical and clinical phases, is inefficient and ineffective in various ways (Harden, 2000). The persistence of the separate '-ologies' has contributed to the content overload, with rapidly accumulating knowledge in each separate field encouraging each discipline to specialize to ensure that it is covered in their teaching block. The reductionism of the basic sciences means that they are increasingly focused on cells and molecules, rather than whole animals, and the ever more technologically sophisticated university teaching hospital is an unfamiliar and challenging learning environment for the new clinical student familiar with the 'safer' environment of the classroom. In the absence of vertical integration of the Flexnerian curriculum, this led to an enhancement of the so-called preclinical–clinical divide (GMC, 1993; Parsell and Bligh, 1995), making it harder than ever for students to reorganize their knowledge from a disease-focused to a problem-focused framework necessary for its application in the clinics (May, 2015). Fortunately, in parallel with the call for more professionally oriented and better balanced clinical curricula, progress in our understanding of student learning and the process of development from novice to expert has allowed the breadth of core knowledge, skills and attitudes to be incorporated into pedagogically sound frameworks (May and Silva-Fletcher, 2015) that ensure that the 4–6 years (depending on whether this is an undergraduate or postgraduate qualification) are used both more effectively and efficiently.

1.1 Active Learning

It is well recognized that while a small number may theorize and mentally extrapolate beyond what they are hearing, if a cohort of students is placed in a traditional lecture, the vast majority will adopt a more passive approach to note taking and memorizing (Biggs, 1999). Those in the latter group need to be actively engaged in various tasks and problem solving to ensure that they

© CAB International 2018. *Veterinary Clinical Skills Manual* (eds N. Coombes and A. Silva-Fletcher)

start to integrate their knowledge and apply it in a meaningful way (Prince, 2004; Prince *et al.*, 2009; Freeman *et al.*, 2014). This has implications for both cognitive skills, such as critical thinking and the understanding of scientific concepts (Nelson, 1999), and the technical skills associated with surgical and medical therapies (Bradley and Postlethwaite, 2004; Baillie *et al.*, 2010). Active, small-group learning provides the context for the realization of all three major categories of learning – behaviourism, cognitivism and social constructivism – recognized in the last century (May, 2017). It stimulates cognitive processes as the learner adapts and applies their knowledge to a problem. It supports the social process that allows individuals to learn from one another and reconstruct their concepts of science and clinical practice as their understanding deepens. With opportunities for repetition of practical tasks, it supports behaviourist responses that lead to automaticity of increasingly complex cognitive and practical processes.

1.2 Deliberate Practice

The idea that individuals are either clever/intelligent/ talented or not, and that there is little that they can do to alter their part in the genetic lottery, is a pervasive and destructive belief that still hampers a student's ability to achieve their full potential (Dweck, 2006). In early adolescence, individuals start to differentiate into two groups: those who have a fixed mindset, see failure in a task as a reflection on them and identify experiences for future avoidance; and those who have a growth mindset, see failure as a challenge to be overcome, and an opportunity for learning that should be sought if they are to make progress (Dweck, 2003, 2007). The fixed mindset develops despite evidence, from a variety of fields of endeavour, that expertise is more related to the hours in which an individual engages in study and practise rather than any initial aptitude for a discipline (Ericsson, 2004). Achievement of solo performance standard on a musical instrument is a good example of this, with those who succeed all devoting in excess of 10,000 h of deliberate (structured/ sequenced) practise to mastery of their instruments, in contrast to less accomplished professional musicians (5000–7500 h) and amateur musicians (2000 h). Behaviourism predicts that more repetition of any task, cognitive or practical, leads to automaticity, which, for simple tasks that are either completed or not, such as

tying a knot, is likely to be a desired end point. However, where, like musical performance, there are qualitative differences in the way in which a task is completed, and where superior performance is only achieved through an iterative process of action and feedback, deliberate practise allows this tendency to automaticity to be overridden and continued improvements to be made (Ericsson, 2009). For complex skills, this deliberate practice may include repetition of individual elements and ensuring that the less successful elements are refined. In domains such as ballet and music, the best ordering of study materials for student development has evolved over hundreds of years; in contrast, in clinical education and scientific research, there is much less consensus over best practice. This emphasizes the need for research on the best approaches for educating clinicians and the development of their teachers (Lynagh *et al.*, 2007; May, 2008, 2017; Silva-Fletcher, 2017).

1.3 Curricular Integration

Historically, professional programmes were populated by the allocation of blocks of classroom time to different departments, with ownership of the content belonging to those separate groups (Harden, 2000). This accounts for the tendency towards overload and the lack of meaningful sequencing of knowledge and skills development. It was up to students to horizontally integrate anatomy, physiology, pathology and pharmacology, navigate the practical–clinical divide (Parsell and Bligh, 1995) and make sense of abnormal biological processes and their treatment (May, 2015). An appreciation of the power of active learning and deliberate practice confirms the superiority of curricular models founded on horizontal integration around systems of the body and vertical integration of concept and skills development (GMC, 1993; Harden, 2000) that avoid cognitive overload (van Merriënboer and Sweller, 2010).

1.4 Anxiety and Learning

An individual's capacity to learn is affected by their emotional state. In particular, when placed in a group, anxiety causes them to focus their mental processes more on social survival than any learning opportunities that the particular context provides (Rogers, 1969).

Until recently, progress in a professional curriculum meant that students often moved from the anonymity of the large-group learning environment of the lecture theatre to the small groups of clinical rotations, at the same time as struggling to cross the preclinical–clinical divide. The busyness of increasingly commercial university-owned clinics, together with the complexity of the clinical environment, could make this transition a very anxious one for many students (May, 2015), particularly those with a tendency towards a fixed mindset (Bostock *et al.*, 2018). This process has been likened to learning to swim by being dropped, as a non-swimmer, into a pool with a mixture of others with ranging degrees of swimming expertise. Some might learn to survive individually; others might be helped by more advanced colleagues (Wearn and Bhoopatkar, 2005). Either way, a considerable amount was left to chance and the novice learner's survival instincts. Sequencing of learning so that it encourages understanding and mastery (van Merriënboer and Sluijsmans, 2009), providing opportunities for rehearsal and gaining fluency in basic techniques before moving on to the more complex (Ericsson, 2009), and integrating bridges between the classroom and the workplace, in the form of safe environments in which to observe and practice technical skills (May and Silva-Fletcher, 2015), are all likely to contribute to confidence that the transition can be accomplished and a reduction in anxiety.

1.5 The Veterinary Clinical Skills Centre

Veterinary Clinical Skills Centres (CSCs) are based on facilities similar to those created by medical schools to develop technical skills in their students. In 2001, the Royal Veterinary College (RVC), University of London, secured external funding for a series of visits by faculty from several UK veterinary schools to medical CSCs in Dundee, Sheffield and London. These were in support of a feasibility study to decide what was needed and whether it would be practical to convert the medical model for the CSC to the veterinary context. This led, during the course of 2002, to the identification of space for redevelopment (a large, redundant clinical research area that was tiled and had a washable floor) and the creation of the RVC's first pilot CSC, which, like the medical CSCs on which it was based, provided relevant learning opportunities in a 'safe'

environment, in a systematic way, that ensured important curriculum outcomes were achieved by all students and not left to chance, and provided a foundation that students could 'use as a springboard from which to achieve the best possible learning from subsequent clinical experience' (Bradley and Bligh, 2005). It was immediately popular with students, for whom it had huge face validity, as they recognized that it focused on skills that they were actually going to have to perform as vets. This first facility provided a model for the development of improved facilities at other schools in the UK and internationally and led, through the Higher Education Funding Council for England's initiative to create Centres for Excellence in Teaching and Learning, to the RVC's Lifelong Independent Veterinary Education (LIVE) Centre (Pirkelbauer *et al.*, 2008), incorporating two purpose-designed clinical skills laboratories, as well as rooms for learning communication skills and facilities that support computer-aided problem solving.

1.6 Feedback

Important to successful learning in the CSCs is the ability to role-model skills for learners, observe their performance and provide timely and meaningful feedback (Bradley and Bligh, 2005). Technical skills development invites behavioural feedback of a type that contributes to improved future performance. The acknowledgement of student effort rather than praise of student 'talent' is important for all learners in helping them to adopt a growth mindset in their professional development (Dweck, 2007). Feedback that provides compliments is liked by students (and increases satisfaction scores on feedback forms), but does not improve future performance. In contrast, feedback focused on student activity leads to improved future performance at the expense of student satisfaction (Boehler *et al.*, 2006), demonstrating that we do not always like what is good for us.

1.7 Effectiveness of Clinical Skills Centres

CSCs incorporate a range of models, from the very basic that provide a framework for learning to tie surgical knots, through simple manikins (life-sized models) that support the development of skills in venepuncture and catheterization, to much more sophisticated simulators, such as the 'haptic cow' (Baillie *et al.*, 2010), that aid the development of manual palpation skills. In the early days of simulator development, fidelity of the model to the real patient was viewed as important. However, it is now clear that a basic model or a more advanced simulator only needs to be 'real' enough to draw the learner into a relevant learning experience. Similar learning gains are achieved for high- and low-fidelity simulators in auscultation, critical care and basic surgical skills (Norman *et al.*, 2012). An important caveat in this regard is the assessment of many CSC-acquired skills through *in vitro* 'shows how' methods (objective structured clinical examinations, or simulator-based assessments), rather than through assessment of their transfer to clinical contexts, and thus the fact that early evaluations of CSC effectiveness were based on comparisons of those assessments with structured or no skills training (Lynagh *et al.*, 2007). However, there is increasing evidence that skills do transfer to the clinical context, through evaluations of simulators such as the haptic cow (Baillie *et al.*, 2005).

1.8 Aggregation of Technical and Other Professional Skills

Proficiency in technical skills is most easily achieved for simple, isolated skills. However, a criticism of the reductionism of the CSC approach is the way in which skills learning and their assessment through objectively structured clinical examinations (OSCEs) fails to encourage and evaluate student proficiency in a complete surgical procedure (for instance, neutering of cats) or the handling of all aspects of a clinical case (May and Head, 2010). In line with understanding of the development of expertise, this has led to the integration of role playing with technical skills training. In medical education, adding these extra elements did not detract from technical skills development and led to significant improvement in patient–physician communication (Nikendei *et al.*, 2007), and these types of integrated learning experiences were also significantly more valued by participating students (Nikendei *et al.*, 2005). A similar integrated skills scenario focused on a farm visit and a pregnancy assessment in a cow has been researched in veterinary education. Students reported positive effects on their confidence

and knowledge, as well as their communication and technical skills (Baillie *et al.*, 2010). The challenge created by the facilitator taking on the role of farmer was seen as 'putting them on the spot' and provoked some anxiety. However, this was seen as 'not a bad thing', as this experience was 'so important for the real world'.

Conclusions

The CSC provides many opportunities to incorporate best practices in learning and teaching, in relation to 'active learning', deliberate practice, sequencing of skills and a safe environment in which to experience challenging and anxiety-revealing scenarios, in a way that supports the development of understanding and avoids excessive cognitive loads. Important to this is facilitator understanding of underpinning pedagogies and appreciation of the way in which CSC-supported learning fits into an integrated curriculum and bridges the classroom–clinic divide. This requires facilitator training and the recruitment of individuals as facilitators who are student focused and can empathetically accommodate all types of learner. Like in many medical CSCs, the RVC's experience is that trained veterinary nurses (in the US, veterinary technicians) excel as CSC facilitators and are seen as approachable by veterinary students. This means that timetabled CSC learning opportunities are well attended and 'drop-in' sessions continue to be popular with clinical students, depending on their needs, throughout their final year of veterinary education.

References: Baillie, S., Crossan, A., Brewster, S., Mellor, D. and Reid, S. (2005) Validation of a bovine rectal palpation simulator for training veterinary students. *Studies in Health Technology and Informatics* 111, 33–36.

Baillie, S., Crossan, A., Brewster, S.A., May, S.A. and Mellor, D.J. (2010) Evaluating an automated haptic simulator designed for veterinary students to learn bovine rectal palpation. *Simulation in Healthcare* 5(5), 261–266. https://doi.org/10.1097/SIH.0b013e3181e369bf.

Biggs, J. (1999) What the student does: teaching for enhanced learning. *Higher Education Research & Development* 18(1), 57–75.

Boehler, M.L., Rogers, D.A, Schwind, C.J., Mayforth, R., Quin, J., Williams, R.G. and Dunnington, G. (2006) An investigation of medical student reactions to feedback: a randomised controlled trial. *Medical Education* 40(8), 746–749. https://doi.org/10.1111/j.1365-2929.2006.02503.x.

Bostock, R., Kinnison, T. and May, S.A. (2018) Mindset and its relationship to anxiety in clinical veterinary students. *Veterinary Record*, submitted for publication.

Bradley, P. and Bligh, J. (2005) Clinical skills centres: where are we going? *Medical Education* 39(7), 649–650. https://doi.org/10.1111/j.1365-2929.2005.02210.x.

Bradley, P. and Postlethwaite, K. (2004) Setting up and running clinical skills learning programmes. *The Clinical Teacher* 1(2), 53–58. https://doi.org/10.1111/j.1743-498X.2004.00039.x.

Christakis, N.A. (1995) The similarity and frequency of proposals to reform US medical education. Constant concerns. *Journal of the American Medical Association* 274(9), 706–711.

Dweck, C.S. (2003) Ability conceptions, motivation and development. In: Tomlinson, P., Dockrell, J. and Winne, P. (eds) *BJEP Monograph Series II, 2: Development and Motivation*, Vol. 2. The British Psychological Society, Leicester, UK, pp. 13–27.

Dweck, C.S. (2006) *Mindset: How You Can Fulfil Your Potential*. Random House, New York.

Dweck, C.S. (2007) Boosting achievement with messages that motivate. *Education Canada* 47(2), 6–10.

Ericsson, K.A. (2004) Deliberate practice and the acquisition and maintenance of expert performance in medicine and related domains. *Academic Medicine* 79(10), S70–81.

Ericsson, K.A. (2009) Discovering deliberate practice activities that overcome plateaus and limits on improvement of performance. In: Willamon, A., Pretty, S. and Buck, R. (eds) *International Symposium on Performance Science*. Association Europienne des Conservatoires Academies de Musique at Musikhochschulen, Utrecht, The Netherlands, pp. 11–21. Available at: http://www.performancescience.org/ISPS2009/Proceedings/Rows/003Ericsson.pdf (accessed 26 February 2018).

Finnerty, E.P., Chauvin, S., Bonaminio, G., Andrews, M., Carroll, R.G. and Pangaro, L.N. (2010) Flexner revisited: the role and value of the basic sciences in medical education. *Academic Medicine: Journal of the Association of American Medical Colleges* 85(2), 349–355. https://doi.org/10.1097/ACM.0b013e3181c88b09.

Flexner, A. (1910/2002) Medical education in the United States and Canada. *Bulletin of the World Health Organization* 80(7), 594–602, extracted from *Bulletin Number Four* (1910) of The Carnegie Foundation for the Advancement of Teaching, New York.

Freeman, S., Eddy, S.L., McDonough, M., Smith, M.K., Okoroafor, N. *et al.* (2014) Active learning increases student performance in science, engineering, and mathematics. *Proceedings of the National Academy of Sciences of the United States of America* 111(23), 8410–8415. https://doi.org/10.1073/pnas.1319030111.

GMC (1993) *Tomorrow's Doctors: Recommendations on Undergraduate Medical Education*. General Medical Council, London.

Harden, R.M. (2000) The integration ladder: a tool for curriculum planning and evaluation. *Medical Education* 34(7), 551–557.

Lynagh, M., Burton, R. and Sanson-Fisher, R. (2007) A systematic review of medical skills laboratory training: where to from here? *Medical Education* 41(9), 879–887. https://doi.org/10.1111/j.1365-2923.2007.02821.x.

May, S.A. (2008) Modern veterinary graduates are outstanding, but can they get better? *Journal of Veterinary Medical Education* 35(4), 573–580.

May, S.A. (2013) Veterinary ethics, professionalism and society. In: Wathes, C.M., Corr, S.A., May, S.A., McCulloch, S.P. and Whiting, M.C. (eds) *Veterinary and Animal Ethics*. Wiley-Blackwell, Oxford, pp. 44–58.

May, S.A. (2015) Creating the consummate professional: historical and contemporary perspectives (based on the BEVA John Hickman Memorial Lecture 2014). *Equine Veterinary Education* 27(9), 489–495. https://doi.org/10.1111/eve.12319.

May, S.A. (2017) Learning concepts and theories, and their application to educational practice. Chapter 4 in: *Veterinary Medical Education: A Practical Guide*. Wiley Blackwell, Hoboken, New Jersey, USA.

May, S.A. and Head, S.D. (2010) Assessment of technical skills: best practices. *Journal of Veterinary Medical Education* 37(3), 258–265. https://doi.org/10.3138/jvme.37.3.258.

May, S.A. and Silva-Fletcher, A. (2015) Scaffolded active learning: nine pedagogical principles for building a modern veterinary curriculum. *Journal of Veterinary Medical Education* 42(4), 332–339. https://doi.org/10.3138/jvme.0415-063R.

NAVMEC (2011) *Roadmap for Veterinary Medical Education in the 21st Century*. North American Veterinary Medical Education Consortium, Washington, DC.

Nelson, C.E. (1999) On the persistence of unicorns: the trade-off between content and critical thinking revisited. In: Pescosolido, B.A. and Aminzade, R. (eds) *The Social Worlds of Higher Education: Handbook for Teaching in a New Century*. Pine Forge Press, Thousand Oaks, California, USA, pp. 168–184. Available at: http://celt.miamioh.edu/lillycon/session_files/uploads/2013_no2104_99_PersistenceUnic_Sm.pdf (accessed 18 October 2017).

Nikendei, C., Zeuch, A., Dieckmann, P., Roth, C., Schäfer, S. *et al.* (2005) Role-playing for more realistic technical skills training. *Medical Teacher* 27(2), 122–126. https://doi.org/10.1080/01421590400019484.

Nikendei, C., Kraus, B., Schrauth, M., Weyrich, P., Zipfel, S., Herzog, W. and Jünger, J. (2007) Integration of role-playing into technical skills training: a randomized controlled trial. *Medical Teacher* 29(9), 956–960. https://doi.org/10.1080/01421590701601543.

Norman, G., Dore, K. and Grierson, L. (2012) The minimal relationship between simulation fidelity and transfer of learning. *Medical Education* 46(7), 636–647. https://doi.org/10.1111/j.1365-2923.2012.04243.x.

Parsell, G.J. and Bligh, J. (1995) The changing context of undergraduate medical education. *Postgraduate Medical Journal* 71, 397–403.

Pirkelbauer, B., Pead, M., Probyn, P. and May, S.A. (2008) LIVE: the creation of an academy for veterinary education. *Journal of Veterinary Medical Education* 35(4), 567–572. https://doi.org/10.3138/jvme.35.4.567.

Prince, M. (2004) Does active learning work? A review of the research. *Journal of Engineering Education* 93(July), 223–231.

Prince, M.J., Vigeant, M.A.S. and Nottis, K. (2009) A preliminary study on the effectiveness of inquiry-based activities for addressing misconceptions of undergraduate engineering students. *Education for Chemical Engineers* 4(2), 29–41. https://doi.org/10.1016/j.ece.2009.07.002.

Pritchard, W.R. (1988) *Future Directions for Veterinary Medicine*. Pew National Veterinary Education Program, Institute of Policy Sciences and Public Affairs, Duke University, Durham, North Carolina.

RCVS (1991) *Report of the Working Party on Veterinary Undergraduate Education*. Royal College of Veterinary Surgeons, London.

RCVS (2001) *Veterinary Education and Training: A Framework for 2010 and Beyond*. Royal College of Veterinary Surgeons, London.

Rogers, C.R. (1969) *Freedom to Learn*. Charles E. Merrill, Columbus, Ohio, USA.

Rollin, B.E. (2006) *An Introduction to Veterinary Medical Ethics*, 2nd edn. Blackwell Publishing, Oxford, UK.

Silva-Fletcher, A. (2017) Teaching the teacher. Chapter 31 in: *Veterinary Medical Education: A Practical Guide*. Wiley Blackwell, Hoboken, New Jersey.

van Merriënboer, J.J G. and Sluijsmans, D.M.A. (2009) Toward a synthesis of cognitive load theory, four-component instructional design, and self-directed learning. *Educational Psychology Review* 21, 55–66. https://doi.org/10.1007/s10648-008-9092-5.

van Merriënboer, J.J.G. and Sweller, J. (2010) Cognitive load theory in health professional education: design principles and strategies. *Medical Education* 44(1), 85–93. https://doi.org/10.1111/j.1365-2923.2009.03498.x.

Wearn, A. and Bhoopatkar, H. (2005) Clinical skills centres: where did we come from? *Medical Education* 39(10), 1078. https://doi.org/10.1111/j.1365-2929.2005.02274.x.

The Modern Outcome-based Curriculum and the Role of the Clinical Skills Laboratory

Ayona Silva-Fletcher
The Royal Veterinary College, London

Introduction

'Most educators know that it would make more sense to operate schools on the basis of what students can actually do' (Spady, 1988, p. 5)

Educators have created the clinical skills lab to solve a training problem in health professionals' education. The problem was the incompetent physician or the veterinarian at the end of a long university education. Today, the day-one graduate is less incompetent. Even if they have not performed a full surgery yet, the graduate is equipped with many skills that can contribute towards that competence. This chapter will explore the rationale for changing curricula to foster skills and competence development and how the solution of the clinical skills lab-based training has become the indispensable educational experience for students. The chapter will build on the pedagogical or learning theories introduced in Chapter 1: active learning, deliberate practice and emotions in learning. This chapter also lays the foundation for Chapter 22, which is a wider exploration of simulation-based training.

2.1 Development of Outcome and Competence-based Curricula

The ultimate goal of health professional education is to develop a graduate who can perform as a professional in society. The traditional curricula with a preclinical–clinical divide (Chapter 1) foster the development of a graduate with a sound knowledge base rather than a graduate who is trained to perform. The change in thinking that the curricula should be developed to measure the outcomes of students, rather than the objectives of the curriculum, started during the latter half of the last century in the USA in the schooling system (Bloom, 1968). 'Outcome Based Education (OBE) means organizing for results: basing what we do instructionally on the outcomes we want to achieve' (Spady, 1988, p. 5). This OBE movement was quickly taken up by the medical sector (Harden *et al.*, 1999) and is now well embedded in curriculum development for health professional education. Although there is some criticism for OBE (McKernan, 1993; O'Neil, 1994) that outcomes narrow down the education to a set of specific, achievable and assessable list of tasks, the notion that outcomes can be developed to be broader and adaptable was fostered by the UK General Medical Council (GMC) in 1993. A landmark development by the GMC was publication of '*Tomorrow's Doctors*' in 1993, revised in 2009 (GMC, 2009). This document contained outcomes and standards for undergraduate medical education and is widely used as the core curriculum. Today the outcomes are defined as competences of a 'Day One' graduate. In the veterinary sector, a similar approach was taken by the Royal College of Veterinary Surgeons (RCVS) in the UK: a 'Day-One-competence' (D1C) document with guidelines for minimum essential competences that all veterinary graduates should have upon graduation was published in 2001 and revised later (RCVS, 2014). Today there are similar documents developed by national and international accreditation bodies that govern health professionals' education throughout the globe: Royal College of Physicians and Surgeons of Canada (2005); Scottish Medical Deans Curriculum Group (2008); American Veterinary Medical Association (2010); European Association of Establishments for Veterinary Education (EAEVE, 2009); and global organizations such as the World Organization for Animal Health (OIE, 2013).

© CAB International 2018. *Veterinary Clinical Skills Manual* (eds N. Coombes and A. Silva-Fletcher)

2.2 Day One Competences (D1C) and Day One Skills (D1S)

How feasible is it to develop a curriculum from a list of Day One competences? Competence can be defined as the ability to do something successfully or efficiently. Competence encompasses not only a 'whole act' but also at a level that can be deemed successful or efficient. It is more useful for the curriculum developers to focus on developing 'skills' (at different stages of the training) that can be used for achieving different competences at the end. For example, to be competent in surgery a variety of skills are necessary from scrubbing, gloving and adherence to aseptic procedures to more direct skills in precision incision, suturing and so on. Some of the same skills can be used in achieving competence in disease control and biosecurity. Adherence to aseptic procedures is essential in the prevention of disease spread and maintenance of biosecurity. Therefore skills that can be applied in a range of competences should be targeted in the curriculum. Across the veterinary sector, the trend has been to develop a list of 'Day One skills' (D1S) by individual veterinary teaching institutions as an outcome of the curriculum. These skills can then be aligned with competences to make sure that all the underlying skills are taught during the curriculum.

2.3 Domains of Veterinary Clinical Skills

There is a wide array of skills that can be called 'clinical skills'. Some skills require motor function, whilst others include non-motor cognitive skills. For example, clinical skills may range from procedural tasks such as taking an X-ray or draining an abscess to more cognitive skills such as diagnostic decision making. It is easier to consider skills under different domains or categories. Michels *et al.* (2012), using a group of physicians who teach clinical skills, coded 127 skills into different categories or domains. In other words, these domains can be considered as four major competences (Fig. 2.1). To achieve competence in physical examination, a range of skills are needed. In the veterinary sector this ranges from skills in safe handling and restraint of the animal to performing examinations such as ophthalmic, cardiac and respiratory assessments. The same skills in safe handling and restraint of the animal may be required to be competent in practical clinical procedures and/or treatment and patient management.

These domains are useful in thinking about how to teach the clinical skills. Different learning theories can be used in teaching and practising skills from different domains. The following learning theories are useful in teaching practical/technical skills which can be learned

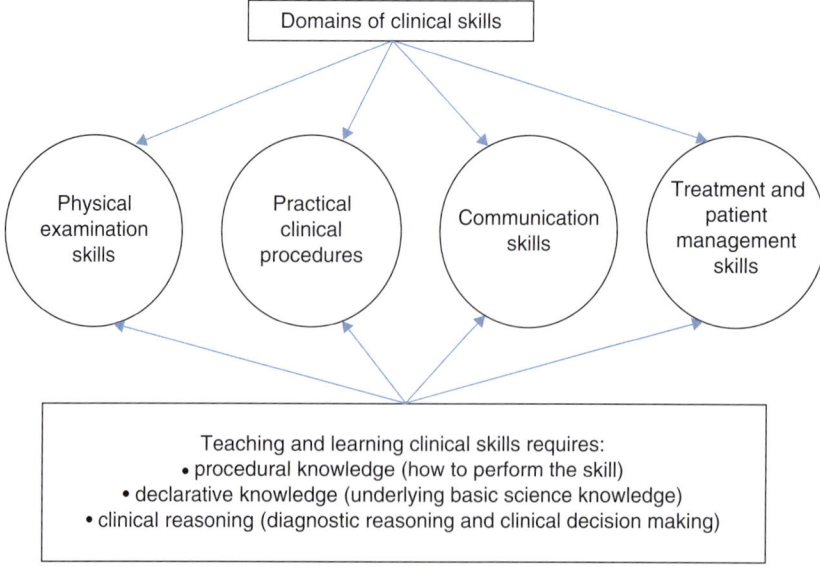

Fig. 2.1. Domains/categories of clinical skills (based on Michels *et al.*, 2012).

and practised in a clinical skills lab. For the purpose of this chapter, only those skills that are taught and practised in a clinical skills lab will be considered here.

2.4 Learning Theories and Teaching Skills

The old 'see one, do one, teach one' adage of skills learning has been detrimental to patients in some situations (Vozenilek *et al.*, 2004) and is no longer considered a practical approach to skills learning. One of the important learning theories that underlie skills teaching is Miller's pyramid of clinical competence (Miller, 1990). Skills learning is described by Miller at four levels: knows; knows how; shows how; and does. Additional levels have been added to demonstrate that underlying knowledge is necessary to learn any skill. As described in Chapter 1, the integration of basic sciences with clinical application is necessary for learning and undertaking a clinical skill.

A more favourable and practical approach to skills teaching is the four-stage approach by Peyton (1998). In this model the student is led through different stages as outlined in Fig. 2.2. A further level on feedback on the skills has been added to improve this approach.

The main teaching models for the acquisition of clinical skills use a sequential and staged approach. Another useful concept for teaching clinical skills is the 'Novice to Master' model (Dreyfus and Dreyfus, 1980). In this five-stage model the mental activities involved in directed skills acquisition are described (Table 2.1). The novice starting from a non-situational point needs an analytical process to monitor and learn the skills. As the novice moves through the levels of competent, proficient and expert to master, the mental processes involved have transitioned from analytical to intuitive and the master no longer needs to monitor the skill. This model is used in the teaching of many skills, from playing musical instruments to more mental games such as chess. The principles and the mental functions involved in developing from beginner to more advanced stages in this model can be applied in clinical skills development.

Peyton's four-stage model

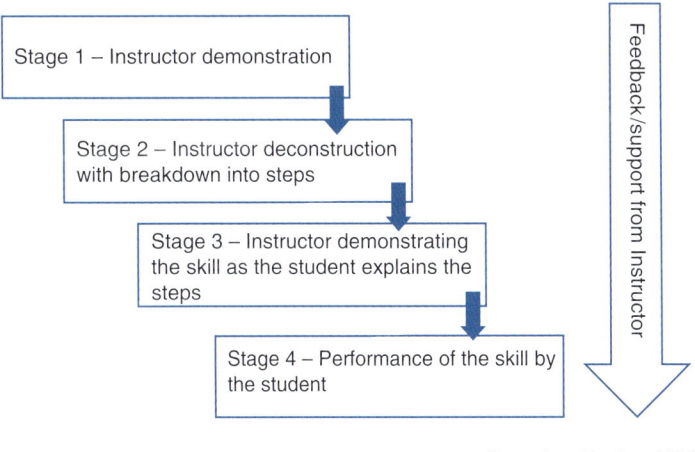

Stage 1 – Instructor demonstration

Stage 2 – Instructor deconstruction with breakdown into steps

Stage 3 – Instructor demonstrating the skill as the student explains the steps

Stage 4 – Performance of the skill by the student

Feedback/support from Instructor

Based on Peyton 1998

Fig. 2.2. Modified Peyton's four-stage approach to technical skills development (based on Peyton, 1998).

Table 2.1. Novice to Expert model (based on Dreyfus and Dreyfus, 1980).

Mental function	Novice	Competent	Proficient	Expert	Master
Reflection	Non-situational	Situational	Situational	Situational	Situational
Recognition	Segmented	Segmented	Holistic	Holistic	Holistic
Decision	Analytical	Analytical	Analytical	Intuitive	Intuitive
Awareness	Monitoring	Monitoring	Monitoring	Monitoring	Absorbed

2.5 Developing a Clinical Skills Lab

'Most students (perhaps over 90 percent) can master what we have to teach them, and it is the task of instruction to find the means which will enable our students to master the subject under consideration' (Bloom, 1968, p. 1). The answer is the clinical skills lab with simulation-based training. There has been a rapid growth in clinical skills labs to train students in essential clinical skills in health professional education. Simulation-based technology is used in these labs without real patients so that students can engage in learning and practising the skill with repetition and feedback (Issenberg et al., 1999). The simulators can include equipment that is used in real clinical situations as well as models (human or animal manikins) for students to learn and practise a skill. These simulators are discussed in great detail in Chapter 23.

The best available evidence suggests that high-fidelity medical simulations facilitate learning if the following conditions are met (Issenberg et al., 2005):

1. Feedback is provided during the learning experience.
2. Learners engage in repetitive practise.
3. The simulator is integrated into an overall curriculum.
4. Learners practise with increasing levels of difficulty.
5. The simulator is adaptable to multiple learning strategies.
6. The simulator captures clinical variation.
7. The simulator is embedded in a controlled environment.
8. The simulator permits individualized learning.
9. Learning outcomes are clearly defined and measured.
10. The simulator is a valid (high-fidelity) approximation of clinical practice.

These conditions underpin clinical skills lab development and maintenance to maximize student learning. Of these, the following practical aspects must be given focus in planning a clinical skills lab.

2.5.1 Feedback

It is useful to develop both formative and summative feedback (Van De Ridder et al., 2008). Formative feedback can be given during informal teaching sessions and the purpose is to offer individual feedback 'at the right time' based on the task just performed. Rudolph et al. (2008, p. 1013) offered a four-step model:

1. Note salient performance gaps related to predetermined objectives.
2. Provide feedback describing the gap.
3. Investigate the basis for the gap by exploring the frames and emotions contributing to the current performance level.
4. Help close the performance gap through discussion or targeted instruction about principles and skills relevant to performance.

Summative assessments offered as pass/fail judgements also offer feedback regarding the level of performance in relation to the skill. Impact of feedback has proved to be positive (McGaghie et al., 2010) but further research is needed to understand the specific feedback models and methods. This will enable the development of feedback standards and guidelines and instructor training.

2.5.2 Deliberate practice

Based on 32 research studies, McGaghie et al. (2010, p. 4) concluded that: 'The evidence is clear … that repetitive practice involving medical simulations is associated with improved learner outcomes. Simulation-based practice in medical education appears to approximate a dose–response relationship in terms of achieving desired outcomes: more practice yields better results.'

Deliberate practice is necessary for a novice to become competent (Ericsson, 2004). The skills lab is an ideal opportunity for deliberate practice. However, it can be very time-consuming and relies on 'highly motivated learners with good concentration'. The integration of skills learning in the curriculum should take all these facts into consideration to optimize the use of the clinical skills lab.

2.5.3 Curriculum integration

The integration of skills development throughout the curriculum is challenging. The skills need to be developed with increasing levels of difficulty to match the students' advancing knowledge. The 'spiral model' of curriculum facilitates this integration, as students can revisit the same skill as they advance through the course (Harden, 1999). The development of a clinical skills lab therefore should be planned in advance (many years sometimes) to achieve effective integration into the curriculum. At the Royal Veterinary College (RVC), the use of simulators is integrated throughout

Table 2.2. A new RVC graduate perspective on how to use the same simulation for different levels of training (developed by Desiree Janine Herrick, author of Chapter 25, this volume).

Clinical skill	Level of skill for different year groups*
Anaesthesia machine set-up and safety check	**Third Year:** Students should become familiar with each component of the anaesthetic machine, and what it is used for. They should have a general understanding of basic anaesthesia **Fourth Year:** Students should begin understanding setting up and checking each component of the machine, what it's used for and the implications for failing to make a proper check **Final:** Students should be confident in preparing and checking all equipment to be used in the delivery of anaesthesia and in patient monitoring. Safely induce general anaesthesia using an appropriate inhalational technique. Safely maintain general anaesthesia using this equipment
Cardiopulmonary cerebral resuscitation	**Third Year:** Students should learn the warning signs of a pending arrest and potential causes **Fourth Year:** Students should begin to understand the steps of basic CPR and feel confident in which equipment is needed **Final:** Students should feel confident understanding and performing basic cardiopulmonary resuscitation
Intravenous catheter placement	**Third Year:** Students should understand what a catheter is, its various parts and what it's used for **Fourth Year:** Students should familiarize themselves with the necessary equipment, understand the anatomy used in the placement and begin to understand the steps in placing IV catheters **Final:** Students should feel confident in placing IV catheters, understanding their maintenance and identifying warning signs of catheter infections
Equine tail bandage	**Third Year:** Students should familiarise themselves with how to approach and safely position themselves by the horse. They should begin to understand the indications for an equine tail bandage and begin to familiarise themselves with how to apply one to the model dock **Fourth Year:** Students should be comfortable safely working around the horse and have the ability to correctly apply and remove a tail bandage to the model dock **Final:** Students need to be able to appropriately apply a neat, firm tail bandage in a safe manner around the horse, understand the importance of its upkeep and when to use one
Obtaining a sterile milk sample from a cow	**Third Year:** Students should familiarise themselves with the proper approach to a cow and how to safely position themselves next to them. They should begin to understand the general process of obtaining a sterile milk sample **Fourth Year:** Students should feel comfortable in approaching a cow safely, obtaining a sterile sample, and understanding the importance of biosecurity of farm work **Final:** Students should feel confident in working around a cow safely, obtaining a sterile sample while paying attention to the details of labelling the sample properly and emphasizing the importance of biosecurity
Ophthalmoscope	**Third Year:** Students should learn the anatomy of the inner eye, and the normal appearance of these structures during an eye exam. They should understand the difference between direct and indirect ocular exams and should begin to learn how to handle and use an ophthalmoscope **Fourth Year:** Students should feel comfortable properly using an ophthalmoscope at different settings for an ocular exam. They should understand how to read the settings in relation to their exam **Final:** Students should be confident in assessing how to use an ophthalmoscope at appropriate settings during an ocular exam. They should be able to recognise common ocular lesions during their assessment
Equine radiology positions and use of machine	**Third Year:** Students should familiarize themselves with the most common projections used in equine radiography and the accompanying equine anatomy **Fourth Year:** Students should understand the focus of radiographic positioning and become familiar with the use of the machine, the rules of safety when using it and radiographic anatomy **Final:** Students should be confident in setting up the standard projections of the equine limb, know the rules and regulations regarding radiography safety, and understand common faults found in radiography

*The different year groups described in this table are based on the BVetMed undergraduate veterinary degree at the Royal Veterinary College, which is a 5-year programme. Students start their training in the clinical skills lab from 3rd year. Final-year students are in their 5th year.

the curriculum and students at different stages of learning can learn skills that are appropriate to the stage of the curriculum. Table 2.2 outlines how the same simulations are used by students in different year groups based on the learning outcomes at the stage of their learning.

2.6   The Safe Learning Environment

The essence of a clinical skills lab and simulation-based practice is the safe learning environment for students. Anxiety and fear affect learning, as has been discussed in Chapter 1. The veterinary clinical environment has the added stress of having to handle and restrain an animal that can be in pain, distress or itself in fear. The physical strength of the veterinarian or the veterinary nurse against the animal's power has to be taken into account. In addition, the place of diagnosis and treatment can be under field conditions, in a barn or another place that is exposed to (harsh) weather conditions. Although the clinical skills labs cannot simulate all of these conditions, the opportunity for the student to practise the technique itself in a safe environment until they become competent in performing the task is immensely valuable. Reducing the anxiety and fear with safety and sense of belonging aids learning (Maslow's 'hierarchy of needs' (Maslow, 1954)). The other main advantage of a clinical skills lab is the opportunity for repeated practice. In an outcome-based education, there is an inevitable need for educators to accommodate the differences in learning rates inherent in any group of students. The clinical skills lab provides this space for students to make mistakes and learn from these mistakes.

2.7   Assessment in the Clinical Skills Lab

The assessment of clinical skills is another challenging task. In the veterinary field, this is particularly difficult as assessing students under 'real clinical' situations can introduce unpredictability due to patient behaviour, which can affect the validity and the reliability of the assessment. The clinical skills lab is immensely useful here, as high-fidelity simulators can be used in high-stakes assessments. Chapters 21 and 22 explore the role of the clinical skills lab in student assessment in greater detail.

2.8   Conclusions

Veterinary clinical skills labs are becoming an essential feature in competence-based veterinary curricula. Much of the research and evidence is built on Issenberg *et al.* (2005) conditions. Some prominent features and best practices include feedback, deliberate practise, curriculum integration, outcome measurement, simulation fidelity (low to high, multi-mode), skill acquisition and maintenance, mastery learning, transfer to practice, team training and high-stakes testing. Instructor training in both teaching and assessment in the clinical skills lab is another essential aspect that must be developed to make the clinical skills lab a place of unsurpassed learning.

References: American Veterinary Medical Association (2010) North American Veterinary Medical Education Consortium, National Meeting 1: Report. Available at: http://aavmc.org/ data/files/navmec/navmecmeeting1report.pdf (accessed 19 October 2017).

Bloom, B.S. (1968) Learning for mastery. *Evaluation Comment* 1(2), 8–18.

Dreyfus, S.E. and Dreyfus, H.L. (1980) *A Five-Stage Model of the Mental Activities Involved in Directed Skill Acquisition.* Storming Media, Washington, DC.

Ericsson, K.A. (2004) Deliberate practice and the acquisition and maintenance of expert performance in medicine and related domains. *Academic Medicine* 79 (Suppl. 10), 70–81.

European Association of Establishments for Veterinary Education (EAEVE) (2009) European System of Evaluation of Veterinary Training (ESEVT). Available at: http://www.eaeve. org/fileadmin/downloads/SOP/ESEVT__Uppsala__SOP_ May_2016.pdf (accessed 17 October 2017).

General Medical Council (GMC) (2009) Tomorrow's Doctors. Available at: http://www.gmc-uk.org/10a_annex_a.pdf_ 25398162.pdf (accessed 17 October 2017).

Harden, R.M. (1999) What is a spiral curriculum? *Medical Teacher* 21(2), 141–143.

Harden, R.M., Crosby, J.R. and Davis, M.H. (1999) An introduction to outcome-based education. *Medical Teacher* 21(1), 7–14.

Issenberg, S.B., McGaghie, W.C., Hart, I.R. *et al.* (1999) Simulation technology for health care professional skills training and assessment. *Journal of the American Medical Association* 282, 861–866.

Issenberg, S.B., McGaghie, W.C., Petrusa, E.R., Gordon, D.L. and Scalese, R.J. (2005) Features and uses of high-fidelity medical simulation that lead to effective learning: a BEME systematic review. *Medical Teacher* 27, 10–28.

Maslow, A. (1954) *Motivation and Personality*. Harper, New York.

McGaghie, W.C.S., Issenberg, B., Petrusa, E.R. and Scalese, R.J. (2010) A critical review of simulation-based medical education research: 2003–2009. *Medical Education* 44(1), 50–63.

McKernan, J. (1993) Perspectives and imperatives: some limitations of outcome-based education. *Journal of Curriculum and Supervision* 8(4), 343–353.

Michels, M.E., Evans, D.E. and Blok, G.A. (2012) What is a clinical skill? Searching for order in chaos through a modified Delphi process. *Medical Teacher* 34(8), e573–e581.

Miller, G.E. (1990) The assessment of clinical skills/competence/performance. *Academic Medicine* 65(99), S63–S67.

O'Neil, J. (1994) Aiming for new outcomes: the promise and the reality. *Educational Leadership* 51(6), 6–10.

Peyton, J.W.R. (1998) *Teaching and Learning in Medical Practice*. Manticore Europe, Rickmansworth, UK.

RCVS (2014) Day One Competences Statement. Available at: https://www.rcvs.org.uk/document-library/day-one-competences-statement/ (accessed 17/10/2017).

Royal College of Physicians and Surgeons of Canada (2005) The CanMEDS 2005 Physician Competency Framework. Available at: http://www.ub.edu/medicina_unitateducaciomedica/documentos/CanMeds.pdf (accessed 17 October 2017).

Rudolph, J.W., Simon, R., Raemer, D.B. and Eppich, W.J. (2008) Debriefing as formative assessment: closing performance gaps in medical education. *Academic Emergency Medicine* 15(11), 1010–1016.

Scottish Medical Deans Curriculum Group (2008) Available at: http://www.scottishdoctor.org/resources/scotdoc3.pdf (accessed 17 October 2017).

Spady, W.G. (1988) Organising for results: the basis of authentic restructuring and reform. *Educational Leadership* 46(2), 4–8.

Van De Ridder, J.M.M., Stokking, K.M., McGaghie, W.C. and Ten Cate, O. (2008) What is feedback in clinical education? *Medical Education* 42, 189–197.

Vozenilek, J., Huff, J.S., Reznek, M. and Gordon, J.A. (2004) See one, do one, teach one: advanced technology in medical education. *Academic Emergency Medicine* 11, 1149–1154.

World Organization for Animal Health (OIE) (2013) Veterinary Education Core Curriculum. Available at: http://www.oie.int/Veterinary_Education_Core_Curriculum.pdf (accessed 17 October 2017).

Introduction

Nichola Coombes and Ayona Silva-Fletcher

The Royal Veterinary College, London

'What matters is not just what students know, but how they use it.'

Sternberg *et al.* (2007, p.143)

Based on outcome-based competence models, veterinary curricula are increasingly moving towards 'skills' development to ensure that undergraduates are competent in what they are expected to do at the end of their training. Developing skills require 'hands-on' practice. It is not always easy to provide hands-on practice to all students and therefore clinical skills centres (CSCs) are immensely useful to offer a safe environment in which to practise skills using simulators and models. Training in the clinical skills lab is not a substitute for training with live animals or in a clinical practice, but the correct approach and techniques can be practised over and over again in this safe simulated environment. Once technique is mastered, the student can try the skill on a live animal. The additional benefit of this training is on the welfare of the animal. As the students are not trying to practise new skills on live animals straightaway, the pain, suffering and stress caused to the animal can be minimized.

Today CSCs are also used for skills assessment. Traditional practical tests have been improved using objectively structured clinical examination (OSCE) and other variations of this assessment type where the student's mastery of the skill is assessed using simulators and models. Although very time consuming and resource heavy (one examiner per student per skill), the examiners can observe the techniques, approaches and specific skills of individual students and this is therefore a valid and reliable assessment method. For more details regarding assessments in the CSC, see Section 8, Chapters 21 and 22.

This chapter gives an overview of the range and scale of CSCs that are used in different parts of the world. Most CSCs described in this chapter are new and in the following sections the authors from these CSCs describe the background that led to development, scope and how they are used in teaching and assessment.

Reference: Sternberg, R.J., Reznitskaya, A. and Jarvin, L. (2007) Teaching for wisdom: what matters is not just what students know, but how they use it. *London Review of Education* 5(2), 143–158.

The Royal Veterinary College UK, Clinical Skills Centre

Nichola Coombes

3.1 Background

In September 2004, the first veterinary CSC in the world opened its doors to undergraduate students at the Royal Veterinary College (RVC) UK. The idea, borrowed from the medical world, was to provide an accessible learning suite, but without the pressures of the clinical environment. It has four dedicated staff who encourage a relaxed and friendly environment for learning practical skills and is used by around 1000 undergraduate and postgraduate RVC veterinary and nursing students each year. It is used for teaching, OSCEs and many free-access 'drop-in' sessions.

Originally the CSC was placed in a disused bovine theatre, but following its success with the students it

© CAB International 2018. *Veterinary Clinical Skills Manual* (eds N. Coombes and A. Silva-Fletcher)

was moved to purpose-built accommodation in the Lifelong Independent Veterinary Education (LIVE) Building opened by Princess Anne in February 2007. LIVE is a unique Centre for Excellence in Teaching and Learning at the RVC that was set up with the help of a £4.5 million grant from the UK Higher Education Academy. The RVC is split across two campuses, one in Central London (Camden campus) and one 16 miles away in Hertfordshire (Hawkshead campus). The CSC is based at the Hertfordshire Campus and comprises two laboratories, three communications skills rooms, staff offices and a computer suite (Fig. 3.1).

3.2   How Does It Work?

Veterinary undergraduate students first attend the CSC sessions in their 3rd year and continue in their 4th and 5th years. There are ten × 1 h–timetabled sessions in the CSC for 3rd year veterinary undergraduate students. For veterinary nursing students CSC sessions start in year 1 and continue to years 2 and 3. All students are initially taught in small groups on how to perform clinical skills. They are then able to return after these taught sessions and practise the skill again in their own time, with the confidence that the staff in the CSC will be on hand to help should they encounter difficulties, or want reassurance that what they are doing is correct. Students can practise aspects of many different veterinary topics, such as anaesthesia, radiography, lab skills, bandaging, cannula placement, fluid therapy, animal handling and theatre skills.

3.3   Developing Teaching Aids in the CSC

Members of the CSC team have authored 'skills help sheets' for each of the stations, which are available in the CSC labs. These are no more than four A4-size pages and comprise simple bullet points of key information with clear photographs in a standardized format, much akin to a 'how-to' recipe for the skill, but they are not a repeat of the lectures on the subject attended by the students. A total of 52 skills stations are available to students within the CSC.

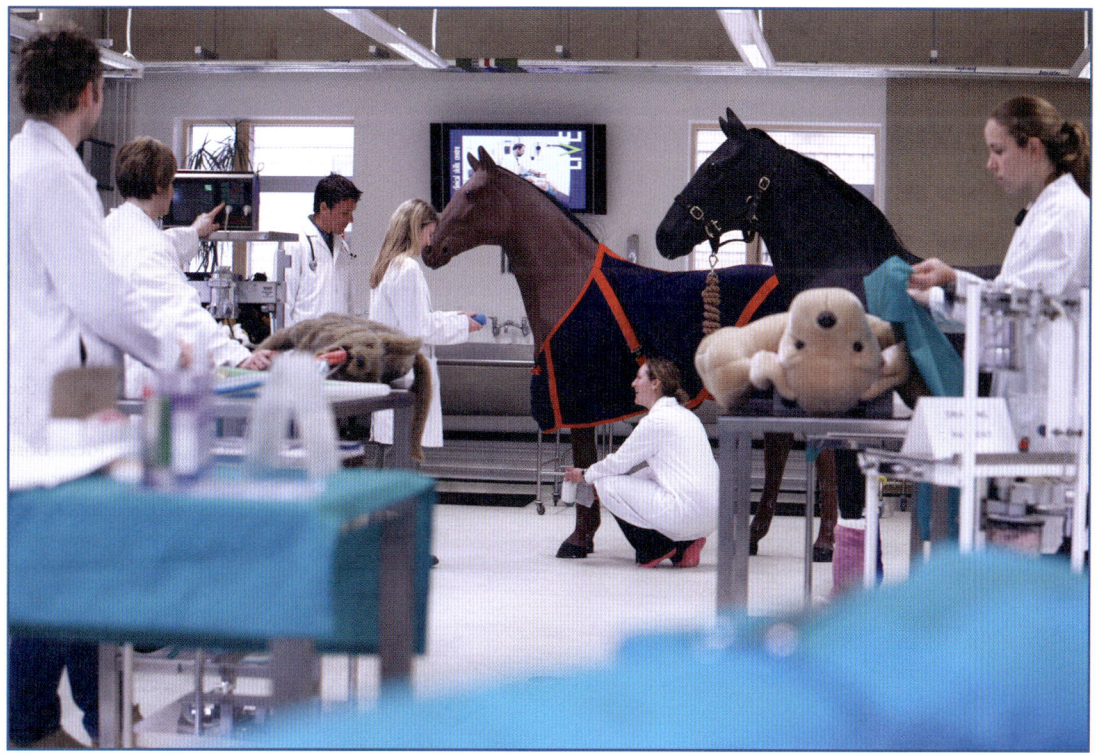

Fig. 3.1. Students practising clinical skills at the RVC's CSC with the aid of video (on screen on the wall).

There are videos, which complement practical teaching sessions not just in the CSC but also in the RVC's three teaching hospitals, and which include animal handling skills. The videos and skills sheets are all available on 'Learn' – the RVC's virtual learning environment.

The staff are known for their patient, approachable and informal attitude towards their students, both in group practical sessions and on a one-to-one basis. In fact, the CSC is often the first port of call when students have a problem of any nature. We feel that, despite the enormous amount of information available online or in books, there is nothing as powerful as the face-to-face contact of teacher and student in skills training.

Our aim is to encourage both veterinary and nursing students to achieve greater confidence in their practical skills, allowing them to feel more integrated into a veterinary team and thus maximize their learning in the workplace.

Lincoln Memorial University College of Veterinary Medicine, Clinical & Professional Skills Program

Julie Williamson and Stacy Anderson

3.4   Background

Lincoln Memorial University, located in Eastern Tennessee, accepted its first veterinary class in 2014. The 4-year Doctor of Veterinary Medicine curriculum is based upon the philosophy of clinical immersion that recognizes that medical knowledge must be developed side-by-side with clinical and professional skills. With this in mind, hands-on skills training begins in the first semester for our students and continues throughout the entire curriculum.

3.5   Facilities

Three large animal buildings were constructed to house the clinical skills program: the ten-stall Equine Stable, the 9000 sq ft (836 m²) Equine Teaching Center (which is equipped with 16 stocks) and the 11,000 sq ft (1022 m²)

Bovine Teaching Center (with headlocks for 96 cows and a workshop space for constructing teaching models). The 43,000 sq ft (3995 m²) Small Animal Clinical Skills Center includes a large clinical skills laboratory, 24-table surgical suite, 18 dental stations, clinical pathology laboratory, diagnostic imaging suite, and clinical skills practise room with models and supplies available for students to work on their skills independently 24 h a day. The professional skills program utilizes small group spaces on campus, including ten state-of-the-art communications suites where students hone their skills by interacting with simulated clients (Fig. 3.2).

3.6   Curriculum

Veterinary students complete 18 credit hours of clinical and professional skills training, divided among their first 3 years of veterinary school, before entering the clinical phase of their training in their 4th year. Students are taught skills and supervised while practising them on models, cadavers or live animals, depending on the nature of the skill and the level of the student. Laboratory sessions develop skills in topics from entry-level to more advanced skills (vertical integration) and are timed to align with students' didactic education in similar topics (horizontal integration).

First-year laboratory sessions focus on handling, restraint and physical examination skills on the common domestic species as well as introducing basic surgery skills such as ligation and suturing. During their second year, students are taught aseptic technique, continue to develop their surgical skills, complete a model ovariohysterectomy and practise techniques they are learning about in their didactic courses such as pathology, theriogenology and anaesthesia. Third-year laboratory sessions include specialty physical examinations, procedure labs and live animal dental and surgical care, spanning large animal, small animal and exotic species. Each semester, students practise professional skills in communication and leadership.

The clinical and professional skills program utilizes approximately 30 veterinarians and eight veterinary technicians as instructors and raters. Most laboratory sessions have one instructor per 8–12 students to facilitate individualized training, and frequent in-lab assessments provide each student with feedback and scores from each laboratory session. Objective structured clinical examinations (OSCEs), surgical skills examinations and directly observed procedures are used to mark a

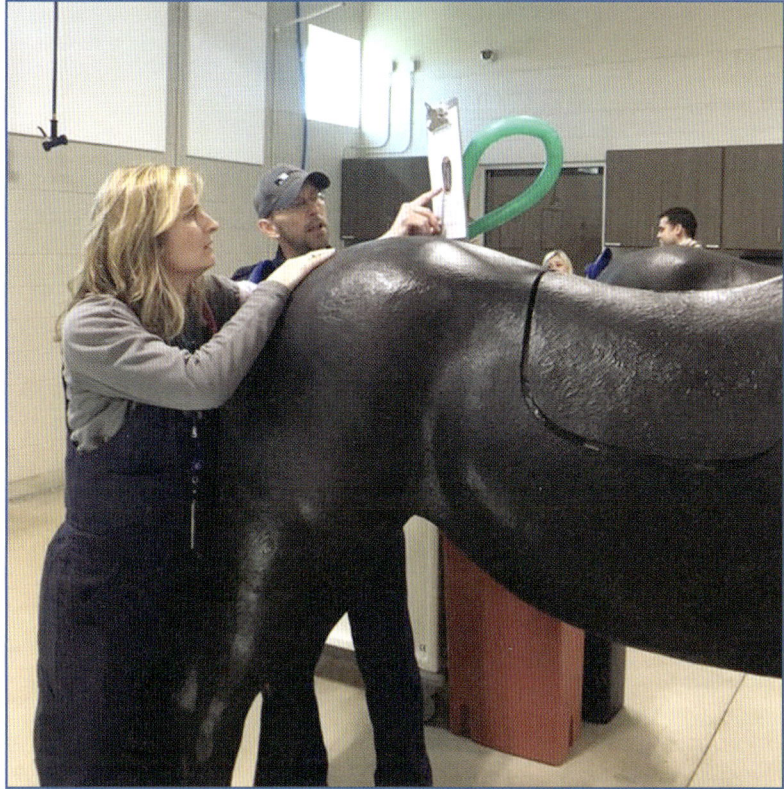

Fig. 3.2. A student learns to perform rectal palpation during a colic laboratory in the Lincoln Memorial University College of Veterinary Medicine, USA.

student's progress through the course of each semester. Because clinical and professional skills are progressive, all assessments are cumulative.

3.7 Resources

In a flipped classroom model, students are assigned to read resources, watch instructional videos, or complete clinical case assignments before coming into laboratory sessions. These resources are available on the students' e-learning platform and can be accessed and reviewed before, during or after the laboratory session to supplement skills learning. Students are encouraged to practise in groups outside of scheduled laboratory sessions in the clinical skills practice room or at home.

Instructors are provided with training in veterinary education topics, including how to simplify tasks for teaching novice students, how to adjust to different student learning styles, how to recognize and approach struggling learners, how to provide corrective feedback that encourages rather than disheartens the learner, and how to assess student skill fairly. Training sessions are offered weekly before each new laboratory session, monthly during veterinary education rounds and yearly during an institutional workshop.

3.8 Model Creation and Research

In keeping with the '3Rs' animal use principles of Replacement, Reduction and Refinement, the clinical skills program utilizes a variety of models for students to perform skills. In addition to using models during laboratory sessions, students are also provided with models to facilitate almost unlimited practice of important techniques at their own convenience, which assists them on their path to mastery. The program uses commercially available models as well as ones that are built in the college's model workshop. This workshop, affectionately dubbed the 'Mad Scientist Lab' due to the preponderance of odd materials it accumulates during model creation, is staffed by a full-time technician who assists instructors wishing to develop new models to support their teaching.

The creation of new models and adoption of novel teaching methods has revealed areas of research pertinent to many veterinary educators who seek to improve their students' practical skills. Faculty has investigated topics including how the use of different surgical skills models may improve student skill, how the assignment of instructors to certain areas of the skills lab may influence student learning and how to improve the reliability of skills assessments. The faculty partners with researchers at other veterinary schools whenever possible to extend the scope of their research.

3.9 Aims

Our primary aim is to support veterinary students on their path to becoming competent, confident veterinarians. We also seek to develop alternative educational methods that spare animal use; to achieve a better understanding of how to teach and assess clinical and professional skills in a progressively more efficient and effective manner; and to cooperate with other veterinary schools worldwide to advance this facet of the profession.

Clinical Skill Center at School of Veterinary Medicine, Mongolian University of Life Sciences

B. Otgontugs and N. Odontsetseg

3.10 Background

In order to respond to the global and social requirements for veterinary graduates, the School of Veterinary Medicine (SVM), Mongolian University of Life Sciences (MULS), had worked on curriculum renovation for 3 years trying to reflect international and national demands

before its implementation from the 2015/2016 academic year. The curriculum renovation started with the help of the Animal Health Project (AHP) of the Swiss Agency for Development and Cooperation (SDC), which was implemented from 2012 to 2016.

3.11 How Does It Work?

Before developing the new curriculum, Day One competences (D1C) were listed. Students must obtain practical D1C skills. Therefore, with the support of SDC AHP and other MULS projects to support teaching and research, three types of clinical skills centre (CSC) were launched in 2016:

1. A room of 120-student capacity dedicated to the CSC. This room is equipped with sewing pads, animal models, anatomy visuals, instruments to detect urine and blood indicators and hygiene testing reagents and instruments for animal-derived products. This room is mostly used for the practical sessions for Years 2 and 3 students (Fig. 3.3).

2. A CSC with large-animal examination stalls, treatment room and animal fencing covering an area of 60 m² constructed and used for clinical teaching. This enables training on live animals. This facility is used for undergraduate practical sessions on animal handling, diagnostics, internal medicine, gynaecology, obstetrics and surgery.

3. A field teaching station established in Ulziit Microdistrict, 30 km from SVM. Ulziit is the closest location where people own pastoral livestock as well as racing horses and dairy, poultry and pig farms. Intensive farms and racing horses need more veterinary care than the nomadic livestock. The SVM aims to make a contract with the farmers and herders on veterinary services. This will help undergraduate students to do clinical practice under the guidance and supervision of teachers. According to the plan, around 20–30 students per day will work in this station. Also this station can be used for continuous training and research. The aim is to develop it further to make it a comprehensive infrastructure for research-teaching-services-production.

Even though these CSCs have just started their functions, we can see some progress in the teaching technology. We think that these CSCs will help in developing not only clinical skills, but also the students' professional attitude.

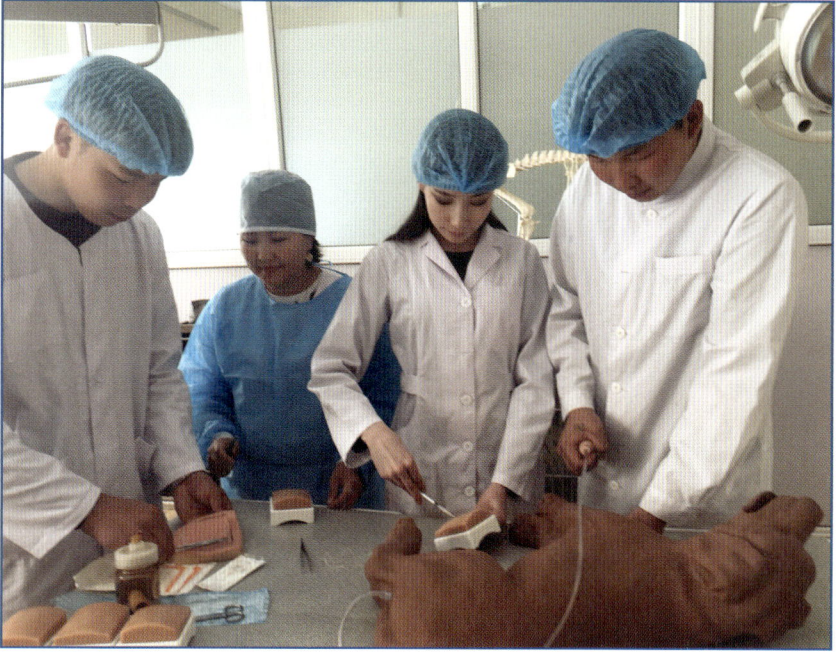

Fig. 3.3. Students practising clinical skills under the guidance of a tutor at the Mongolian Veterinary School.

Veterinary Clinical Skills Laboratory, Faculty of Veterinary Medicine and Animal Science, University of Peradeniya, Sri Lanka

Aruna Amarasinghe and M.L.A.N.R. Deepani

3.12 Background

The Faculty of Veterinary Medicine and Animal Science (FVMAS) of the University of Peradeniya, Sri Lanka, is the only higher educational institute that offers a degree programme leading to a Bachelor of Veterinary Science (BVSc). At present, about 100 students register for the course each year. All the graduates from the faculty have been gainfully employed, primarily in the public sector (i.e. animal production and health, public health, wildlife and zoo animal sectors), with more and more venturing into the private sector (i.e. private practice, marketing, business management, etc.).

As identified in the recent self-evaluation report of the FVMAS, one of the major deficiencies of the undergraduate training programme had been the inadequate training in clinical sciences. This was primarily due to lack of suitable clinical facilities and lack of orientation of clinical teachers to impart clinical skills to the students. From the feedback received from current veterinary undergraduates, past graduates and employers, the lack of practical exposure and poor skill development were identified as the number one priority areas in improving the quality of veterinary graduates and also as a fundamental requirement in enhancing their employability. According to the BVSc curriculum revised in 2000, the current Veterinary Science study programme had given significant weight to teaching and assessing the knowledge domain. Less emphasis was given to imparting and evaluating the skills domain, whereas the attitude domain was rarely addressed and evaluated. Time allocated for the undergraduate teaching programme, shortage of staff, lack of required number of field cases during a stipulated time and logistic reasons, etc. contributed to the above inadequacies. Veterinary undergraduates needed to develop fundamental skills and competences to cater for the demand for veterinary services in many animal species. However, achievement of this goal was a daunting task within the limited time of eight semesters (4-year course duration). In particular, the difficulty of executing and giving practical exposure to clinical cases covering all the domestic animal species and giving required hands-on experience to develop skills was a frequently discussed topic among all the stakeholders in this discipline. It was necessary, therefore, to devise alternative methods to impart enough skills to veterinary students of the FVMAS.

In 2013, Sri Lanka's Ministry of Higher Education, with the help of World Bank funding, launched a programme called 'Higher Education for the Twenty-First Century' (HETC) with a view to improving higher education institutes in Sri Lanka. In response to a call from the HETC, an innovative project proposal was submitted by the FVMAS and the proposed 'CLIP' (Clinical Learning Improvement Program) was able to secure US$250,000 of competitive funding for the project. CLIP was aimed at covering all three domains during learning and evaluation processes in the veterinary clinical teaching programme at the FVMAS. The proposal was primarily intended to have a clinical skills laboratory to impart essential veterinary skills to the students. Secondly, it was proposed to improve the efficiency and effectiveness of field training programmes that cover both clinical and production aspects.

3.13 Establishment of the Veterinary Skills Laboratory at the FVMAS

The initial objectives of the proposed veterinary skills laboratory were to get the students to master the basic veterinary skills, to maintain uniformity in student exposure to fundamental veterinary skills, to maintain uniformity in student evaluation in their practical skills, and to develop interactive learning and teamwork among students and bring out the excitement of a novel teaching and learning facility.

The FVMAS opened its newly established veterinary skills laboratory for students' use in June 2015. The facility was initiated with the development of ten skill stations using imported simulators. In parallel with this, a workshop was held to create awareness among the academic staff on the use of the skills lab facility for

undergraduate teaching and evaluation on the same day. Also, a series of workshops were conducted to introduce the new facility to the entire veterinary student community of the FVMAS and the students were given a chance to experience the models. Excellent feedback was received from the students following these introductory workshop sessions. As suggested in the project proposal, some of the simulator models were designed and developed by the veterinary students as their final-year projects and the necessary guidance and funds were supported by the project. Currently, the facility is being used by veterinary students (Fig. 3.4) and we are in the process of integrating the facility into the formal curriculum for teaching and assessment process with the proposed curriculum revision. The facility is also being used by the Sri Lanka College of Veterinary Surgeons (SLCVS) for its Continuous Professional Development programmes for veterinarians, generating some income to the facility. This income is being utilized to maintain and develop the facility after the project ended in 2016. The lab was developed under the generous support of HETC/QIG/R2/2/PDN/VET Science grant of the Ministry of Higher Education of Sri Lanka.

Department of Veterinary Medicine, University of Cambridge, Queen's Veterinary School Hospital Pauline Brown Clinical Skills Centre

Catherine J. Wager

3.14 Background

The Queen's Veterinary School Hospital Pauline Brown Clinical Skills Centre opened in January 2015. It consists of a large multifunctional skills rehearsal space, a diagnostic imaging room and a teaching consultation room (Fig. 3.5). A full-time Clinical Skills Centre Facilitator oversees the day-to-day running of the Centre, with the support of technicians and the academic lead for clinical skills, Dr Jacqueline Brearley.

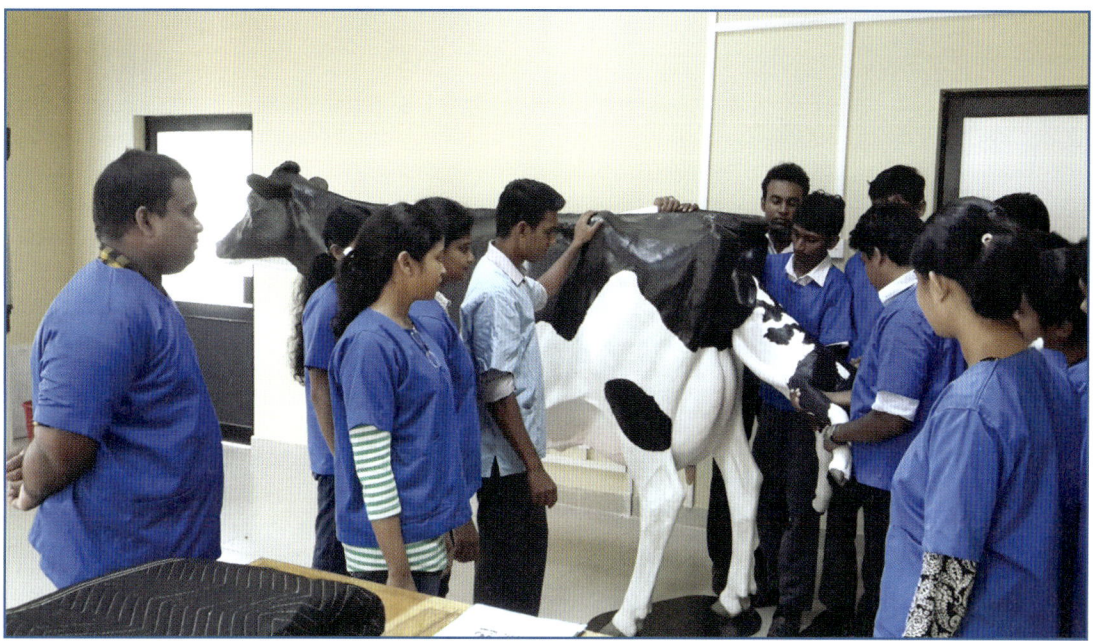

Fig. 3.4. Students receive training on a cow dystocia simulator in the CSC lab in Sri Lanka.

The Centre was funded by the University of Cambridge Veterinary School Trust, also known as Camvet, who continue to lead fundraising campaigns for the additional resources required as the Centre grows. A University of Cambridge Learning and Teaching Innovation Fund grant enabled the acquisition of 15 tablet devices and the production of a library of clinical skills videos to support the students as they develop their Day One competences. Access to these videos is through the Centre's virtual learning environment, allowing students to view them as needed, including remotely when completing extramural studies rotations with veterinary practitioners.

The Centre is available to students studying veterinary medicine at Cambridge throughout the entirety of their course in a variety of ways, including time-tabled access, lunchtime workshops and one-to-one tutorials. Additionally, a 24-hours-a-day, 7-days-a-week, anytime-access drop-in usage policy exists. This allows students to rehearse skills at the times that best suit them and also fosters a culture of student ownership of the Centre, with the aim of enhancing student engagement with the facility.

The Centre is also available to staff members and postgraduate students. It accommodates both in-house and external continuing professional development events and plays an active role in outreach and engagement activities.

3.15   How Does It Work?

One of the principal remits of the Centre is to enable veterinary students to practise the wide range of practical skills needed by new graduates. Over 40 skills, relating to a range of species and disciplines, are available. Each skill is accompanied by a detailed, step-by-step illustrated instruction booklet, whilst the video library of skills demonstrations continues to grow.

In addition to the wide range of teaching models and simulations, small animal handling can be practised with live animals. Dogs belonging to Centre staff spend time in the Centre during the day and it is felt that their presence is a valuable contribution to student welfare. Large animal handling skills can also be practised at the same Department site with the assistance of a dedicated technician. This allows students to build on skills they have been introduced to in the Centre through simulation, by providing access to cows and horses in a realistic situation.

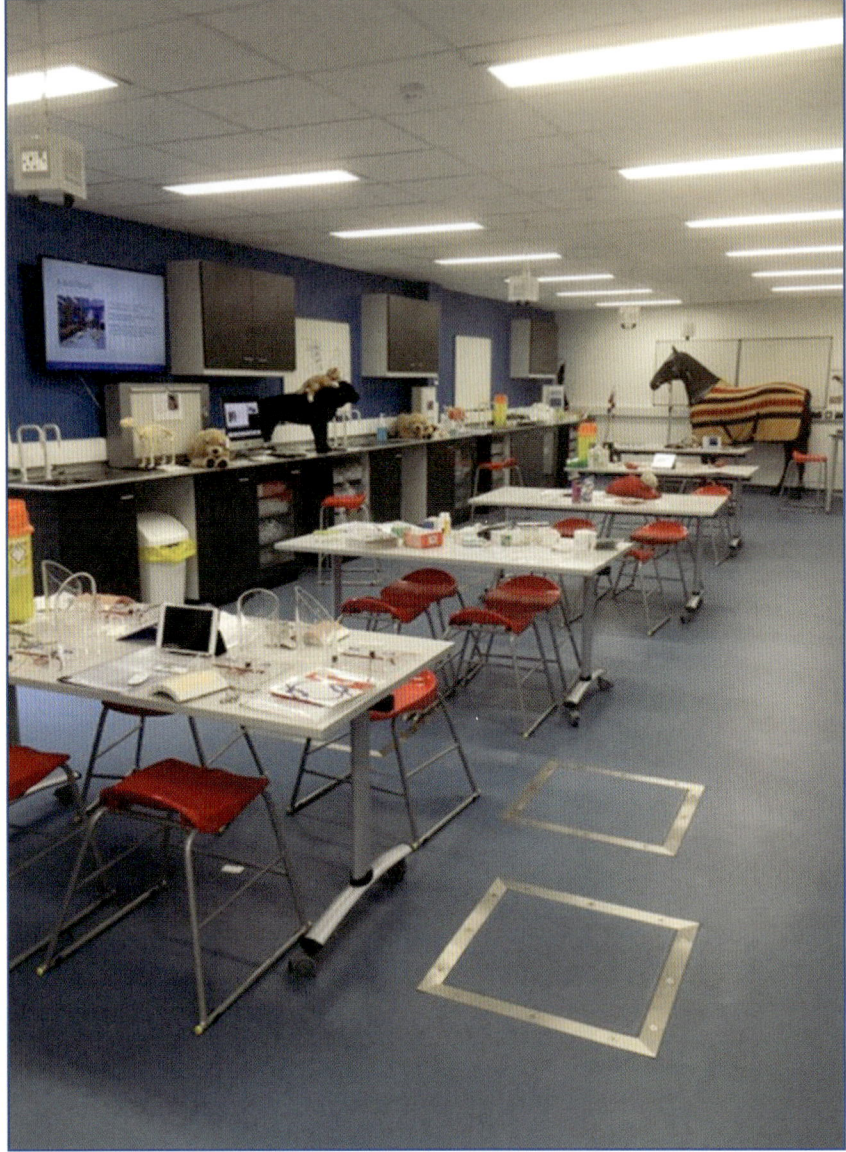

Fig. 3.5. The Clinical Skills lab at the Cambridge Vet School, UK.

Clinical skills teaching is embedded into the curriculum, from basic animal handling for first-year preclinical students, to a series of termly rotations in the first and second clinical years of the course. These rotations start with sessions dedicated to task-based training using bench-top models and progress to the rehearsal of clinical skills in sequence, through case-based scenarios. Additional dimensions of these simulations include clinical decision making, simulated client communication and use of local documentation, as preparation for final-year hospital rotations. Students complete the scenarios with the supervision and assistance of teaching staff.

The Centre also facilitates the assessment of practical skills at key points throughout the course and supports students in all aspects of their assessment preparation.

3.16   The Future

In its continuing development and expansion, the Centre is dedicated to contributing to the growing evidence base for veterinary clinical skills. This includes assisting with the supervision of student elective projects involving both the creation and validation of clinical skills teaching aids. These projects epitomize the Centre's aims of being a student-owned, evidence- and research-based clinical skills teaching facility.

Today, the centre is accessible for both veterinary and nursing students free of charge 7 days a week up until 10.30pm. The Manager of the Clinical Skills Centre is available for hands-on tutorials and questions Mondays and Thursdays until 6pm. In addition to offering drop-in access 7 days a week, the centre works with the teachers of clinical sciences to set up specific training sessions as needed as part of the regular teaching curriculum. Each year, KTC opens its doors to 280 veterinary students and 180 nursing students.

Kliniskt Träningscentrum (Clinical Teaching Centre) at the Department of Clinical Sciences at the Swedish University of Agricultural Sciences

Britt Coles, Desiree Karlsson and Pia Haubro Andersen

3.17   Background

The first Swedish educational centre to offer clinical training for veterinary students was opened in 2009. It was then housed in a smaller space adjacent to the equine clinic in the old Animal Hospital building of the Swedish University of Agricultural Sciences (SLU) in Uppsala. This new centre, Kliniskt Träningscentrum (KTC), offered students a space where they could practise their clinical skills without the immediate stress of a real clinical setting, yet with the opportunity to learn practical skills with the help of various medical modules, dummies and educational software (Fig. 3.6). When the Animal Hospital moved into brand new facilities in 2014, KTC moved with it. The additional funds that came with relocating all nursing students from the SLU Skara campus to the Uppsala campus as well, that same year, made the acquisition of additional KTC teaching materials possible. These additional materials were very much appreciated by the students visiting the new and greatly improved larger space.

3.18   How Does It Work?

SLU in Uppsala offers the country's only programme in veterinary medicine. The programme is 5½ years long. The first 3 years are theory based and the subsequent 2 years are focused on practising the clinical skills based on that theoretical foundation. The last 6 months are dedicated to the veterinary students writing master's theses in veterinary medicine. The veterinary students are introduced to KTC in the 3rd year of their programme.

The university also offers the country's only programme in veterinary nursing. This programme is 3 years long. Even though the first year has an emphasis on theory, the nursing students are introduced to the training centre that same year. The centre plays a continued cardinal role in their education as the last 2 years of the veterinary nursing programme have an emphasis on clinical skills. Half of the last term is spent writing up a bachelor's thesis in veterinary nursing.

KTC offers a variety of opportunities for the students. They include:

- Case scenarios. Jerry is a stuffed animal in sudden need of cardio-respiratory resuscitation. Subsequently, Jerry offers an excellent opportunity to practise team-building under artificial stressful conditions by simulating an emergency case without risking the welfare of a live patient.

- Training of proper procedures for scrubbing in for surgery and other hygiene procedures.

- Surgery dummies and other training modules for both basic and advanced invasive surgical procedures.

- Computer-based interactive training modules, including the Glass Horse.

- A permanent set-up of four cameras that can film the students in different training scenarios, with subsequent playback and feedback.

- Skills stations offering opportunities on how to take blood samples and inject medications intravenously, intramuscularly and as an epidural.

- Techniques and methods for examining and diagnosing various conditions that can be practised on full-scale animal models as well as smaller dummies. One of the large-scale models is a fibreglass horse used for training on wound care, blood sampling and the administration of injections.

In its current form, the centre offers a much-needed space for students to enhance their clinical skills at their own pace in an ethical and supportive environment, with and without the supervision of trained staff, thus making the space cost effective in the long run.

Jordan University of Science and Technology (JUST), Faculty of Veterinary Medicine, Clinical Skills Laboratory

Zuhair Bani Ismail and Ehab Abu-Basha

3.19   Background

The Veterinary Clinical Skills Laboratory (CSL) located in the Faculty of Veterinary Medicine at Jordan University of Science and Technology (JUST), Jordan, was established in 2015. It is the only veterinary clinical skills centre in Jordan as well as in the Middle East. The mission of the centre is to provide a venture for hands-on clinical and diagnostic learning in the Faculty of Veterinary Medicine Program at JUST. Not only does the CSL offer an advanced learning environment,

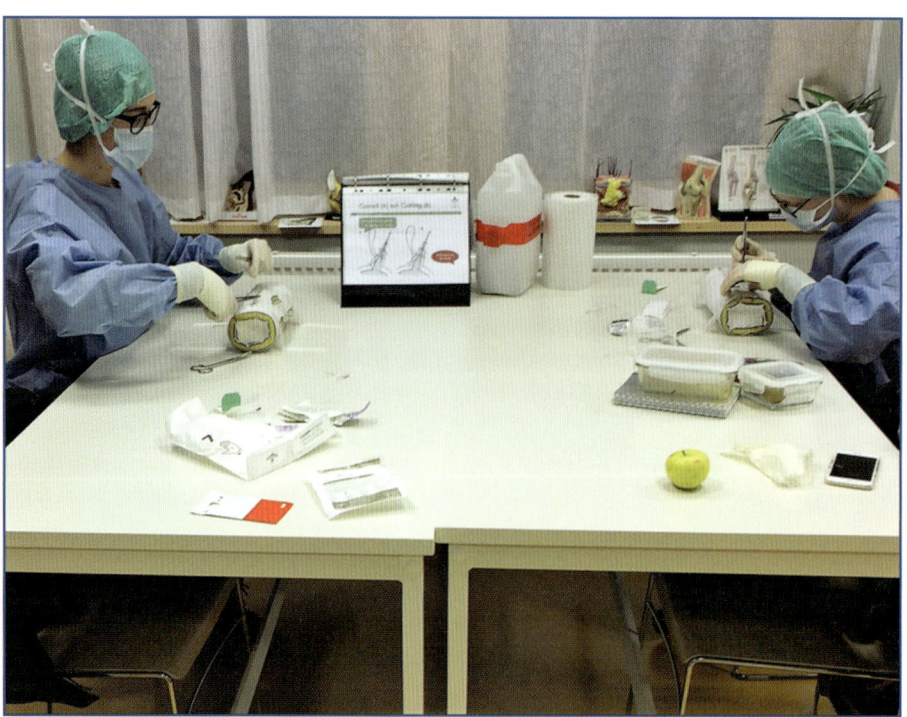

Fig. 3.6. Two students practising suturing skills at the clinical training centre in Uppsala, Sweden.

but it also provides students with the opportunity to expand their understanding of the interactions between animal and human health.

The CSL is open all day long during the week to veterinary undergraduate students. Both 4th and 5th year veterinary students have the opportunity to attend the centre to perform many hands-on experiences and develop essential clinical skills, including use of suture materials, suturing techniques, knot tying techniques, surgical instrument identification, handling and care, hypodermic needles and intravenous catheters (Fig. 3.7). Students can practise blood withdrawal from small animals using animal models (dolls), placing intravenous catheters in small animals using models, blood smear preparation and examination, and performing urine and faecal analysis. The CSL also provides models for fracture repair using various internal and external fixation techniques, models for placing distal limb bandages in small and large animals, and rectal palpation models for cows' and mares' reproductive examinations. The students also practise surgical scrubbing, gowning and gloving techniques in the centre. The CSL contains several models of large and small animal inhalational anaesthesia machines so that students can gain experience in operating and maintaining them. Business management and communication skills are included in the centre as an integral part of the self-learning programme using many videos that have been made available. There are also videos demonstrating many of the clinical skills such as general physical examination and handling of different animal species, and different diagnostic techniques such as endoscopy, ultrasound, radiology and biopsy. In addition, the centre contains many preserved (whole and dissected) animal specimens and multiple bone specimens that students can use to learn veterinary anatomy.

3.20 How Does It Work?

The CSL is supervised and kept well-maintained by one of our most dedicated staff members, who is a skilled veterinarian with wide clinical expertise in both large and small animal practices. During 2016, over 200 students used the centre at least once per semester to practise different skills. The centre is also used for teaching a general veterinary surgery course (2 credit hours), veterinary anaesthesiology course (1 credit hour), general theriogenology courses (several courses), parts of the clinical examination course (2 credit hours) and objective structured clinical exams (OSCEs).

Practical sessions are typically scheduled every week according to registered practical courses. A Faculty member (course coordinator), a CSL supervisor and a teaching assistant attend the practical sessions to supervise the students. Students can also attend the centre in their free time to gain further experience after they coordinate with the CSC supervisor.

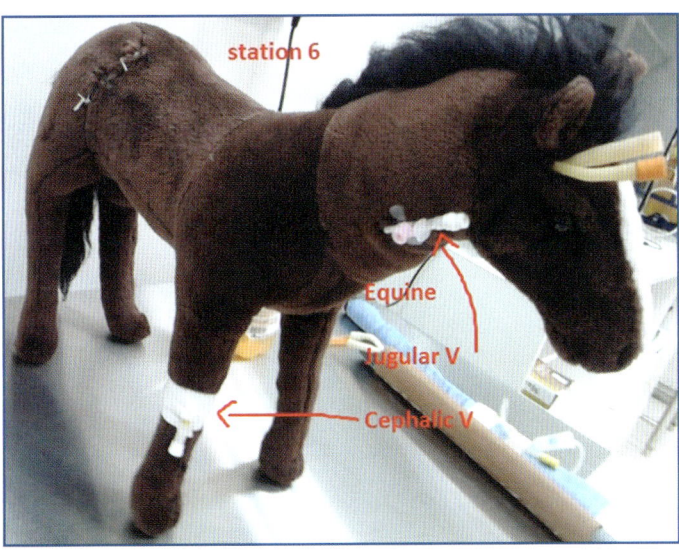

Fig. 3.7. An equine model developed in Jordan to practise intravenous injections.

3.21 Developing Teaching Aids in the CSL

The Faculty of Veterinary Medicine is in the process of developing a clinical skills log book and clinical skills list that all students have to sign off before graduation. A significant portion of this list will be executed and signed by the CSL supervisor. The CSL supervisor has developed clear instructions for each skill station as a guide to the students while performing the skills. These instruction notes are placed in a clear location next to the designated skill station in the centre. Step-by-step guidance showing how the skill is performed is also photographed in consequence and placed on the wall above each station.

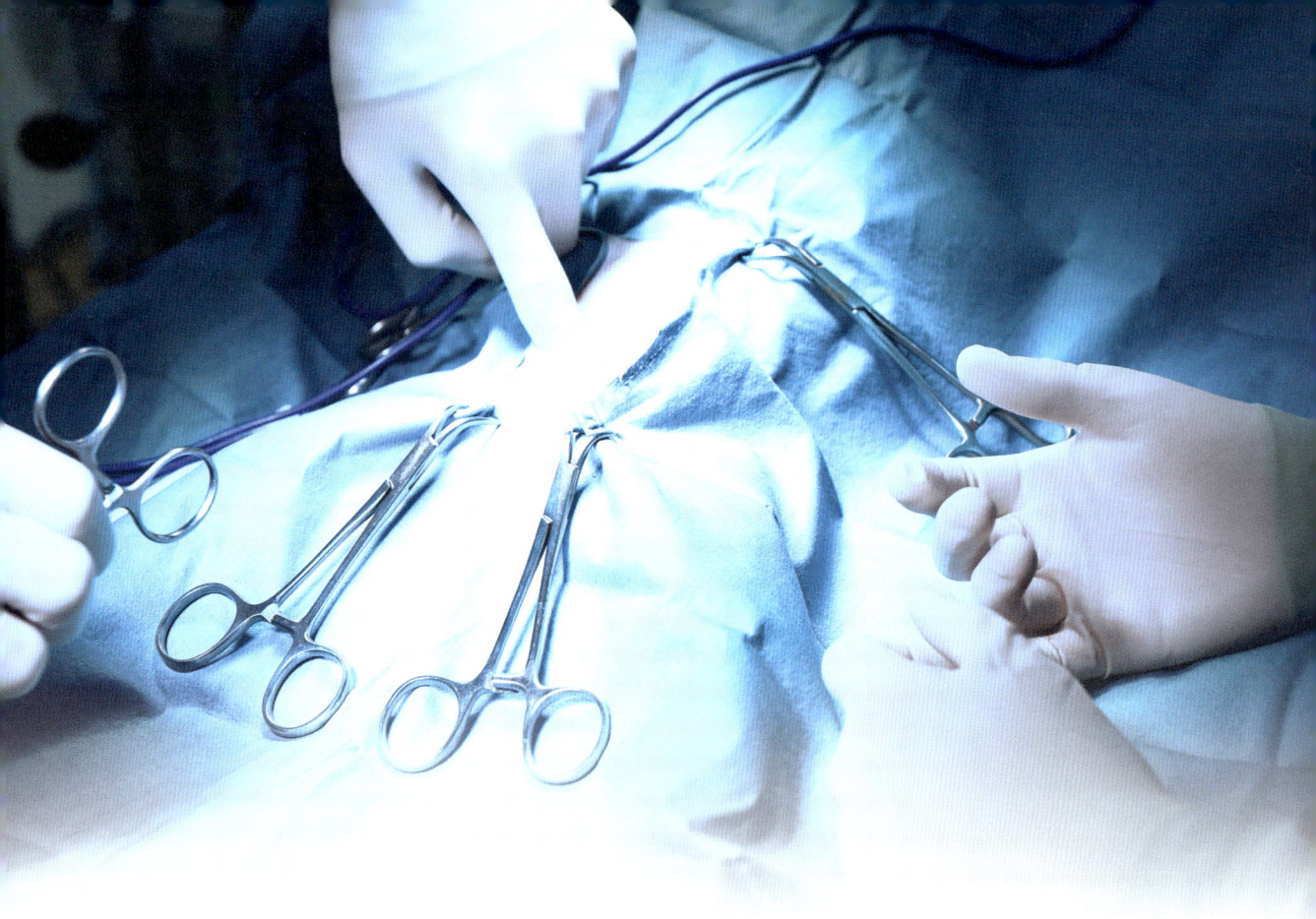

Surgical Theatre Skills

Section Editor: Fiona Brown

Introduction

Performing surgery requires different skills: maintaining asepsis from start to finish, including a meticulous approach in using the relevant instruments, materials and the closure of the incision. In this section you will be introduced to different stages of surgery, from preparation to finish and how to initiate and maintain asepsis of the instruments, the patients and the surgical assistant or the surgeon. Details of how to use the instruments in the closure of incision wounds will be given in detail so that you can practise these skills in a safe environment.

Within this section there are three chapters:

Chapter 4: Theatre Practice

Chapter 5: Surgical Instruments

Chapter 6: The Fundamentals of Suturing

Within each chapter you will find pictures and tips about how to practise relevant basic Day One skills. Each chapter will also detail key points for each set of skills and point out the health and safety considerations, which are critical to good practice.

An overview of all the learning outcomes is presented below and the more detailed learning outcomes are presented under each chapter.

Learning objectives

After studying this section, students should be able to:

- Demonstrate skills in asepsis during surgical scrubbing, drying of hands, gowning, gloving and draping a patient in readiness for surgery.
- Identify general surgical instruments and the type of materials they are made of.
- Perform as a surgical assistant using appropriate instrument handling skills.
- Understand and perform the sterilization process.
- Understand the differences between different types of knots, handle surgical instruments appropriately and match the suture materials to the tissue.
- Start and finish continuous patterns.

What You Will Use

Clinical skills sheets (SS)

Eleven clinical skills sheets will be used in this section. Reference will be made to each skill sheet at the relevant point within the chapter. Clinical skills sheets for the following accompany this section:

SS 4.1 Surgical scrub

SS 4.2 Hand drying

SS 4.3 Gowning

SS 4.4 Closed gloving

SS 4.5 Open gloving

SS 4.6 Draping using the four-quadrant technique

SS 5.7 Opening a sterile instrument pouch

SS 5.8 Instrument handling and selection

SS 6.9 One-handed tie, right-hand method

SS 6.10 Two-handed tie (the bird's beak version)

SS 6.11 Instrument suture – square knot or surgeon's knot

Videos (V)

Thirteen videos will be used in this section and reference will be made to each video at the relevant point within the chapter. Videos will be hyperlinked and the following accompany this section:

V 4.1 WHO hand wash

V 4.2 Surgical gowning (fabric gown)

V 4.3 Surgical gowning (paper gown)

V 4.4 Closed gloving

V 4.5 Open gloving

V 4.6 Draping (4-drape)

V 6.1 One-handed tie

V 6.2 Two-handed tie

V 6.3 Modified Miller's knot

V 6.4 Slip knot

V 6.5 Aberdeen knot

V 6.6 Simple interrupted suture

V 6.7 Simple continuous suture

4 Theatre Practice

Fiona Brown
The Royal Veterinary College, London

Learning objectives

By the end of this chapter, students should be able to demonstrate:

- Aseptic awareness.
- Surgical scrubbing.
- Drying of hands in an aseptic manner.
- Gowning and gloving aseptically.
- Draping a patient ready for surgery.

The student's aseptic awareness should mean that they are ready to act as a scrub assistant, a circulating assistant and/or later as a surgeon.

Clinical skills sheets (SS)

Six clinical skills sheets will be used in this chapter and these can be found at pages 37–48. Reference will be made to each skills sheet at the relevant section within the chapter. The details of the clinical skills sheets used are as follows:

SS 4.1 Surgical scrub
SS 4.2 Hand drying
SS 4.3 Gowning
SS 4.4 Closed gloving
SS 4.5 Open gloving
SS 4.6 Draping using the four-quadrant technique

Videos (V)

Six videos will be used in this chapter to demonstrate how to perform the clinical skills and these are:

V 4.1 WHO hand wash
V 4.2 Surgical gowning (fabric gown)
V 4.3 Surgical gowning (paper gown)
V 4.4 Closed gloving
V 4.5 Open gloving
V 4.6 Draping (4 drape)

Introduction

An awareness of aseptic technique is essential to anyone working in a clinical veterinary practice, so all surgical and nursing students will be expected to demonstrate that they are competent from their first day in practice.

Veterinary students will be given the opportunity to carry out surgical operations under direct supervision when on their compulsory extramural studies (EMS) placements in practice, and student nurses will also be learning how to help to prepare and assist during these surgical procedures when on their clinical placements away from the classroom.

These aseptic techniques can be easily rehearsed away from the clinical environment. The student can perfect these skills in their own timeframe until they are ready to apply them to real-life surgical situations. The underlying principles are essential, no matter what environment you work in, and it is important that these skills are practised, perfected and applied throughout the student's time before qualifying. The techniques will soon become second nature when the student veterinary surgeon or nurse is given the opportunity to apply them for real in the operating theatre.

Of course, all veterinary environments are different with regard to what facilities and equipment are available, but as long as all underlying principles are observed, there is room for a range of techniques and adaptations using directly transferable skills: they can be made to fit any environment.

© CAB International 2018. *Veterinary Clinical Skills Manual* (eds N. Coombes and A. Silva-Fletcher)

The methods described here have been taught within the Royal Veterinary College Clinical Skills Centre with a view to fully supporting and complementing the clinical training received by undergraduate students when in the teaching hospitals belonging to the college, whilst on EMS and clinical placements.

Peer learning together

- These skills are best practised when working in pairs, one person acting as a circulating assistant and the other as the lead surgeon.
- Make sure to swap roles to ensure that you have a clear understanding of different roles in practice.

Once learnt in the skill centre laboratory it's important to maintain these high standards when starting to apply these principles to surgical skills (see Chapter 6) so the student's skill is constantly being reinforced and applied.

When you start visiting the clinical skills centre to practise your surgical skills like suturing and surgical knots and ties, get into the habit of scrubbing, gowning and gloving first and it will become second nature.

4.1 Aseptic Technique: Personal Awareness

Anyone who enters the environment of an operating theatre needs to have an understanding of the importance of asepsis, which is taking appropriate action to avoid microbial contamination of surgical incisions. Circulating staff (those not gloved and gowned) should not touch or lean over sterile fields, taking care when moving around scrubbed personnel and sterile equipment. Any student practising these skills outside of the clinical environment and within the simulated environment of a skills laboratory should have an awareness of this and undertake to perform the skill as if in a sterile operating environment, thereby ensuring this awareness becomes second nature.

4.2 Roles Within Theatre

The term 'staff' is used to describe all people in the operating theatre. In reality, this commonly includes veterinary surgeons (VSs) and Registered Veterinary Nurses (RVNs) but often includes student vets and nurses. It is also important that other members of the practice are aware of good aseptic practice, as care assistants and receptionists may occasionally visit the theatre. It is not uncommon for veterinary practices to have visitors such as work experience students and therefore it is important that they are made aware of how to move about the theatre and what to touch and what not to touch.

4.2.1 Circulating staff

These are staff members, most commonly RVNs, whose role is to assist the surgical team. They open sterile packaging, secure scrubbed personnel into their gowns, fetch additional equipment, select and open suture material packets, keep a record of swabs and instruments, operate and monitor equipment such as suction machines and may have a role in monitoring anaesthesia.

4.2.2 Scrubbed personnel

These are the staff members who are gowned and gloved and so are considered sterile. This can include the surgeon, surgical assistant/nurse, and for bigger practices may include someone whose role is to take responsibility for the surgical instrument trolley (see Chapter 5).

Any scrubbed personnel should avoid turning their backs on the sterile field, keeping their arms and hands above their own waist level at all times in front of their body to ensure that they never inadvertently contaminate themselves or the surgical field.

4.2.3 Working together

When preparing for surgery, you need to rely on others to help you don gowns and gloves, so it is very important that you are able to take instruction but also to direct people clearly.

As you will be working as a team, it is important to ensure that you are happy with your role and if necessary discuss before scrubbing what is expected of you so that your responsibilities are clearly defined.

It is essential that any breach in sterility (or potential breach) is reported immediately and acted upon, therefore replacing equipment, changing gloves and re-scrubbing if necessary.

The opening of equipment packaging is a prime example of where contamination occurs. Both the scrubbed and non-scrubbed assistant need to take responsibility here to ensure that they do not touch each other. The assistant should check that the sterile pouch (see 'Sterilization' in Chapter 5) is not damaged and is in date. If acting as a circulating (unscrubbed) assistant in practice, or when practising with your peers, ensure when opening sterile pouches that you present the gloves or surgical instrument in such a way that minimizes any contamination. This is not a moment to rush: the circulating assistant needs to take time to present the equipment so that it is easily grasped and the scrubbed personnel need to take care as they take the instrument, gown, glove or drape that they do not touch the unsterile surface of the packet or the scrubbed assistant. The role of the scrubbed assistant is covered in more detail in Chapter 5.

Before your first time scrubbing up, try to find the time to watch a surgical team prepare for surgery. Watch how they work as a team, the different roles they take on and how they move around each other.

4.3   Attire

There is a potential for the surgical team to contaminate the surgical wound during the procedure. Every realistic step within the realms of the facilities available should be taken to minimize microbial contamination.

To reduce contamination from the outside environment, it is prudent for anyone entering the surgical environment to be appropriately clothed and ideally this should include changing out of outside clothes and shoes into clothing designated for the surgical environment, such as scrub suits and theatre-specific footwear. Surgical scrubs are ideal; they are easily identifiable as theatre attire, are comfortable, easily washed and changed if they become dirty, and can also be of different colours to signify the different roles of the theatre

team. After all, once a mask and hat is worn, it can become difficult to tell who is who. Appropriately cleaned comfortable footwear is also advised.

Removing all jewellery, avoiding artificial nails, covering the hair and wearing masks helps to reduce microbial contamination.

4.4   Scrubbing Up

The surgical scrub is the process by which the surgical team wash their hands and arms in order to significantly reduce the number of bacteria (both transient and residual skin bacteria). Gloves should always be worn during the surgical procedure, to ensure a sterile barrier, but a thorough scrubbing approach significantly reduces a potential contamination risk should a glove's integrity be breached during the procedure.

The ideal properties of a scrub solution include detergent/soap to remove surface dirt, oil and some surface bacteria. To be aseptic we need to take this one step further and destroy the micro-organisms. For this we rely on antiseptics and so an antimicrobial solution is chosen. Examples include: povidone–iodine and chlorohexidine gluconate.

What is the difference between disinfectants and antiseptics?

Disinfectants and antiseptics both work by destroying and removing micro-organisms but they are used in different ways.

- Disinfectant kills micro-organisms in the environment, such as walls and floors.
- Antiseptic action is on the skin.

A methodical approach is adopted by taking into account the contact time required for the antimicrobial soap to take effect, whilst also ensuring that all the skin surfaces are covered.

Contact times vary between products, but are generally a 5-min first scrub of the day, followed by 3-min scrubs subsequently. Newer waterless solutions are becoming more common, such as Sterilium. They have a short contact time (only 1.5 min) and have many advantages over the traditional scrub solutions, including reducing damage to skin as they do not require the use of a scrubbing brush. They do need to be used with pH-neutral detergents prior to application to remove gross dirt and a standard clinical hand wash should be performed to facilitate this.

 SS 4.1 for details of surgical scrub procedure

 V 4.1 for a demonstration of the WHO hand wash procedure

V 4.1 video.cabi.org/rizxx

 Breaking sterility

Sterility may be broken by touching the tap after scrubbing (turning the tap off by hand), so make sure you use your elbows if necessary.

 A variety of adaptations may be seen in practice with alternative antimicrobial soaps, waterless alcohol-based antiseptic solutions, pre-packaged scrub brushes/sponges and brushless approaches, but the important thing to remember is that the basic principles remain the same.

 Many clinical skills centres will have access to a light box where you can assess the efficacy of your scrubbing technique. These will fluoresce the skin where contact with the product has been achieved.

4.5 Drying Hands

After the surgical scrub, you will need to dry your hands and arms in order to put the sterile gloves on. If you are using a product such as Sterilium, hand drying is not necessary as it evaporates quickly.

Some disposable gown packs include a disposable paper towel, one for each hand.

If you have only one towel to use, it helps to mentally divide the towel into four quarters – one quarter for each hand and each arm.

 SS 4.2 for details of clinical hand drying

 V 4.1 for a demonstration of the WHO hand wash procedure

V 4.1 video.cabi.org/rizxx

4.6 Gowning

Gowns allow you to cover the body with a sterile field; this allows you to lean close to the surgical site whilst reducing the chance of contamination. The clean, dry gown will be folded or rolled and presented sterilized in either a box or a sterile bag. An assistant is required to open the packaging and then to secure the scrubbed person into the gown. This assistant and scrubbed person must ensure that they only touch the inside (unsterile) surface of the gown. Once gowned, only the area above the waist is considered sterile, so hands must remain raised and it helps to keep hands clasped together.

4.6.1 Colour coding

- Disposable drapes and gowns are usually blue.
- Reusable drapes and gowns are usually green.

 SS 4.3 for details on how to gown in a sterile manner

 V 4.2 on surgical gowning (fabric gown) and **V 4.3** on surgical gowning (paper gown)

V 4.2 video.cabi.org/rhfqi

V 4.3 video.cabi.org/icvoj

4.7 Gloving

As it is impossible to sterilize a person's skin, it is the wearing of sterile gloves that acts as a sterile barrier between the surgeon and the patient. Gloves are available in different sizes and can be made of different materials to suit individual needs (such as allergy/sensitivity). It is important that your gloves fit correctly and are in close contact with your skin to allow for good dexterity and feeling. Too large and they will get in your way and be potentially dangerous; too tight and you risk loss of sensation and swelling.

- Closed gloving reduces the risk of accidental contamination as the hands remain inside the gown at all times.

- Open gloving is an alternative method but you are limited in the sterile field, especially if gloving without a surgical gown being worn.

 SS 4.4 for details on how to carry out closed gloving and **SS 4.5** for open gloving

 V 4.4 for closed gloving and **V 4.5** for open gloving

V 4.4 video.cabi.org/pxdwh

V 4.5 video.cabi.org/gpoip

4.8 Draping

Draping the surgical area allows you to reduce the contamination risk from the patient or from the environment and is performed once the surgical area has been clipped and prepped with a surgical scrub solution such as povidone or chlorhexidine. Some practices may choose a fenestrated drape, either with pre-cut holes, or surgeons may cut their own in a disposable paper drape. The benefits of using a fenestrated drape are that draping is quick, but unless the drape is very large it limits the size of the sterile field. A classic four-drape technique allows for a large sterile field but also the freedom to enlarge the incision area if needed. With the inclusion of gowns on the surgical team, this creates a continuous sterile field.

 SS 4.6 for details on how to perform the four-drape technique

 V 4.6 for draping (four-drape technique)

V 4.6 video.cabi.org/acngn

4.8.1 Reusable fabric or disposable paper?

Many practices use disposable gowns and drapes. Disposable items cost more to purchase over time but they remove the need for laundering and the staffing costs involved in their preparation for use. Disposable gowns have the advantage of not only being water resistant but also having a waterproof coating, reducing the risk of strike-through contamination should the area become wet. They also have a wraparound design where more of the body is covered.

Paper drapes tend to be larger than the fabric ones. As an additional level of protection, plastic adhesive drapes applied to the skin can be used.

Regardless of which type you may see in practice, practising the skill with fabric gown/drapes allows you to re-roll the same gown or fold the same drapes again and again to perfect your technique. Once you are confident with what you can and cannot touch, try the technique with a paper version; although the paper gowns secure in a slightly different way the basic principles are the same. Paper drapes are much the same but they can be a little slippery, so it is doubly important to secure them to the patient as soon as two touch, to avoid them sliding on to the floor.

 Reflect back on this chapter.

- Are you happy with the different roles in theatre?
- Can you explain the role of the circulating staff?
- Can you open an instrument package for a scrubbed colleague without breaking sterility?
- Can you scrub using different techniques?
- Can you gown and put on surgical gloves?
- Can you drape a patient using a four-drape technique?

Further Reading: Fossum, T.W. (2013) Part 1: General Surgical Principles. In: *Small Animal Surgery*, 4th edn. Elsevier Mosby, St Louis, Missouri, USA.

Hamilton, M.H. (2012) Sterilization and disinfection. In: Baines, S., Libscomb, V. and Hutchinson, T. (eds) *BSAVA Manual of Canine and Feline Surgical Principles*. BSAVA, Gloucester, UK, pp. 8–21.

McHugh, D., Young, A. and Johnson, J. (2011) Theatre practice. In: Cooper, B., Mullineaux, E. and Turner, L. (eds) *BSAVA Textbook of Veterinary Nursing*, 5th edn. BSAVA, Gloucester, UK, pp. 738–773.

Clinical Skills Sheet

4.1. Surgical scrub

Task:

Carry out a 5-minute surgical scrub in preparation for surgery using a sterile scrub brush from the wall-mounted scrub container.

Method
Remove watches, bracelets and rings – put somewhere safe!
Turn on the taps – to produce a steady flow of water at a comfortable temperature.
Keep hands higher than elbows – wet hands and arms thoroughly.
Use elbow to depress soap dispenser and apply 2–3 pumps of antimicrobial soap on to free hand (either chlorhexidine or povidone-iodine if you are allergic to 'Hibiscrub'). 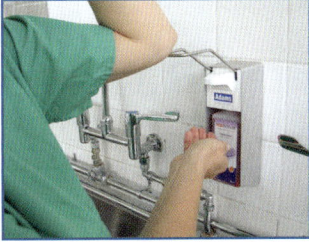
Work into a lather over both hands and forearms as far as the elbow. 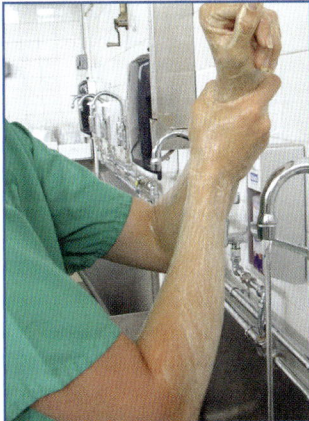
Use elbow to depress lever on the wall-mounted scrub container – remove one scrub brush. 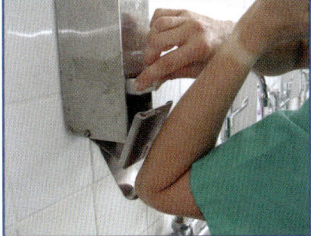

Method
Clean under nails with short nail-cleaning bristles, under running water. 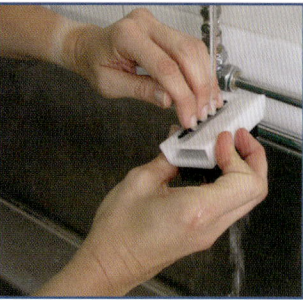
Rinse hands and forearms – keeping hands higher than elbows.
Apply 2–3 pumps of antimicrobial soap – work into lather on hands and forearms up to the elbows.
Note the starting time.
Both hands: for approx 4 minutes (or at least 10 strokes of the brush on each plane) • Scrub the nails. • Scrub all 4 planes of each finger. • Scrub the palm of the hand. • Scrub the back of the hand.
Use hands or brush to spread soap up forearm – *two-thirds* of the way to the elbow.
Repeat a short scrub* procedure for each hand.
Spread soap up the forearm – *halfway* up to the elbow.
Repeat a final short scrub procedure for each hand.
Drop scrub brush into sink.
Check clock to ensure that scrub procedure has taken no less than 5 minutes.
Rinse both hands and arms thoroughly under the running water.
Turn off the taps with elbows.
Continue to keep hands higher and stand over the sink to allow most of the water to run off into the sink.
Keep hands higher than elbows throughout.
Both hands scrubbed for appropriate length of time.
Do not touch any article with hands or forearm.

*A **short scrub** means simply that, i.e. not scrubbing the planes of your fingers/hands for 10 scrubs, but 2–4, as long as you use the time efficiently.

© RVC

Clinical Skills Sheet

4.2. Hand drying

Task:

You have scrubbed your hands in preparation for a surgical procedure. Now dry your hands and put on a surgical gown.

Method
Ask your assistant to open the gowning box on the table in front of you.
Remove the towel from the box, taking care not to drip water on the gown beneath it, or touch the outside of the 'sterile' box.
Grasp the towel whilst keeping your hands higher than your elbows.
Step back from the table.
Allow the towel to unfold, holding on to one corner.
Hold a quarter of the towel over your right hand and use this quarter to dry your fingers, palm and back of your left hand. 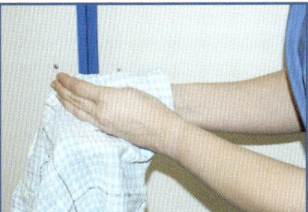
Move your right hand across to the 'second' quarter (the one to the left of the first) and dry your left forearm – *work in one downward direction from your wrist to your elbow – do not return to your wrist once your elbow has been reached!* 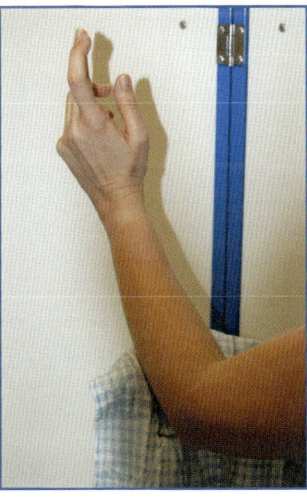 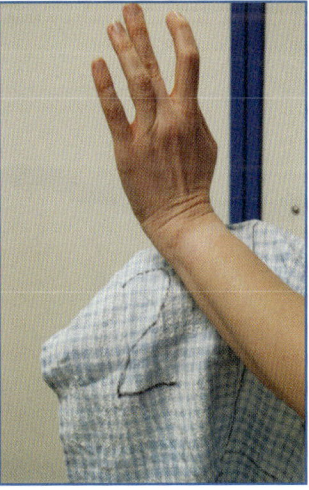

Method
Once the first hand and arm are dry, bring the dry hand diagonally across to the opposite end of the towel. 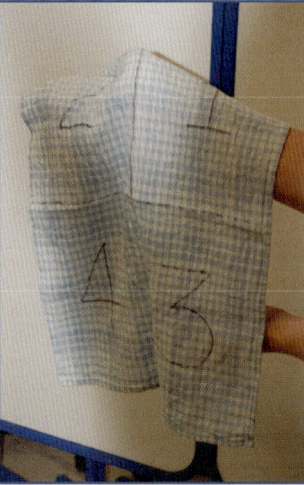
Hold the 'third' quarter of the towel over your left hand and dry the fingers, palm and back of your right hand. 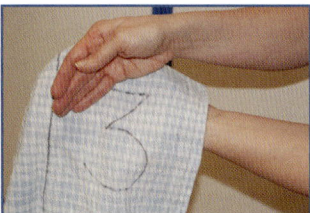
Move your left hand down to the last quarter.
Use the last quarter of towel to dry your right forearm – *work in one downward direction from your wrist to your elbow – do not return back to your wrist once your elbow has been reached!* 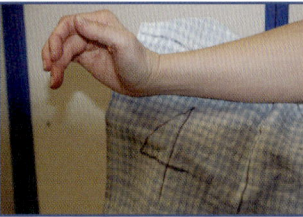
Drop the used towel into a proper receptacle or on to a 'dirty' bench surface if a receptacle is not provided (not on to floor!).
Do not lower your hands below your waist level throughout.
Question: What is the aim of scrubbing the skin prior to putting on a gown and gloves?
Answer: To remove any gross dirt and to reduce as much as possible the number of micro-organisms on the skin. The scrub solution should have a prolonged effect in suppressing the levels of organisms on the skin once underneath surgical gloves.

© RVC

Clinical Skills Sheet

4.3. Gowning

Task:

You have scrubbed and dried your hands in preparation for a surgical procedure. You must now put on a surgical gown.

Method
Ask a non-sterile assistant to open the box containing the gown.
The sterile gown (folded inside out) should be grasped at the shoulders and removed from the box, being careful to touch only the inside of the box and outer (inner) surface of the gown. Lift the gown out of the box, away from the table/nearby surfaces and allow it to fall open away from the body. 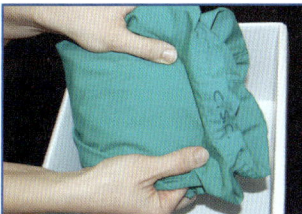
Guide both arms into the sleeves of the gown. If closed gloving, ensure that your hands are retained within the sleeves of the gown. No attempt should be made to pull the gown over the shoulders. 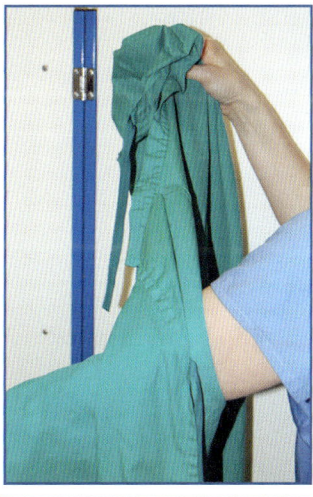 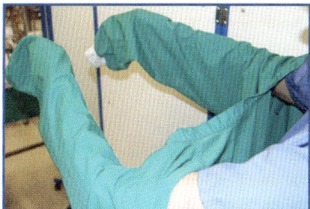
An unscrubbed assistant should then be instructed to pull the back of the gown over the shoulders (touching only the inside of the gown) and fasten the back/neck ties, again being careful to touch only the inside of the gown.

Method
With the hands retained within the sleeves, bend slightly to pick up the waist tie/s and pass these to the assistant without coming into contact with him/her.   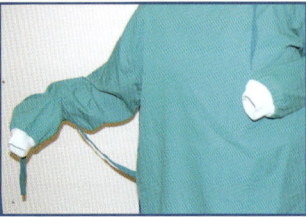 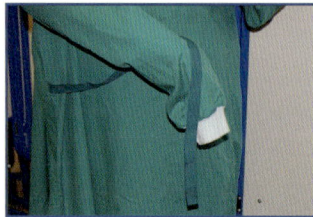
Ask the assistant to fasten waist tie/s at the side (side-tying gown) or back (back-tying gown).   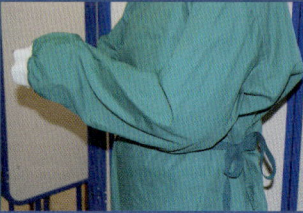
Keep hands within cuffs of the gown.
Hands and arms should be held out in front of the body, above the waist.

© RVC

Clinical Skills Sheet

4.4. Closed gloving

Task:

You have scrubbed and dried your hands and put on a sterile gown. You must now put on a pair of gloves using the closed gloving method.

Method
Keep both hands within the cuffs of the gown. 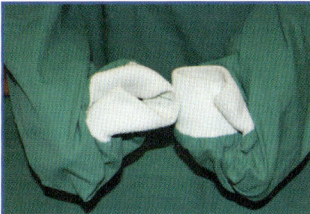
Ask an unsterile assistant to select an appropriate size of glove and instruct them to open the glove packet (without touching the inside of the packet).
Take the inner glove packet (without touching the outer packaging), turn it around and drop it on to the table. Unfold packaging to expose gloves (fingers of the gloves should be pointing towards you). 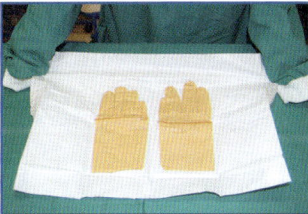
With either hand first, pick up the appropriate glove by the rim. Left hand should select the glove on the right or right hand should select the glove on the left. 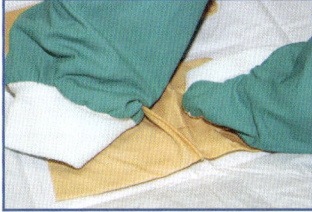
Turn your hand over so your palm is facing upwards. The glove should be lying on your palm and wrist with the fingers of the glove pointing down towards your elbow. 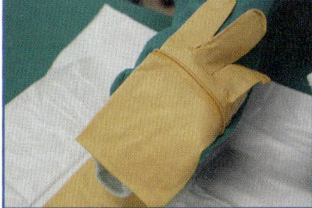

Method
Grasp the uppermost rim of the glove with the other covered hand and in one movement pull the glove over the first hand. 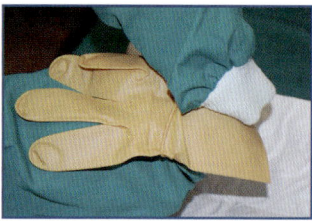 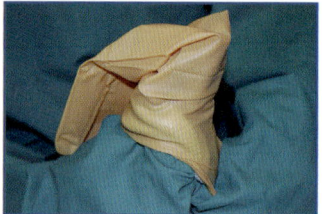
Ensure the rim of the glove entraps the cuff of the gown. 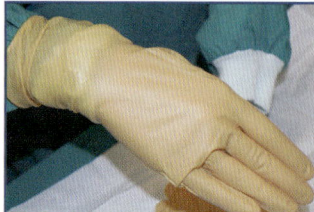
Pick up the remaining glove by the rim with the ungloved hand and turn the hand over so the glove lies on the palm and wrist. 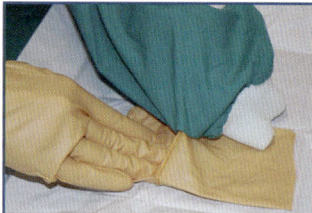
Grasp the uppermost rim of the glove with the other gloved hand and in one movement pull the glove over the second hand. 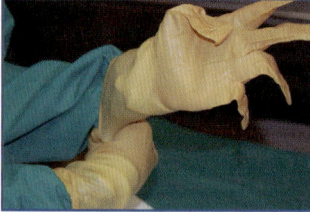
Ensure the rim of the glove entraps the cuff of the gown and adjust the fingers and cuffs as necessary to ensure a snug fit.
Clasp the hands together and ensure that the hands remain above the waist after gloving is completed. 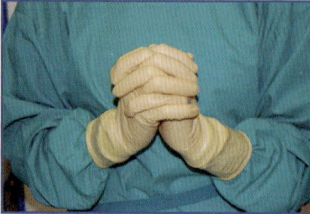

© RVC

Clinical Skills Sheet

4.5. Open gloving

Task:

You have scrubbed and dried your hands and put on a sterile gown. You must now put on a pair of gloves using the open gloving method.

Method
If you are wearing a gown, push both hands through the cuffs of the gown (this may have been done earlier). Ask an unsterile assistant to select an appropriate size of glove and instruct them to open the glove packet (without touching the inside of the packet).
Take the inner glove packet (outer packaging not touched).
Drop the inner glove packet on to the table and unfold the packet to expose the gloves (glove fingers should be pointing away from you).
Pick up the first glove touching only the inner folded down surface. Remember to put right glove on right hand and left glove on left hand. 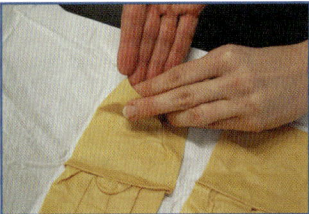
Pull the glove halfway on to the first hand, leaving the cuff folded back and hooked over the thumb. 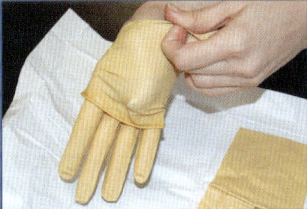
Slide the gloved fingers under the cuff of the other glove (outer surface). 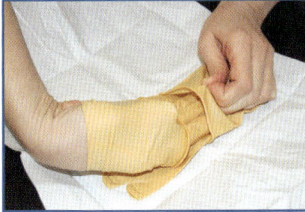

Method
Slide fingers of the ungloved hand into the fingers of the second glove and with one smooth movement, pull the glove onto the hand. 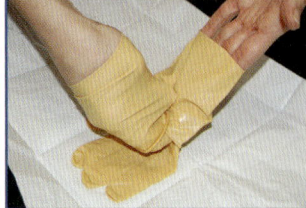 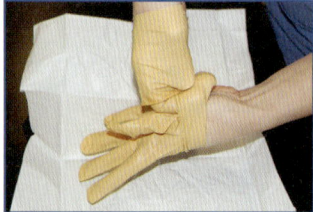
If you are wearing a gown, pull the folded cuff of the glove over the cuff of the gown.
Place fingers of the entirely gloved hand under the cuff of the first, semi-gloved hand and unhook the thumb. 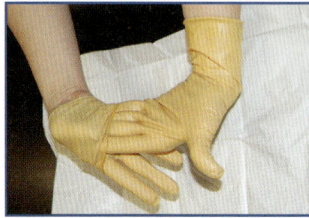
If you are wearing a gown, pull folded cuff of the glove over the cuff of the gown.
Adjust your fingers within each glove to ensure a comfortable fit.
Clasp hands together and ensure that hands remain above the waist after gloving is completed. 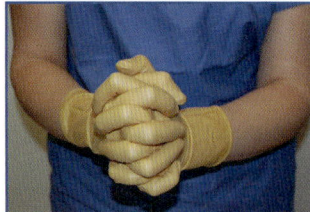
Question: Some gloves are lubricated with a fine starch powder that is put on to assist the wearer in the gloving procedure. • What are the potential disadvantages of this? • How can this be overcome?
Answer: The powder can cause a foreign body inflammatory response that may interfere with wound healing and possibly cause adhesions. A way to overcome this would be to wash off the powder with sterile water and wipe over with a sterile towel before commencing or assisting with surgery.

© RVC

Clinical Skills Sheet

4.6. Draping using the four-quadrant technique

Method
Assume that the skin has already been cleansed; you should be wearing sterile gloves and gown.
Ask assistant to open the drape box without touching the contents.

1st drape
- Grasp the first drape firmly so it doesn't fall open, lifting it out of the box.
- Take hold of the two *upper* corners of the drape – one corner in between the thumb and forefinger of each hand.
- Step away from the table to allow room to open the drape fully; allow drape to drop open by extending arms outwards
- Fold over approx 10–15 cm of the top of the drape *away* from yourself

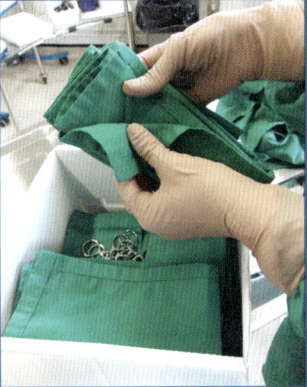

Hold the drape at the folded corners and rotate the wrists inwards, wrapping the drape around your hands (*so that your hands are covered by the drape – see picture*).
Therefore there is no possibility of breaking sterility when placing the drape on the animal.

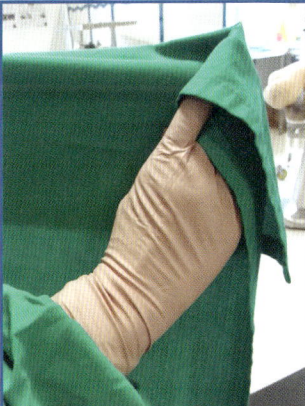

Approach the table and lay the first drape laterally (*down the length of the animal along one side*).
Lay the drape so that the folded edge lies parallel to and about 5 cm lateral to the midline
Observe your hands whilst releasing the corners of the drape, taking care *not* to touch the animal with your gloved hands.

Method
Do not adjust drape towards the incision site once placed: you would be breaking sterility – moving from 'unclean' to 'clean'.

2nd drape
- Retrieve from the box, open and fold the top 10–15 cm over as before.
- Bring your hands together (to make the drape smaller) and move around to the opposite side of the patient.
- Open up your hands and lay the 2nd drape as before, opposite the 1st drape.
- Release and observe one hand at a time.

Retrieve the **3rd drape** from the box, open and fold over as for the 2nd drape.

Walk around the patient and lay the 3rd drape caudally to cover the unclipped fur (making the drape smaller whilst walking around).

It is up to you which order you place the drapes in. However, as soon as there are two drapes touching each other, you must place a towel clip as below to prevent them from slipping off the animal.

Towel clips
- Pick up and separate from each other.
- Attach the 1st towel clip – place tips diagonally across one corner of the drapes.
- Pick up a small fold of skin through the drape and close the clip.

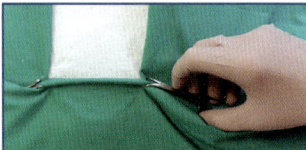

As per the picture, tuck the towel clip under the drape (*to prevent them becoming entangled in any suturing material during surgery*).
- Attach the 2nd towel clip – as above, to the other corner of the drapes.

Retrieve the **4th drape** from box, open and fold over as for the other drapes.

Lay this drape cranially. (Student may 'fly' this drape if access is difficult, e.g. anaesthetic machine is in the way. This means that as you open your arms to lay the drape down, you use this momentum to 'fling' the drape over the head end of the patient.)

Attach the final two towel clips in the remaining corners of the drapes and tuck under the drapes.

Essential points:
- Ensure *all* towel clips are attached to skin *and* drapes.
- **If at *any time* you reposition a towel clip for a firmer placement and it has entered the body cavity, it is no longer sterile, so discard it and use another towel clip.**
- Ensure that drapes cover all of the unclipped fur and that no 'long' fur is poking out of the fenestrated area.

© RVC

5

Surgical Instruments

Alison Young
The Royal Veterinary College, London

Learning objectives

By the end of this chapter, students should be able to:

- Understand the choice of material for the manufacture of instruments.
- Identify general surgical instruments.
- Aseptically open and accept sterile surgical instruments and kits.
- Maintain and provide surgical instruments as a surgical assistant.
- Understand and perform the sterilization process.

 Clinical skills sheets (SS)

Two clinical skills sheets will be used within this chapter and they can be found at pages 54–59. References will be made to each skills sheet at the relevant section within the chapter. The details of the clinical skills sheets used are as follows:

SS 5.7 Opening a sterile instrument pouch
SS 5.8 Instrument handling and selection

 Health and safety key points to be aware of in this chapter

- Sharps.
- Disposing of sharps.
- Trolley layout and the passing of instruments to prevent injury to other members of the team.
- Sharps and consumables count to prevent incidents of foreign objects being left within a patient.

Introduction

Surgical instruments are required for every surgical procedure. Some have multiple uses, others are specific to individual surgeries or surgeons. They are available from a number of sources and made with a variety of materials.

Surgical instruments, of a good quality, are expensive to purchase. However, they will be used repeatedly for many years if they are well cared for and used correctly (i.e. for the role for which they were designed). The cost per use is therefore reasonable when the instruments are well maintained. If instruments are not cared for, or not maintained properly, then they may cause more trauma to the patient's tissue during surgery. This can, in turn, lead to haemorrhage and surgical site infection. This could have a serious impact on the patient's outcome.

Veterinary students will see a vast array of surgical instruments during their rotations and placements in practice. There are many instruments that are common-place and others that may only be seen in specialist settings. Depending on the institution in which the veterinary or nursing student is trained, there are many names for basically the same instrument, which can be confusing at times.

Identifying instruments, their names and use can be done theoretically with books, websites and product catalogues. However, practical application of handling and using these instruments will help greatly with understanding their function. This does not always have to be done in a clinical environment; practising away from the pressured situation is beneficial. Seeing the instrument used correctly and in a surgical situation can help to cement the student's knowledge.

Within this chapter you will find pictures and tips about how to conduct basic Day One instrument handling skills. Each section also details 'Key Points' for each set of skills, which are critical to good practice.

© CAB International 2018. *Veterinary Clinical Skills Manual* (eds N. Coombes and A. Silva-Fletcher)

This chapter will cover the following:

- What instruments are made of and why that guides our choice when purchasing.
- General recognition and use.
- Aseptic provision and use – opening a kit.
- Surgical assistant role.
- Sterilization.

5.1 Manufacturing of Instruments: Common Materials

- Stainless steel is probably the most common material for surgical instruments. It has great strength with high resistance to corrosion.
- Tungsten carbide inserts can be added into the tips of stainless steel instruments to increase the strength and resistance to wear. They are often identified by their gold-coloured handles.
- Chromium-plated carbon steel is cheaper than traditional stainless steel. These instruments will not last as long as stainless steel instruments and may rust and blister when in contact with chemicals and saline.
- Titanium is a much more expensive material than the other options. Commonly used in ophthalmic instruments, as their dull appearance also reduces glare when used under an operating microscope. They are also much lighter in weight to hold, which helps with delicate surgery.

5.2 Identifying General Instrumentation and Instrument Sets

Instruments can be kept in surgical packs or sets containing multiple instruments, or as individually packed items. Instrument sets often contain items that would be used for a specific surgery (e.g. bitch spay, dog castration) or they may be more generic (e.g. soft tissue, abdominal, orthopaedic, etc.). The contents of the sets will be dependent on the operating veterinary surgeon or team. They will vary between practices and so before

starting a surgery or assisting as a veterinary student it would be advantageous to review the list of the instruments contained within the pack and ensure that you are familiar with them all.

 Have photographs and names of the instruments in the general sets for revision purposes before the surgery. Use your clinical skills centre to see instruments in real life.

5.3 Aseptically Open and Accept Surgical Kits and Instruments

Before any instrument set or pouch is opened, the integrity of the packaging must be inspected to ensure that it has not been damaged and sterility breached. The contents should be confirmed with the surgical team and the sterilization expiry date and process indicator checked.

Some practices use multi-layer materials during the sterilization process. The outer layer is used as a dust layer and so is removed by the circulating member of the team. When opening the inner layer, care must be taken by non-sterile members of the team not to touch the contents or inside surface of the packaging (see Chapter 4).

 A common mistake

When opening an individual instrument pouch, items can slip and fall to the side. If the instrument touches the side of the pouch it is deemed to be contaminated and therefore needs re-processing before use.

As a scrubbed surgical assistant, it will be expected that you are able to take items passed from the circulating team member. Taking time and care during this process is important to ensure that items are not contaminated, especially when only one is available and surgical and anaesthetic time would be increased for the patient if an instrument has to be re-processed.

SS 5.7 for details of how to open a sterile instrument pouch

5.4 Maintain and Provide Surgical Instruments

Veterinary students will often be scrubbed surgical assistants during their training period and this will continue once qualified in some situations. Aseptic technique to be a scrubbed member of the team is covered in Chapter 4.

Having a well laid-out surgical instrument trolley with good organization of instruments and equipment helps to make the surgery more efficient. This is important to reduce anaesthesia and surgical time for the patient. There is no standardized rule for the layout of the trolley: personal preference of the surgeon or trolley assistant is often used. Instruments with similar functions or types can be grouped together for ease of identification and choice.

It is important that one person organizes the trolley and has instruments set out in an order they find logical and intuitive for easy and efficient passing of instruments. The scrubbed assistant should check the integrity of the equipment as it is opened and perform a consumable count as the trolley is laid out.

Items that are regularly used should be set out for the assistant or surgeon to reach easily. Instrument handles facing the surgeon allows the assistant to pick up and pass into the palm of the surgeon's hand. Instruments should be passed with a reasonable amount of force to allow the surgeon to know the item is within their hand by feel alone.

 SS 5.8 gives details of how to select, handle and pass instruments

Care must be taken when placing and removing instruments from the trolley. Scalpel blades and suture needles are sharp and instruments should not be placed on top of these as they may cause injury to the team. Less commonly used items that are clean/unused should remain in the tray that the kit was processed in on the trolley. Items that have been used should not be placed back into the tray, to prevent contamination. The only exception to this rule may be the storage of scalpel blades on handles. To prevent a break in asepsis if the scalpel blade punctures the trolley drape, it may be stored in the metal tin of the surgical kit.

At the end of the surgery the inventory carried out at the beginning of the surgery should be repeated. Instruments with small detachable parts, such as retractors, should be checked to ensure all parts are present. Swabs should be counted twice to prevent a miscount being recorded. Sharps, such as scalpel blades and suture needles, should also be counted on to and off of the trolley. These items should be removed and stored separately, in a metal bowl, until they can be safely disposed of in an appropriate bin. This will help to prevent injury to the team that will clean and process the instruments ready for the next procedure.

5.5 Sterilization Process

At the end of the procedure, instruments should be separated and any specialized or delicate instruments removed to prevent damage. Processing should start immediately at the end of the surgery where possible. Blood and saline are corrosive to surgical instruments and can cause pitting and damage if not removed quickly. Rinsing or soaking in water helps to remove this; hot water should not be used as it causes coagulation of proteins.

 If it is not possible to fully clean the instruments immediately, placing them in a bowl of cold water or placing a wet towel over them helps to prevent blood and saline drying out on the instruments until it is possible to process them properly.

For manual cleaning, all items should have ratchets opened and disassembled where possible. A soft brush can be used for joints, ratchets and serrations. After this initial clean the items should be placed in an ultrasonic bath containing an appropriate detergent. Ultrasonic baths are very useful at removing debris from hard-to-reach areas such as box joints. Instruments should then be rinsed and have instrument lubrication applied to moveable parts.

Alternatively, washer/disinfectors are available. Instruments are loaded into baskets straight from the surgical trolley. They are designed to decontaminate items prior to sterilization through cycles that clean, disinfect using high temperatures and then dry. They use de-ionized water and so damage to instruments is reduced and there is no need to lubricate moving parts.

After cleaning and before packaging, all instruments should be inspected to ensure that they are fully functional, joints are not misshapen and ratchets are able to hold position, etc. If any instruments were reported to be blunt during the surgery, they should be cleaned and then removed from the surgical pack to prevent them being re-processed and placed back into the system.

5.5.1 Packing of instruments for sterilizing

Packaging of instruments and surgical kits may have small differences between individual practices but the principles of the procedure remain the same. Items that may damage or pierce the packaging during the process should be covered or double wrapped to prevent this.

When packaging items, thought should be given to how the item will behave when opened in a surgical environment. Loose items or those with a propensity to flick out when opened should be double bagged so that the internal bag can be taken by the scrubbed member of the team to open securely on the instrument trolley aseptically.

 Instruments should be placed into sterilization pouches with the handles at the end of the packet where the peel end opens to allow the scrubbed team member to remove them safely.

5.5.2 Sterilizing instruments

There are various methods of sterilization. Some, but not all, will be available for use within the veterinary practice. There are advantages and disadvantages for all and these are shown in Table 5.1.

It is very important to ensure that the sterilization process has been successful and there are many methods to monitor this.

- Physical or mechanical monitors – show that the parameters have met the manufacturer's guidelines. Examples include graphs, charts, digital displays and printouts. This only shows if the machine has performed correctly; it does not allow for other factors, e.g. correct packaging and loading.

Table 5.1. The advantages and disadvantages of common methods used in sterilizing instruments.

Method of sterilization	Advantage	Disadvantage
Autoclave - steam under pressure	• Most commonly used method in veterinary medicine • Quick turnaround time for instruments • Non-toxic	• Potential for injury for user if not maintained or used correctly • Not suitable for heat-sensitive items
Ethylene oxide	• No damage to heat-sensitive items	• Toxic – hazardous to personnel (carcinogenic?) • COSHH regulated • Long cycle time (12–24 h) • Long airing time prior to use (24 h)
Hydrogen peroxide gas plasma	• Quick turnaround time for equipment (28–60 min cycle time) • No damage to heat sensitive items (<50°C)	• Cannot be used for some materials – paper, wood, fabric • Cannot be used for closed or items with long lumen (>30 cm)
Gamma irradiation	• Used for single-use items • Long lifespan of sterilized items • No damage to heat-sensitive items	• Specialist equipment required • Hazardous to personnel

- Chemical indicators – usually heat- or chemical-sensitive inks that change colour when a specified time, temperature and pressure have been achieved. Can be used internally or externally, often stickers applied to packets. There are six classes of chemical indicators.

- Biological indicators – the most accurate method, demonstrates lethality within a particular load.

5.5.3 Expiration dates

The timeline guides to the storage of processed items vary, depending on how the item was sterilized:

- Autoclave – 1 year
- Ethylene oxide – 6 months
- Hydrogen peroxide – 1 year

Many manufacturers are now moving towards not having an expiry date for mass-used consumables that are sterilized with gamma irradiation. There is more of an approach that it remains sterile unless the packaging is breached.

Conclusion

The sterilization process can be time consuming and is often seen as less important than the surgical procedure itself. However, without reliable and thorough practices observed in the sterilization process, instruments would not be available and no amount of complicated surgery could be performed. Time should be scheduled into the day to allow this to happen effectively and efficiently.

Further Reading: McHugh, D., Young, A. and Johnson, J. (2011) Theatre practice. In: Cooper, B., Mullineaux, E. and Turner, L. (eds) *BSAVA Textbook of Veterinary Nursing*, 5th edn. BSAVA, Gloucester, UK.

Reuss-Lamky, H. (2010) Beating the 'bugs'; sterilization is instrumental. *Veterinary Technician* 32(11), E1–E8.

Veerabadran, S. and Parkinson, I.M. (2010) Cleaning, disinfection and sterilization of equipment. *Anaesthesia and Intensive Care Medicine* 11(11), 451–454.

Ward, A. (2007) Instrumentation and sterilization. In: Martin, C. and Masters, J. (eds) *Textbook of Veterinary Surgical Nursing*. Elsevier, St Louis, Missouri, USA, pp. 299–331.

Clinical Skills Sheet

5.7. Opening a sterile instrument pouch

Please note that the technique used in this skills sheet is also very relevant if you are opening syringe and needle packets, sterile glove packs, urinary catheters/drains as well as surgical equipment.

Method
Ensure your hands are clean and dry before handling the package to minimize the risk of contamination.
First examine the bag for any visible damage. 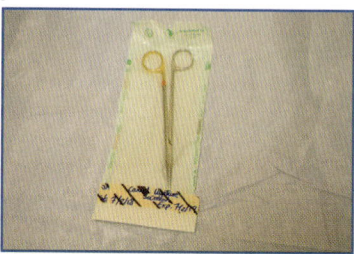
Check the date of expiry. 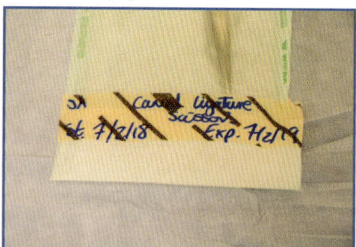 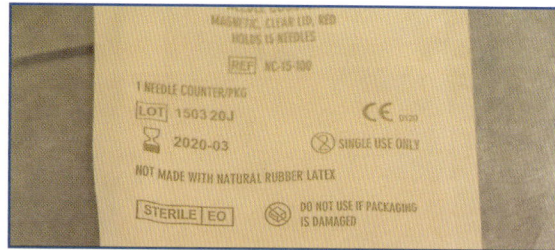
Check the sterility status of the package by looking for the sterility marker. **Sterile** (see how the indicator is brown): 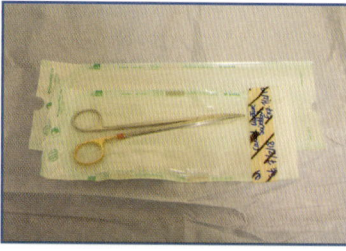 **Unsterile** (see how the indicators haven't changed colour): 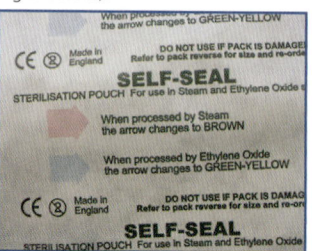

Method
Using thumbs of both hands, loosen the corners of the pouch (the peel end). 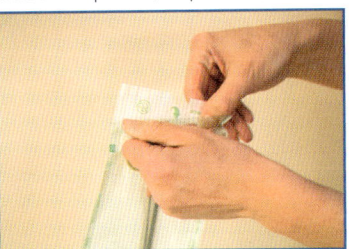
Slowly and smoothly start to peel the package sides away from each other, exposing the inside of the package to the sterile personnel. 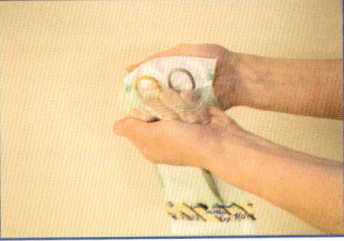
Take care not to touch the inside of the pouch as you offer the instrument to the sterile personnel, also taking care not to touch the instrument or the sterile person. 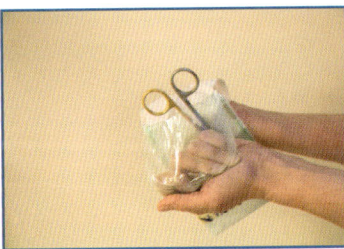 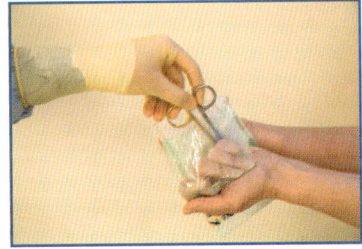
The sterile personnel firmly grasps the instrument, touching only the inside of the pouch, and removes it and places it safely on the instrument trolley until ready for use. 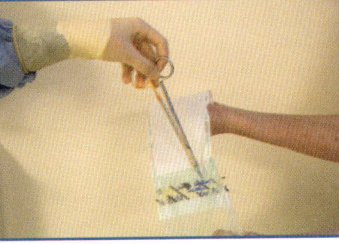
Watch closely for any breach of sterility.

Method

Question:

What would you do if there was a breach in sterility during instrument exchange?

Answer:

- If the packet was damaged or if the unsterile assistant touched the instrument or inside of the packet (but not the surgeon), then a new sterile instrument would have to be obtained.
- If the surgeon breaks sterility during the instrument handover by touching either the assistant or the outside of the package, then neither the instrument nor the surgeon is sterile, the instrument must be discarded and the surgeon will have to re-glove and/or re-gown/scrub, depending on the nature of the breach.

The unsterile assistant then disposes of the packet into the waste bin.

© RVC

Clinical Skills Sheet

5.8. Instrument handling and selection

Task:

Working in pairs, take it in turns to assume the role of a surgeon and assistant/scrub nurse. The surgeon reads the list of instruments (choose from attached lists A, B, or C) and the assistant must pass the correct instrument in the correct grip. Students may also find it helpful to describe the function as they pass the instrument.

Method

Passing surgical instruments

Needle holders

Depending on the surgeon's preference, needle holders may be passed ready loaded with suture material.

If loaded, grasp the needle ¼ to ½ way along the eye in the tip of the needle holder's jaws. Close the jaw on the 1st or 2nd ratchet.

Pass the instrument with the needle pointing upwards, placing the rings into the surgeon's palm ready for use. Take care to ensure that any suture strand is kept free and doesn't drag over the sterile field.

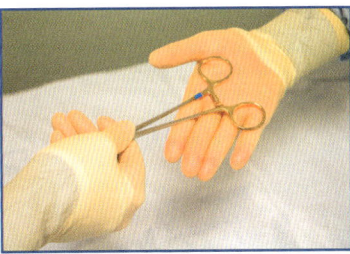

Artery forceps

Should be passed with any point upwards, jaw clamped in the first ratchet for security.

The handles should be pressed firmly into the hand.

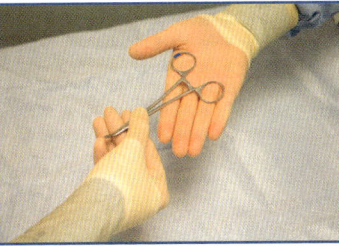

Thumb forceps

Passed in a finger-grip way so that the surgeon can receive into a pencil grip.

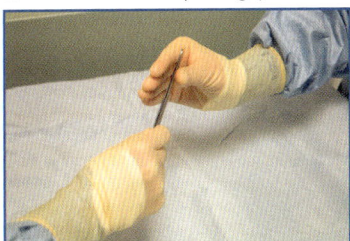

Method

Scalpel handle with blade attached

Passed with the blade pointing towards the assistant and away from the surgeon receiving into a pencil grip, protecting both from the blade.

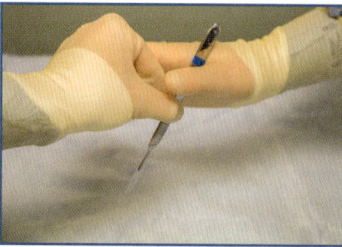

Alternatively the scalpel can be passed in a tray in order to avoid any chance of accidental injury (this is becoming more of a protocol in the NHS).

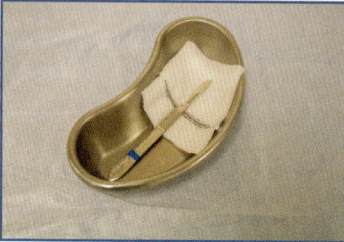

Once the blade has been placed on the handle the scalpel should not be placed back on the instrument trolley itself but placed into a metal tray to avoid the risk of accidently stabbing the drape and breaching sterility.

Holding instruments

Ringed instruments (scissors, forceps, needle holders)
Held with thumb and ring finger, with index finger along the shank to stabilize the instrument.
Top view:

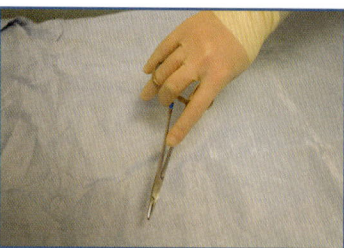

Underside view:

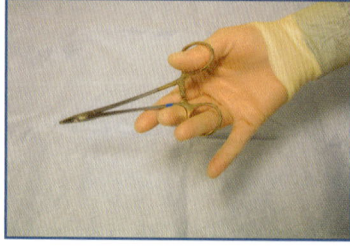

Scissors are always brought to the surgical site or to suture material with the blades closed, then used carefully cutting with tips only.

Method

Scalpel
Held in pencil grip.

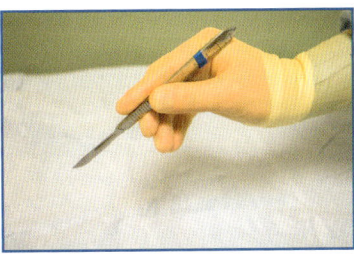

Thumb forceps
Held in pencil grip.

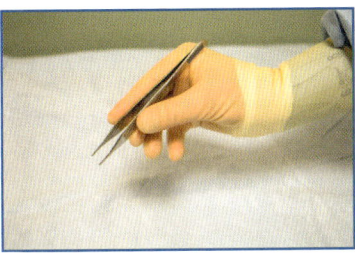

List A	List B	List C
Mayo-Hegar needle holder	Gillies needle holder	Olsen-Hegar needle holder
Halstead mosquito forceps (curved)	Halstead mosquito forceps (curved)	Halstead mosquito forceps (curved)
Debakey thumb forceps	Jean thumb forceps	Treve forceps
Mayo scissors	Metzenbaum scissors	Dressing scissors
Number 3 scalpel handle	Number 4 scalpel handle	Number 3 scalpel handle
Gelpi retractor	Backhaus towel clip	Allis tissue forceps

© RVC

6

The Fundamentals of Suturing

Nicola Jayne Kulendra

The Royal Veterinary College, London

Learning objectives

By the end of this chapter, students should be able to:

- Understand the differences between different types of knots.
- Tie a square knot, surgeon's knot, modified Miller's knot, slip knot and an Aberdeen knot.
- Handle surgical instruments appropriately.
- Understand the differences between suture materials that influence the choice in different types of tissue.
- Choose an appropriate needle.
- Start and finish continuous patterns.
- Be aware of the technique for suturing in a drain.

Clinical skills sheets (SS)

Three clinical skills sheets will be used in this chapter and these can be found at pages 73–91. References will be made to each skills sheet at the relevant section within the chapter. The details of the clinical skills sheets used are as follows:

SS 6.9 One-handed tie, right-hand method

SS 6.10 Two-handed tie (the bird's beak version)

SS 6.11 Instrument suture – square knot or surgeon's knot

Videos (V)

Seven videos are used in this chapter to demonstrate how to perform the clinical skills. They are:

V 6.1 One-handed tie
V 6.2 Two-handed tie
V 6.3 Modified Miller's knot
V 6.4 Slip knot
V 6.5 Aberdeen knot
V 6.6 Simple interrupted suture
V 6.7 Simple continuous suture

6.1 Basic Knot Techniques

Knots are used to ligate vessels and to start and finish suture lines. On a basic level, a knot binds two pieces of suture material together and the aim of tying a knot is to create a secure bond between two pieces of suture.

Knots can be created by hand ties or using instruments. Generally, hand ties are used for vessel ligation and instrument ties are used for suturing tissue. The main advantage of an instrument tie is that it can be used when the free suture end is short.

- The two knots used most commonly are the square knot and the surgeon's knot.
- Slip knots include the granny knot and half-hitch. These are most often tied by mistake but a half-hitch can be very useful when placing a ligature in a deep body cavity or around a large bulk of tissue where you would lose tension with a simple square knot.

Knot hints and tips

How many throws?

- After completing a knot, more throws are needed.

© CAB International 2018. *Veterinary Clinical Skills Manual* (eds N. Coombes and A. Silva-Fletcher)

- The number of throws is dictated by the properties of the suture material and the location and function of the knot.
- Generally, four throws are necessary for interrupted surgical knots (Marturello *et al.*, 2014).
- For continuous suture patterns: to start the suture, an additional one to two throws are placed and an additional two to three throws are required to finish the suture, as the final knot consists of three strands of material (Rosin and Robinson, 1989).
- The knot security properties of the suture material also affect how many throws to place. Multifilament materials such as polyglactin 910 (Vicryl) and silk have superior knot security compared with monofilament materials like nylon or polydioxanone (PDS).

6.1.1 One-handed tie, two-handed tie or an instrument tie

A one-handed tie is used when you have restricted space within a body cavity. One hand is exteriorized from the abdomen to maintain tension on one suture. The two-handed tie is used when you cannot achieve this tension and is used more in large-animal surgery. The one-handed tie is usually performed with the right hand as 'dominant', but it can be performed with either hand, which can improve dexterity.

 In order to follow the steps in performing these ties, please follow the clinical skills sheets **SS 6.9** for one-handed tie, right-hand method and **SS 6.10** for two-handed tie.

 V 6.1 One-handed tie and **V 6.2** Two-handed tie

V 6.1 video.cabi.org/uauey

V 6.2 video.cabi.org/gdkhw

6.1.2 Square knot

A square knot consists of two throws and can be created by performing a one-handed tie, two-handed tie or an instrument tie. This knot is used to start and finish most suture patterns, including both interrupted and continuous patterns. A basic square knot consists of two throws placed in opposite directions. It is important to apply tension evenly to avoid creating a half-hitch or slip knot. Failure to reverse directions of the hands results in a granny knot. Granny knots are less secure than a square knot as they are prone to slipping. The main disadvantage of a square knot is a slight loss of tension between placing the first and second throws, which can lead to a loose suture. This can be a problem when ligating a large ovarian pedicle, for example; therefore it is more prudent to use a slip knot (half-hitch), surgeon's knot or a modified Miller's knot. Steps for creating square knots and granny knots are summarized in Box 6.1.

 In order to follow the steps in performing a square knot, please refer to the clinical skills sheets **SS 6.9**, **SS 6.10** and **SS 6.11**, which detail these knots performed by hand and with instruments. After practising the knots using the clinical skills sheets, use Box 6.1 and perform a self-assessment.

6.1.3 Surgeon's knot

A surgeon's knot is formed by placing one strand of suture through the loop twice on the first throw of a square knot (Box 6.2). All subsequent throws are regular square knots. It can be performed using a one-handed tie, two-handed tie or instrument tie. The main advantage is that it does not lose tension for subsequent throws compared with a square knot because of the friction created by the double loop of the first throw. It has a few disadvantages, namely extra bulk, asymmetry and the potential for unravelling. Therefore, it is only used in situations where the tension is too great for a square knot. It is also not compatible for all suture materials as it can cause fraying (e.g. catgut).

6.1.4 Modified Miller's knot ('strangle knot')

This is a variation of the traditional Miller's knot, which was used to tie bags of flour and grain. The main advantage

Box 6.1. Steps to performing a square knot and a granny knot.

Square knot	Granny knot
1. Cross the ends of the suture to form a loop around the vessel. 2. Wrap one end (short end) by passing it under the other end (long end) and through the loop to form the first throw. 3. Pass the short end under the long end and through the loop to complete the second throw. 4. Tightening the knot results in a square knot. 5. Place more throws.	1. Cross the ends of the suture to form a loop. 2. Wrap one end (long end) by passing it under the other end (short end) and through the loop to form the first throw. 3. Passing the short end underneath the other end and through the loop creates a granny knot.

Box 6.2. Steps to performing a surgeon's knot.

1. Cross the ends of the suture to form a loop.
2. Wrap one end by passing it under the other end **twice** and through the loop.
3. Pass the one end under the other end and through the loop to complete the second throw.
4. Tightening the knot results in a surgeon's knot.
5. Place more throws.

Box 6.3. Steps to performing a modified Miller's knot.

1. Pass the suture around a pedicle twice. Do not let the loops cross. The short end should be on the bottom or right-hand side of the loops and the long end at the top or left side.
2. Hold the long end, short end and two loops in the non-dominant hand.
3. Pass the needle holders underneath the loops from bottom to top (or right to left) and grab the short end of the suture.
4. Tightening the knot results in a Miller's knot.
5. Place more throws.

is the creation of friction, which is very useful in tying a knot over a large pedicle (e.g. to ligate an ovarian pedicle during a bitch spay). For that reason, it has become known as the gold standard of surgical knots (Ortills *et al.*, 2014).

The knot is formed by passing a suture around the pedicle twice to create two loops (Box 6.3). The free end of the suture is then passed over and under the two loops. This is then tightened and more square knots are applied on top as necessary. It is easiest when performed with surgical instruments.

6.1.5 Slip knot (half-hitch)

This is a variation of the square knot and is another type of friction knot, useful in situations of high tension. The only difference between performing a slip knot (Box 6.4) and a square knot is the tension between the strands. The first throw of a square knot is performed loosely. The second throw is created and all the tension is placed in the long end of the suture; the short end is held loose. The long end is pulled tight.

 Please watch the video **V 6.3** on performing a modified Miller's knot. After practising the knot using the video, use Box 6.3 and perform a self-assessment

V 6.3 video.cabi.org/inmnp

 Please watch the video **V 6.4** on performing a modified Slip knot. After practising the knots using the video, use Box 6.4 (without pictures) and perform a self-assessment

V 6.4 video.cabi.org/nlegi

6.1.6 Aberdeen knot

To end a simple continuous suture, either a square knot, surgeon's knot or an Aberdeen knot is required (Box 6.5). The Aberdeen knot has been shown to be superior to a surgeon's knot (Stott *et al.*, 2007) and is relatively simple to perform. Four throws are required to produce a secure knot (Schaaf *et al.*, 2009). In addition, less suture material is required to form an Aberdeen knot, which leads to smaller knots.

 Please watch the video **V 6.5** on performing a modified Aberdeen knot. After practising the knots using the video, use Box 6.5 and perform a self-assessment

V 6.5 video.cabi.org/lrbvx

6.2 Instrument Handling

Careful practice of instrument handling techniques is important prior to performing surgery. Gentle tissue handling and proper use of surgical instruments are essential to follow Halstead's principles.

Halstead's principles

1. Gentle tissue handling.
2. Meticulous haemostasis.
3. Strict aseptic technique.
4. Preserve blood supply to tissue.
5. Eliminate dead space.
6. Appose tissues accurately with minimal tension.

6.2.1 Needle holders

Correct use of the needle holder can minimize tissue trauma and improve suturing efficiency. Needle holders should only grasp the needle and any suture distal to the

---

Box 6.4. Steps to performing a Slip knot.

1. Cross the ends of the suture to form a loop.
2. Wrap one end by passing it under the other end and through the loop. Ensure the loop is left loose.
3. Pass one end under the other end and through the loop to complete the second throw. Do not tighten. Keep all the tension in the longer thread.
4. Pull the longer thread tight whilst holding the short end loosely. Pulling on the long end will move the knot closer to the pedicle.
5. Place more throws.

Box 6.5. Steps to performing an Aberdeen knot.

1. Finish the continuous suture pattern.
2. Pull the final loop of the suture loose.
3. Pull the free end of the suture through the final loop whilst creating a loop with the free end.
4. Pull the new loop created with the free end tight.
5. Place more throws in the same way.
6. To end, pull the free end through the loop completely (do *not* create a new loop).
7. Pull the free end tight and bury the suture by passing it deeply through the tissue and exiting a distance away from the knot (ensure not to cut off knot).

---

knot about to be created. The needle holder weakens the suture material so should not be used to grip parts of the suture that will form the knot or any part of a simple continuous suture between the knots.

There are three ways of holding the needle holders: thumb–ring finger (tripod) grip; modified thenar eminence grip; and the pencil grip (Fig. 6.1a,b,c).

The thumb–ring finger (tripod) grip is most commonly used and allows precise control with regard to opening and closing the instrument using the digits. The index finger is extended to stabilize the instrument and the thumb and ring finger control the ratchet.

The thenar eminence grip allows a simple continuous suture to be placed rapidly as the needle can be grasped easily and removed from the tissue to place the next throw of the suture. The needle holder is held between the thenar eminence (ball of the thumb) and the ring finger. The needle holder is steadied with the metacarpophalangeal joint of the thumb and the tip of the ring finger is used to control the other ring and release the ratchet.

The pencil grip is used only with needle holders that have spring handles such as Castroviejo or ophthalmic instruments and is used for suturing delicate tissue.

6.2.2 Thumb forceps

Thumb forceps are held in the non-dominant hand and grip when their two tines are compressed between the thumb and forefinger (Boothe, 2012). They allow the surgeon to pick up and release tissue quickly during dissection and suture placement. They should be held in a grip like a pencil and not ventral to the palm (Fig. 6.2a,b).

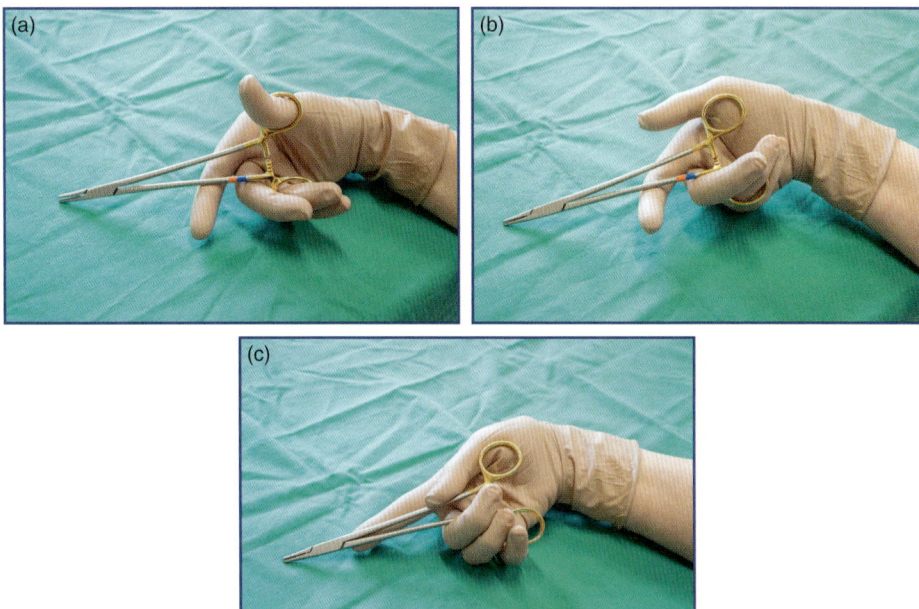

Fig. 6.1. Different needle holder grips: (a) thumb–ring finger (tripod) grip; (b) thenar eminence grip; (c) pencil grip.

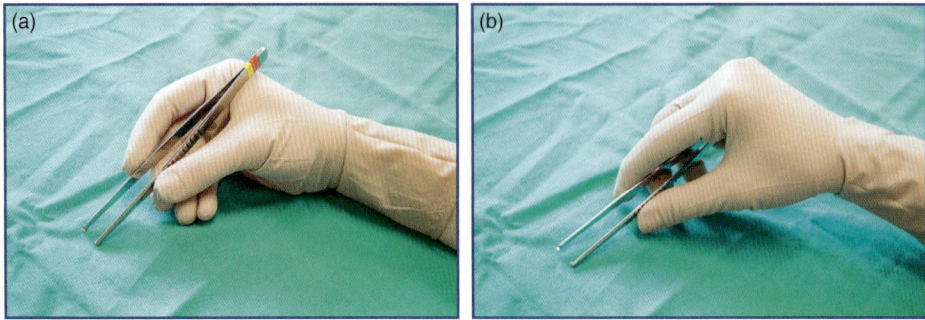

Fig. 6.2. (a) Correct and (b) incorrect 'palm' grip of thumb forceps.

Tissue forceps cause inflammation and so they must be used with great care to reduce tissue trauma. For delicate tissues, forceps with an undulating surface such as Debakey forceps are used. For skin and more fibrous tissue, forceps with a 'rat tooth' tip, such as Adson or Adson-Browns, are preferred.

6.2.3 Scissors

Scissors are held in the dominant hand with the thumb and ring finger in the rings controlling the scissor action and the index finger stabilizing the instrument (this is the same grip as for needle holders). Scissors may be used for sharp or blunt dissection. Sharp dissection involves using the scissors conventionally by pushing the semi-open blades through the tissue carefully. Cutting with the tips involves least trauma to the tissue. Blunt dissection involves inserting the closed tips of scissors into tissue and opening and withdrawing the tips. This breaks down connective tissue and allows the surgeon to identify important structures.

6.2.4 Scalpel

A scalpel is used to make an incision or to pierce a hole in tissue. In small animals, a number 10 or 15 blade is used most commonly to make incisions with the cutting edge and a number 11 blade is used to pierce holes with the tip.

H & S key point

When loading and unloading scalpel blades, always face the cutting edge away from your fingers.

Tips when using a scalpel

1. Make incisions perpendicular to the surface of the skin/organ.
2. Using a scalpel causes less trauma to tissue than scissor incisions.
3. Use smooth movements rather than a sawing action.
4. The aim is to produce a full-thickness incision with one sweep of the blade.
5. Use your non-dominant hand to stabilize the tissue.

There are two ways of holding the scalpel handle: the fingertip grip (Fig. 6.3a) and the pencil grip (Fig. 6.3b). To incise through the skin, a slide cut should be performed. This involves careful control of depth and length of the incision. To enter a hollow viscus or body cavity, a press cut or stab incision should be performed.

6.2.5 Haemostatic forceps

Haemostatic forceps are used to dissect around structures and are particularly useful to isolate blood vessels; dissection should be performed at right angles to the vessel. The tips should always face upwards. A tripod grip is used in the dominant hand with the aim to compress tissue with as little cutting and crushing as possible. Removal of the haemostats can be performed with either hand. Either a tripod grip or a palmed grip can be used. To remove using the palmed grip: grasp one ring with the index finger and thumb and disengage the ratchet by applying pressure on the other ring using the middle and ring fingers (Schmiedt, 2012).

6.3 Suture Classification: Absorbable versus Non-absorbable

Suture can be classified into many categories: absorbable versus non-absorbable, natural (Table 6.1) versus synthetic (Table 6.2), monofilament and multifilament. Absorbable sutures are further separated into those with fast absorption and long absorption times (Chu *et al.*, 1999). Knot security is also a factor to consider. Some materials, such as polypropylene, are inert and cause minimal reaction; others, such as catgut, can incite significant reaction. The advantages and disadvantages of each material must be taken into careful consideration. For example, catgut is cheap and has excellent knot security but it has unpredictable loss of tensile strength and absorption and so its use cannot be recommended.

There are some situations where the healing of a tissue may be compromised because of the presence of infection or vascular compromise following trauma and so a suture with longer loss of tensile strength or a slightly larger size is chosen. Smaller sutures have better knot security.

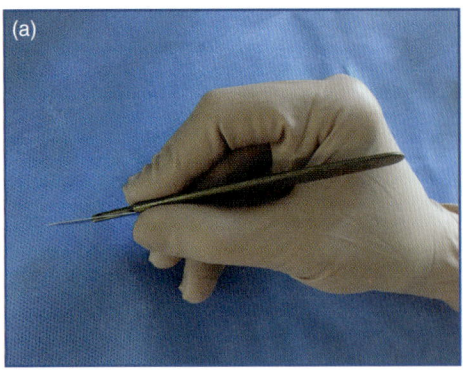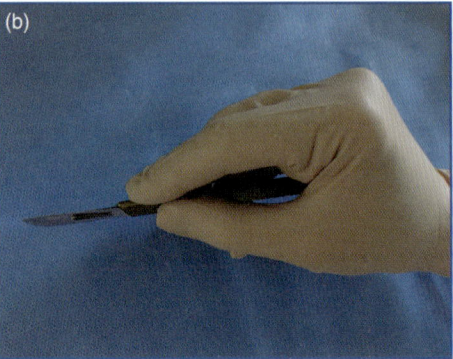

Fig. 6.3. Holding the scalpel handle, using (a) fingertip grip and (b) pencil grip.

Table 6.1. Different qualities of natural suture materials.

Suture (trade name)	Mono- or multifilament	Rate of loss of tensile strength	Time to complete absorption	Reaction	Knot security
Silk (Mersilk)	Multifilament	Gradual over time	n/a	Moderate	Good
Chromic catgut	Multifilament	21–28 days. Unpredictable	90 days	Marked	Good

6.4 Selection of Suture Materials

Selection is mainly down to the preference of each surgeon but there are some principles by which to abide (Table 6.3). A suture is only needed until the tissue has healed. All suture material is foreign and has the potential to cause reaction and act as a nidus for infection. Braided multifilament materials are more prone to bacterial inoculation. Therefore, the suture that is absorbed fastest and has the smallest size is chosen. However, this need is balanced against the requirement for strength that lasts for as long as the tissue takes to heal. It is important to know how long a tissue takes to regain its tensile strength in order to select an appropriate suture. In some cases, such as left arytenoid lateralization procedures (tieback), it is necessary to keep the larynx permanently abducted and so a permanent suture such as polypropylene (Prolene) is used. In other tissues, such as the intestines and bladder, it is important that the suture materials disappear once the tissues have healed, as permanent sutures can cause ulcers or act as a nidus for stone formation, respectively.

 Practical tips to choosing the *size* of a suture material

1. General rule: 3 metric for dogs, 2 metric in cats and small dogs
   a. For delicate tissue, reduce by 1 (e.g. use 2 metric for a Labrador's intestine).
   b. For tough tissue, increase by 1 (e.g. use 3.5/4 metric for the rectus fascia in a Labrador).
2. There are two classification systems for suture materials:
   a. The United States Pharmacopoeia (USP) system, which assigns a size specific to each suture material based on the diameter, tensile strength and knot security. The main disadvantages are that for suture sizes less than 0 (3.5M), the smaller number represents a larger suture size (e.g. 3/0 is smaller than 2/0).
   b. The metric system, where each unit represents 0.1 mm diameter (e.g. 2 metric represents a suture size of 0.2 mm diameter).

Practical tips to choosing the *type* of suture material

1. Fascia such as the external rectus sheath heals slowly
   a. It regains only about 20 % of its strength at 1 month and only 70 % at 9 months.
   b. All the strain is taken by the suture material, therefore long acting absorbable/non absorbable ones are used.

Generally, polydioxanone (PDS) or polyglyconate (Maxon) are good choices as they retain their tensile strength for at least 6 weeks.

2. Skin and fascia heal more quickly, so a suture material that lasts for 2–3 weeks is sufficient, e.g. poliglecaprone 25 (Monocryl) or polyglytone 6211 (Caprosyn).

6.5 Choosing a Suture Needle

The smallest, sharpest needle should be used. It should be grasped in the tips of the needle holders. Most needles are curved, which has the advantage of ease of use in deep cavities. Straight needles can be used without instruments in the skin.

 Handling needles poses a risk of needle stick injuries. Care must be taken to avoid picking needles up with fingers; needle holders should be used to remove needles from tissue.

There are two types of needle:

1. Swaged-on needles are directly attached to the suture material and have many advantages over the

Table 6.2. Different qualities of synthetic suture materials.

Suture (trade name)	Mono- or multifilament	Rate of loss of tensile strength			Time to complete absorption	Tissue reaction	Knot security
Polyglactin 910 (Vicryl rapide)	Multifilament	Strength gone by 2–3 weeks			42 days	Low	Average
Polyglytone 6211 (Caprosyn)	Monofilament	Strength gone by 2–3 weeks			56 days	Low	Average
Polyglcaprone 25 (Monocryl)[a]	Monofilament	*1 week*	50–60 %		119 days	Mild	Average
		2 weeks	20–30 %				
Polyglycolic acid (Dexon)	Multifilament	50 % at 2–3 weeks			90 days	Low	Good
Polyglactin 910 (Vicryl)	Multifilament	50 % at 2–3 weeks			56–70 days	Low	Average
Polydioxanone (PDS II)	Monofilament		*3/0 and larger*	*4/0 and smaller*	182–238 days	Mild	Average
		2 weeks	80 %	60 %			
		4 weeks	70 %	40 %			
		6 weeks	60 %	35 %			
Lactomer 9-1 (Polysorb)	Multifilament	80 % at 2 weeks 30 % at 3 weeks			56–70 days	Low	Average
Polyglyconate (Maxon)	Monofilament	50 % at 4–5 weeks			180 days	Low	Good
Glycomer 631 (Biosyn)	Monofilament	50 % at 5–6 weeks			180 days	Low	Average
Nylon (Ethilon/ Monosof)	Monofilament	Gradual loss over time			n/a	Negligible	Low
Polypropylene (Prolene/ Surgipro)	Monofilament	No loss			n/a	Negligible	Low

[a]Interesting fact: dyed Monocryl is 10 % stronger than undyed Monocryl after 1 and 2 weeks.

Table 6.3. Suture material relative to tissue type.

Tissue type	Suture material choices	Suture size for a cat or small dog	Suture size for a medium- or large-breed dog
Skin	Monofilament nylon (Ethilon/Monosof) Multifilament Nylon (Surgilon/Nurolon/Bralon)	1.5M (4/0)	2M (3/0)
Intradermal/ subcutaneous	Poliglecaprone 25 (Monocryl) Polyglytone 6211 (Caprosyn) Polyglactin 910 (Vicryl) Lactomer 9-1 (Polysorb)	1.5M, 2M (4/0, 3/0)	2M (3/0)
Fascia/muscle	Polydioxanone (PDS II) Polyglyconate (Maxon)	3M (2/0)	3.5M, 4M (0, 1)
Viscera (stomach, intestines, bladder)	Polydioxanone (PDS II) Polyglyconate (Maxon)[a]	1.5M (4/0)	2M (3/0)
Ligating small vessels (e.g. ovarian)	Polyglactin 910 (Vicryl) Lactomer 9-1 (Polysorb)	2M (3/0)	3M (2/0)
Ligating large vessels (e.g. pulmonary arteries, portosystemic shunts)	Polypropylene (Prolene/Surgipro) Silk (Mersilk/Permahand)	2M (3/0)	3M (2/0)
Hernia repair	Polydioxanone (PDS II) Polyglyconate (Maxon) Polypropylene (Prolene/Surgipro)	3M (2/0)	3.5M, 4M (0, 1)
Nerve repair	Polypropylene (Prolene/Surgipro)	1.5M (4/0)	2M (3/0)

[a]In theory, a short-duration monofilament suture such as poliglecaprone 25 is sufficient for suturing viscera as it loses 60% of its tensile strength within 1 week. Normal intestine should have regained enough strength by this stage to prevent leakage. However, it is rare to suture healthy intestine and so the author always uses a long-duration absorbable suture such as polydioxanone (PDS II) for viscera. Poliglecaprone 25 is not suitable for the bladder (Lipscomb, 2012).

eyed needles. They cause less tissue trauma, as the junction between the needle and suture is smooth. They are more likely to be sharper and less likely to fray the suture material, causing damage and loss of integrity

2. Eyed needles have a hole at the end of the needle and require the suture material to be threaded through it. These needles can be reused as long as they are still sharp, otherwise they will cause tissue trauma. Suture material should only pass through the eye once, otherwise the bulk of material will cause a large hole in the tissue. The disadvantages are many compared with swaged-on needles and include the suture material detaching, more tissue trauma and damage to suture material.

Needle points may be cutting or non-cutting.

- Round-bodied needles are used for viscera and organs such as the liver which are more friable.
- Cutting needles are used where the tissue has more collagen and is tougher, such as fascia and skin. The cutting action is provided by a triangular shape to the needle.
  - Tapercut needles are a compromise between a round-bodied and cutting needle.
  - Cutting needles have the cutting edge (tip of triangle) along the concave aspect of the needle.
  - Reverse cutting needles have the cutting edge on the convex aspect of the needle.

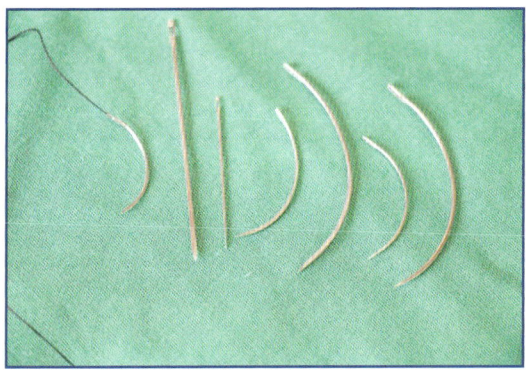

Fig. 6.4. Different types and sizes of suturing needles.

These have the advantage of preventing the suture 'cutting through' the tissue.
○ Spatula cutting needles have a flat top and bottom and are used for very fine suture and mainly in ophthalmic sutures.

Different types and sizes of suturing needles, including a swaged one, are shown in Fig. 6.4.

6.6 Choosing Suture Patterns

Identifying an appropriate suture pattern to close the incision whilst offering maximal support is crucial to the outcome of a surgery. Patterns are classified according to the following criteria:

- Continuous or interrupted.
- How they align the tissue edges: appositional, inverting or everting.
- One-layer or two-layer closure.
- Whether they are tension-relieving patterns.

6.6.1 Continuous versus interrupted patterns

 Please watch the two videos **V 6.6** Simple interrupted suture and **V 6.7** Simple continuous suture

V 6.6 video.cabi.org/nynzu

V 6.7 video.cabi.org/opltl

 Also see **SS 6.9**, **SS 6.10** and **SS 6.11** for basics of suturing

As you watch the videos and look at the skills sheets, note the advantages and disadvantages listed in Table 6.4

Table 6.4 compares the advantages and disadvantages of using interrupted versus continuous patterns.

6.6.2 Appositional versus inverting versus everting patterns

- Appositional sutures hold the tissue in close approximation in the same anatomical layers as they were before they were incised.
- Inverting patterns cause the tissue edges to move into the centre of the lumen of a hollow viscus. They can lead to narrowing of the lumen and should be avoided in small-animal intestinal surgery.
- Everting sutures cause the tissue edges to move outwards.

Table 6.4. The differences between continuous and interrupted sutures patterns.

Pattern	Advantages	Disadvantages
Interrupted	Easier to adjust tension One knot can fail without causing entire line to fail	Use excessive suture material Take longer More knots and suture material
Continuous	Quicker to place Less suture material used More even tension distribution No increased risk of dehiscence compared with interrupted sutures for closure of intestines	Failure of one knot can cause failure of entire line Can cause purse-string effect in hollow organs such as intestine

Choosing one type over another

Generally, appositional sutures are chosen, as there is evidence that they allow superior tissue healing when compared with other patterns. Bringing the tissue into correct anatomical apposition speeds up healing and results in a lower incidence of stricture formation (Radasch *et al.*, 1990; Kirpensteijn *et al.*, 2001). For closure of intestinal wounds, simple interrupted or continuous avoids narrowing of the lumen and stricture formation.

6.6.3 One-layer versus two-layer closure

The majority of incisions are closed with one-layer closure. The stomach separates into two layers on incision and so it lends itself to being closed in two layers. The mucosa and submucosa are closed in one simple continuous layer and the muscularis and serosa are closed in another simple continuous layer. In other situations, where the integrity of the suture line is in doubt, an additional suture line, usually an inverting continuous pattern such as a continuous Lembert pattern, can be performed to augment the original suture line.

6.6.4 Tension-relieving patterns

There are a number of tension-relieving patterns, such as cruciate, vertical or horizontal mattress patterns. As a general rule, wounds should be closed with minimal tension. If there is reliance on tension-relieving sutures to close the skin for example, the wound is at risk of dehiscence.

6.6.5 Starting and finishing continuous patterns

There are some points to consider in starting and finishing continuous suturing. Watch the video **V 6.7** on simple continuous suture and note the steps below

V 6.7 video.cabi.org/opltl

1. Place the needle at one end of the incision and take a bite of at least 5mm of tissue from superficial to deep into the incision at 90 degrees to the tissue.
2. Once the needle exits the tissue, grasp it with the needle holders in the centre of the incision.
3. Pass the needle through the opposite side of the incision from deep to superficial at least 5 mm from the incision edge.
4. Tie a simple interrupted suture. The number of throws depends upon the suture material and the location of the knot. Generally, five throws are sufficient. For the linea alba, six throws are preferable to start and eight are necessary to finish a simple continuous suture.
5. Perform the continuous pattern.
6. To end it, leave the last suture loose and grab it with the needle holders, ensuring that the tension of the entire suture line is sufficient.
7. Tie a simple interrupted suture. NB: Instead of having two free ends, there will be one free end, and one which forms a loop. Ensure that the suture line is not slack by removing any tension from the loop side of the suture.

6.6.6 Starting and finishing intra-dermal continuous patterns

There are some points to consider in starting and finishing intra-dermal suturing. Note the following steps:

1. Place the needle deep into the centre of the incision at one end and pass it into the superficial aspect of the wound.
2. Pass the needle through the opposite side of the incision from superficial to deep into the tissue. This will help to keep the knot buried deep in the tissue when suturing superficial layers like the skin and subcutis.
3. Tie a simple interrupted suture.
4. Perform the continuous pattern.
5. To end it, leave the last suture loose and grab it with the needle holders, ensuring that the tension of the entire suture line is sufficient.
6. Tie a simple interrupted suture. It is useful to perform an Aberdeen knot as there is less suture material left in the wound.

See video **V 6.5** on performing an Aberdeen knot

V 6.5 video.cabi.org/lrbvx

6.7 Suturing in a Drain

6.7.1 Penrose drain

These drains work by capillary action so one end must remain in the incision. The drains exit in a dependent location, so that must be considered prior to placement. They should not exit the incision, as they will be more likely to cause wound breakdown. It is not necessary to anchor the drain inside the wound and doing so can lead to complications such as leaving a piece of drain inside the wound.

Box 6.6. Steps to place a Penrose drain.

1. Prior to wound closure, place Penrose drain with one end in dorsal aspect of wound.
2. Decide where you would like the drain to exit the wound. The most dependent part will optimize drainage.
3. Place a pair of mosquito haemostats from inside the wound and tent the skin at the required drainage point.
4. With your other hand, use a scalpel to incise over the tips of the forceps.
5. Use another pair of haemostats to pass through your incision from outside to in, so the tips end up inside the wound.
6. Grab the end of the Penrose drain with the mosquito haemostats and pull the drain from inside the wound to out.
7. Using monofilament nylon on a needle, take a bite of the skin adjacent to the drain site. The needle should exit through the incision.
8. Take a bite through the Penrose drain.
9. Tie a simple interrupted suture.
10. Place another suture at the drain exit site, 180 degrees to the first suture.

6.7.2 Other drains and tubes

These include, for example, chest drains, active suction drains and feeding tubes. Tubes such as chest drains or oesophagostomy tubes are best secured using Chinese finger-trap sutures, which tighten as the tubes are removed, preventing dislodgement.

Box 6.7. Steps to securing a drain using a Chinese finger-trap suture.

1. Using monofilament nylon on a needle, take a bite of the skin adjacent to the tube.
2. Tie a simple interrupted suture in the middle of the suture, leaving the ends long to tie the suture.
3. Pass the two ends of the suture around the back of the tube and place a double throw.
4. Pass the two ends of the suture around the front of the tube and place a double throw.
5. After every turn, ensure that the suture is sufficiently tight to indent the tube. NB: Too tight will result in occlusion of the lumen of the tube.
6. Repeat steps 3 and 4 until there are 12–16 throws in total.
7. Tie the last throw into a surgeon's knot.

References: Boothe, H.W. (2012) Instrument and tissue handling techniques. In: Tobias, K.M. and Johnston, S.A. (eds) *Veterinary Surgery*. Elsevier Saunders, St Louis, Missouri, pp. 201–213.

Chu, C.C., von Fraunhofer, J.A. and Greisler, H.P. (eds) (1999) *Wound Closure Biomaterials and Devices*. CRC Press, Boca Raton, Florida, USA.

Kirpensteijn, J., Maarschalkerweerd, R.J., van der Gaag, I., Kooistra, H.S. and van Sluijs, F.J. (2001) Comparison of three closure methods and two absorbable suture materials for closure of jejunal enterotomy incisions in healthy dogs. *Veterinary Quarterly* 23(2), 67–70.

Lipscomb, V.L. (2012) Bladder. In: Tobias, K.M. and Johnston, S.A. (eds) *Veterinary Surgery – Small Animal*. Elsevier Saunders, St Louis, Missouri, USA, pp. 1978–1992.

Marturello, D.M., McFadden, M.S., Bennett, R.A., Ragetly, G.R. and Horn, G. (2014) Knot security and tensile strength of suture materials. *Veterinary Surgery* 43, 73–79.

Ortills, A., Rodriguez, J. and Calvo, B. (2014) The Miller's knot as an alternative to the surgical knotting? Characterization of the mechanical behavior. *Journal of the Mechanical Behavior of Biomedical Materials* 38, 154–162.

Radasch, R.M., Merkley, D.F., Wilson, J.W. and Barstad, R.D. (1990) Cystotomy closure. A comparison of the strength of appositional and inverting suture patterns. *Veterinary Surgery* 19(4), 283–288.

Rosin, G. and Robinson, G.M. (1989) Knot security of suture materials. *Veterinary Surgery* 18(4), 269–273.

Schaaf, O., Glyde, M. and Day, R.E. (2009) A secure Aberdeen knot: *in vitro* assessment of knot security in plasma and fat. *Journal of Small Animal Practice* 50, 415–421.

Schmiedt, C.W. (2012) Instrument and tissue handling techniques. In: Tobias, K.M. and Johnston, S.A. (eds) *Veterinary Surgery – Small Animal.* Elsevier Saunders, St Louis, Missouri, USA, pp. 187–213.

Stott, P.M., Ripley, L.G. and Lavelle, M.A. (2007) The ultimate Aberdeen knot. *Annals of the Royal College of Surgeons of England* 89, 713–717.

Clinical Skills Sheet

6.9. One-handed tie, right-hand method

TASK:

Perform a *right*-handed one-handed tie making a square knot.

- You will be using this method when you are space-limited and therefore your *left* hand will be outside the body cavity and your *right* hand will be doing all the work.

- Please note: we are teaching this in a completely simulated way with a sandbag and two colours of string to enable you to understand how to perform this knot adequately.

- You need to be able to do it with your 'eyes closed', as in the real surgical environment it is unlikely you will be able to see what your hands are doing.

Method
Take the upper suture (red) in your **right** hand, over your index finger and thumb, held securely in your palm by your remaining three fingers.   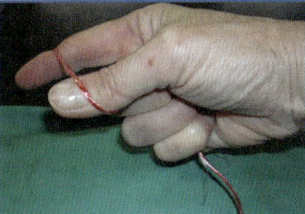
Your **left** hand is holding the lower suture (yellow) vertically upwards *keeping tension on this suture at all times.*   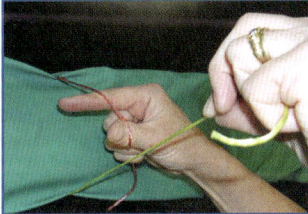
With your **left** hand, place this suture on to the first joint of your **right** index finger   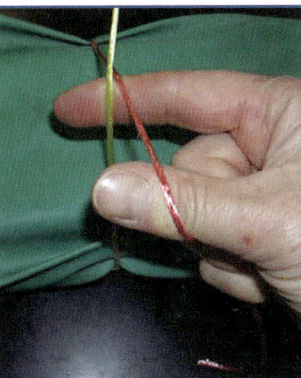

Method

Curl your **right** index finger under the red suture, hooking on to the yellow suture.

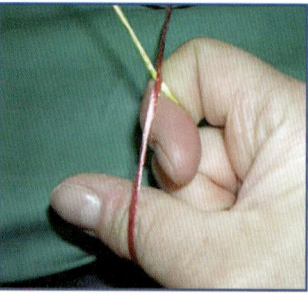

Straighten your index finger over the top of the red suture, pushing it downwards.

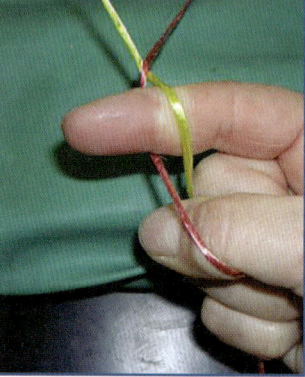

Pull your **right** thumb out of the way and bring it under both sutures to hold on to the red suture against your **right** index finger. Let go of the red suture from your **right** palm.

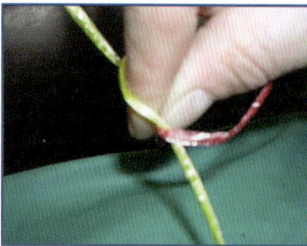

Method

Pull the red suture through underneath the yellow suture in a downwards direction towards your body, at the same time with your **left** hand pulling the yellow suture away from you.

You have now completed the ***first throw*** – keep the tension on both sutures and flat on to the sandbag.

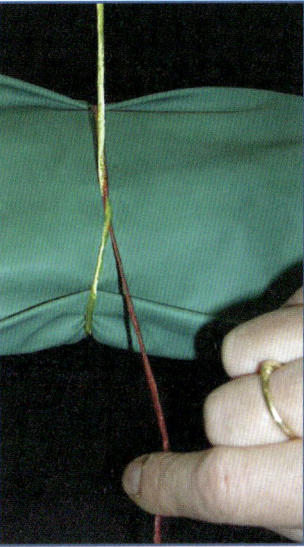

Hold the three remaining fingers of your **right** hand together and wrap them downwards towards the first throw …

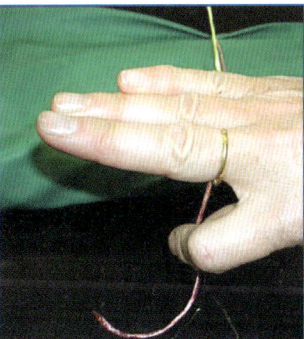

… now rotate your **right** wrist, so that your palm is facing upwards. You still have the red suture firmly in your **right** index finger and thumb, it is now lying across your **right** fingers.

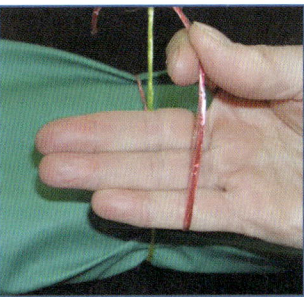

Method

Bring your **left** hand towards your body, which will have the effect of placing the yellow suture against the first joint of your **right** middle finger.

(Hold the yellow suture towards yourself, at tension.)

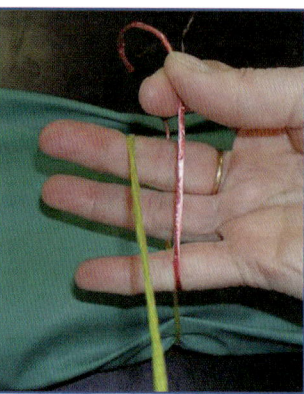

Hook the yellow suture with the middle finger of your **right** hand and draw it underneath the red suture.

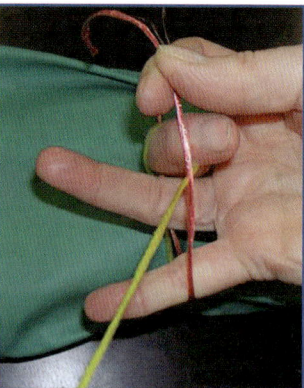

Straighten your middle finger and rotate your hand to pull the finger in a downwards direction through the loop you have created.

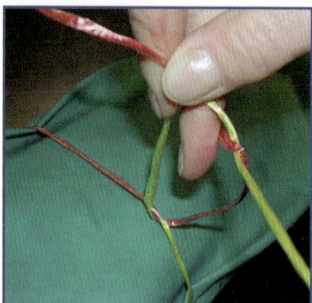

Method

With your ring finger, hold the red suture against the underneath of your **right** middle finger, to secure it.
Then pull it completely through the loop and horizontally away from your body.

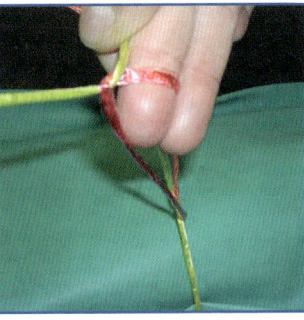

You have now completed the *second throw* and created a **square knot** - well done!
(Also called a reef knot.)

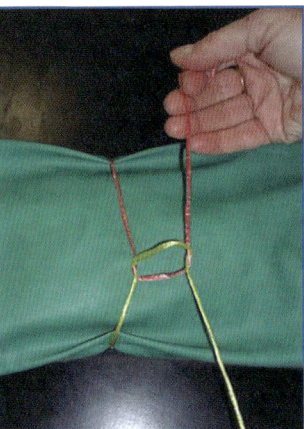

- **You can reverse this method if you are left-handed.**
- You will probably find that as you become more confident with this technique, you will adapt the finger positions to suit yourself more.
- Once you are comfortable with this technique, practice it using suture material whilst wearing surgical gloves.

© RVC

Clinical Skills Sheet

6.10. Two-handed tie
(the 'bird's beak' version)

This method can be used instead of a one-handed tie for blood vessel ligation – if there is adequate 'space' – tending more towards large animal surgery.

(This sheet has been produced after many requests from students, and may seem somehow 'patronizing' but it works.)

During the whole of this procedure, it is very important to maintain tension on the 'suture material' (in this case, coloured string).

Method
Your left index finger and thumb are the 'bird's beak', here shown open. The **red** suture material is coming from the *far side* of the sandbag, over your **left** index finger, into your left palm, where your other three fingers hold it securely. The end of the red suture material should be pointing towards you. 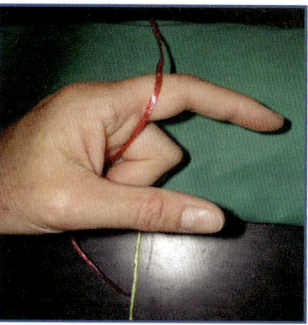
Your **right** hand holds the **yellow** suture vertically, placing this inside the 'bird's beak' shape of your left index finger and thumb. 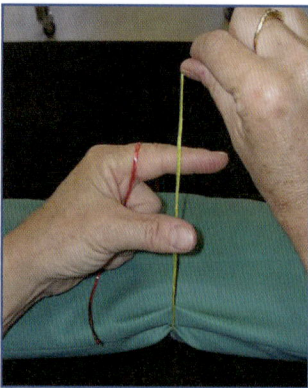

Method

Close the 'beak' with the yellow suture material inside (not holding between finger and thumb).

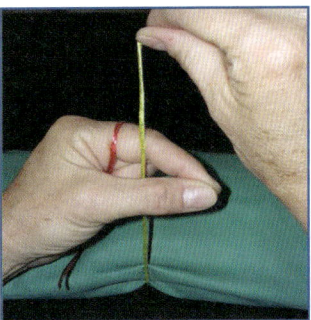

Rotate the pointed end of the beak down between the two sutures towards your left, under the red suture (a).

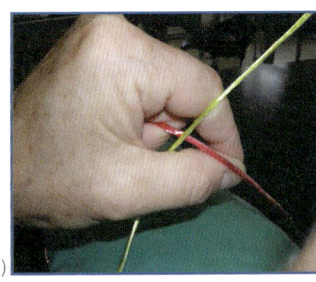
(a)

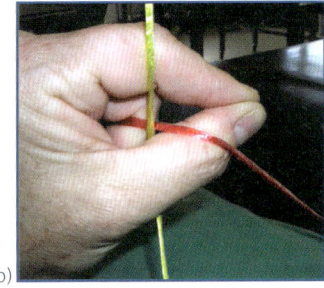
(b)

Continue rotating until the beak points directly away from you.
The red suture now wraps over your thumb (b).

Make sure you maintain a vertical tension throughout on the yellow suture in your right hand.
Lift your left index finger up, opening the 'beak' of your left hand.
With your right hand, move the taut yellow suture on to the tip of your left thumb.

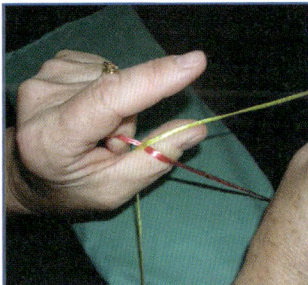

Method
Now reform the 'beak' (by closing your left index finger on to the yellow suture, gripping it between your index finger and thumb).   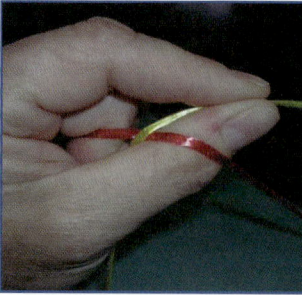
Let go of the yellow suture with your right hand.   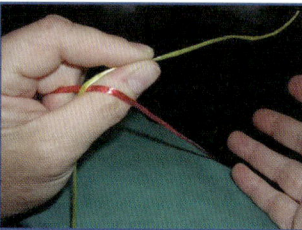
Rotate the pointed end of the beak down between the two sutures towards your right, under the red suture.   The red suture now wraps over your index finger; the yellow suture is coming under the red suture   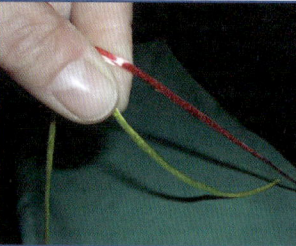
With your right hand, grab the offered yellow suture, pulling it *away* from your body towards the far side of the sandbag, and at the same time pull the red suture in your left hand *towards* your body.   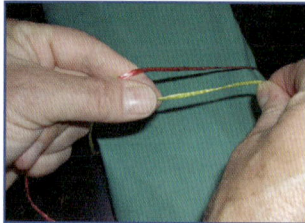

Method

You should now be in this position (***first throw***).
HOORAY!

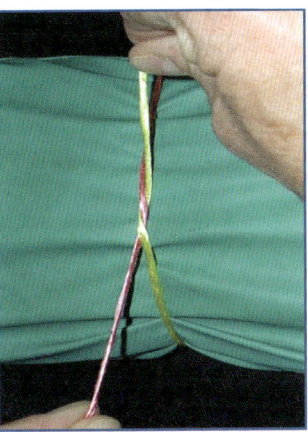

Lift your index finger up out of the way (holding the red suture still in your left palm), rotate your left wrist, moving your thumb down and under the red suture which will in effect make your thumb point away from you with the red suture *wrapped over it*.

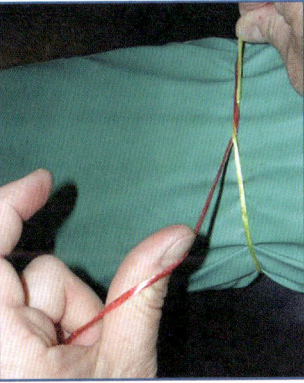

With your right hand, place the taut yellow suture inside the 'beak' shape of your left hand.

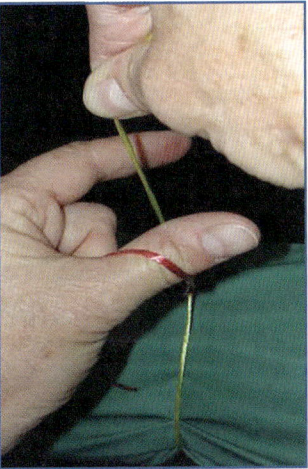

Method

Close the 'beak'.

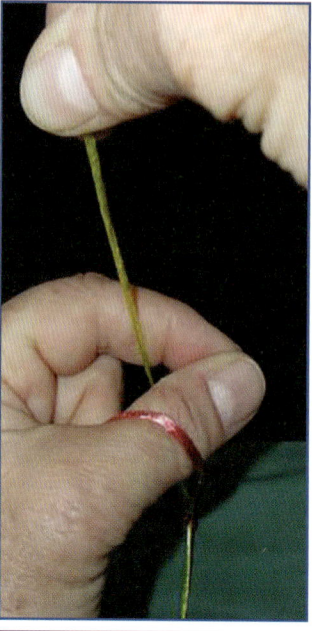

By lifting your left elbow and rotating your wrist, you will push the beak through the loop between the two sutures (c). Continue pushing the beak towards yourself and then to the right. The red suture is now wrapped over your index finger (d).

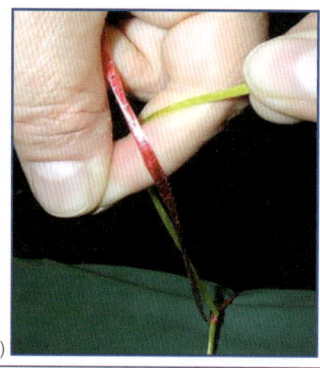

(c)

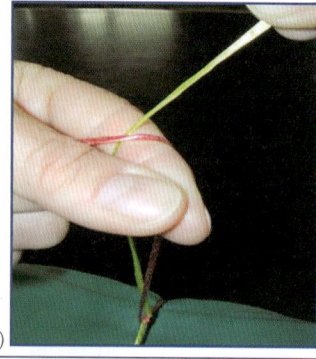

(d)

Make sure you have maintained vertical tension on the yellow suture. Now open your 'beak', laying the yellow suture on to the tip of your index finger.

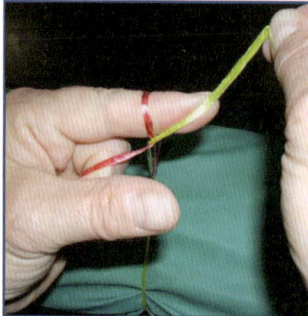

Method

Close your thumb onto the yellow suture, gripping it and reforming your 'beak'.

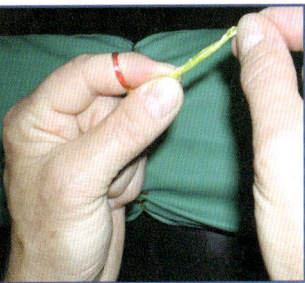

Let go of the yellow suture with your right hand.

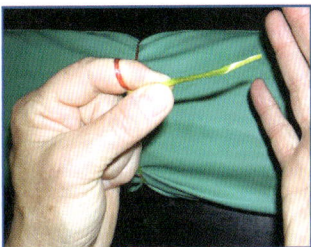

Push your beak back down through the loop (which is formed around your left index finger), continue this rotation until your beak points away from you.

The yellow suture should go under the red suture.

Offer the yellow suture to your right hand.

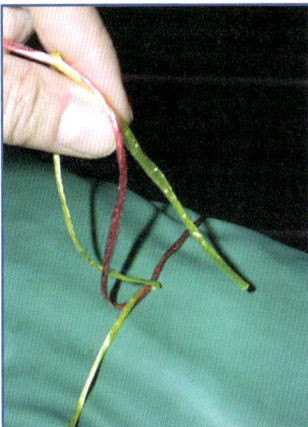

Method

Pick up the yellow suture with your right hand and pull it down *towards* your body, opening the beak at the same time to release the yellow suture.

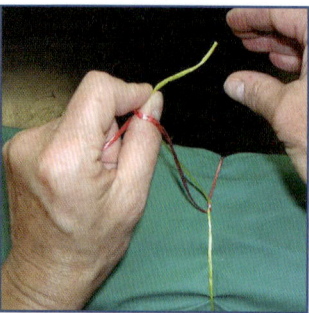

At the same time pull the red suture in your left hand *upwards* and away from yourself, hanging on to it in your left palm still.

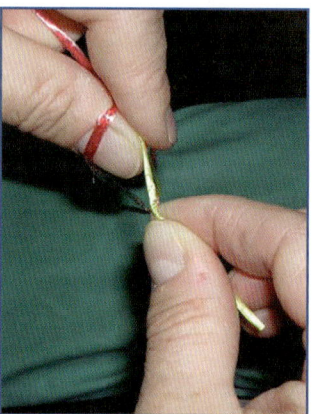 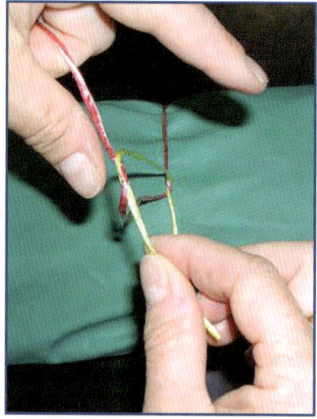

Square knot!

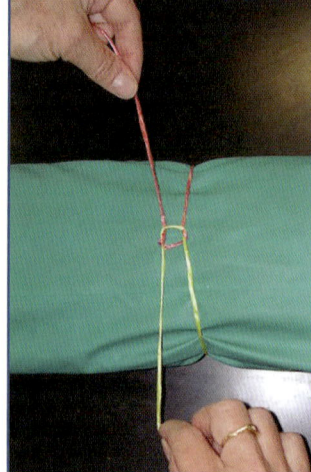

This technique describes how to do the two different throws that make up the **two-handed square knot**. You will, in practice, use several throws – normally at least four, but this depends on the suture material type.

To add additional throws for knot security, you are in effect putting one completed square knot on top of another – you must not just use the second throw repeatedly, as this will make a slip knot.

© RVC

Clinical Skills Sheet

6.11. Instrument suture: square knot or surgeon's knot

Method
Gather your equipment: • Mayo-Hegar needle holder.   • Rat-tooth forceps (Treeves).   • Small Mayo scissors.   • Suture material.   • Needle (size 14 curved triangular cutting for small animal incision closure).   • Suture pad with 'wound' cut into it.   • Suture material.   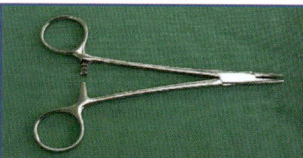
Select the appropriate suture material, either multifilament nylon or monofilament nylon.   Pull up from the reel approx. 30–40 cm length of suture material. Take care not to 'break sterility' when you do so.   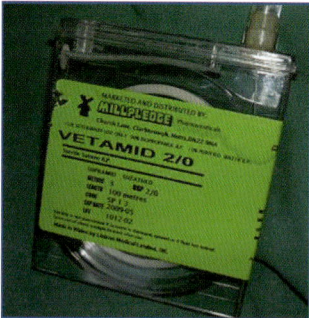
Thread needle – do *not* double thread the suture material through the eye of the needle or tie a knot. (This would cause more trauma to the wound.)
Needle holders are held using thumb–ring finger (4th finger) grip in your 'leading' hand.   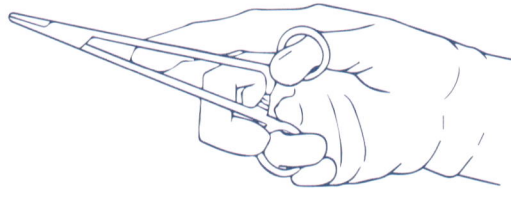

Method

Place the needle between the jaws of the needle holder as follows:
- Have the needle at right angles to the needle holder.
- Grasp the needle at half or two-thirds of its length.
- Grasp in first 3rd of the jaws of the needle holder, towards the tip of the jaws.
- Lock the ratchet of the needle holder.

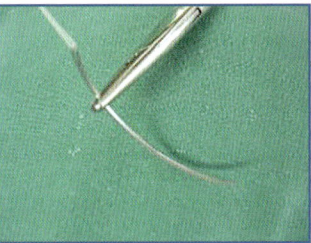

Hold rat-tooth forceps in the other hand using the pencil grip.
NB: To 'palm your instrument', flick it into the palm of your hand and secure with the heel of your thumb. The 'teeth' are facing downwards, (which prevents the suture material becoming tangled in them when performing the 'throws').

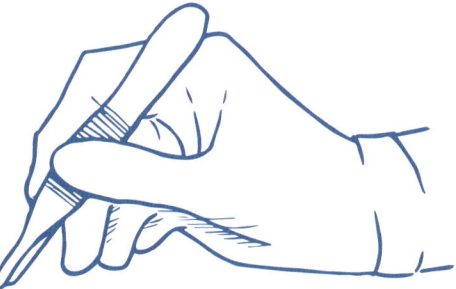

- These forceps are *never* used to handle/grip the needle.
- These forceps are not used to grip the suture material or needle unless they are Adson-Brown forceps.

At one end of the wound, stabilize the skin on the wound's far edge with your rat-tooth forceps.
Note: you are suturing *towards* yourself.
Place the needle approx. 5–7 mm *away* from the incision edge on the FAR side of the incision.
- *The needle should be at a 90° angle to the skin.*

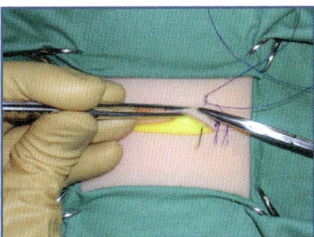

Push needle completely through the skin, aiming it to come up through the incision. (See the footnote at the end of this sheet for the reason.)

Method
Release the needle from your needle holder (whilst still maintaining the grip with your rat-tooth forceps on the far skin edge).

Re-grasp the needle with the needle holder, about a half to one-third away from the eye of the needle as before.
Pull suture through the skin – leaving approximately 5 cm of free end of suture material on the far side of the wound.

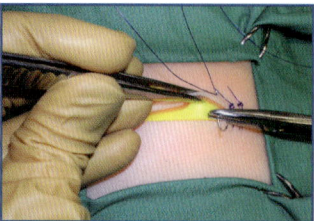

NB: You may need to use your fingers to hold on to the suture material to prevent it from becoming unthreaded from the needle.
If so, 'palm' your forceps prior to holding the suture material near to the eye of the needle.
(You would not need to do this step with swaged-on suture material.)

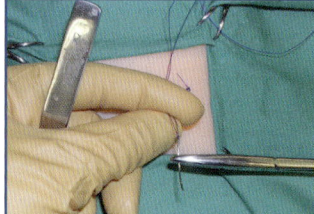

Stabilize the skin on the wound's *near edge* with rat-tooth forceps
- Push the needle up through the underside of the skin.
- It should appear 5–7 mm *away* from the incision edge.

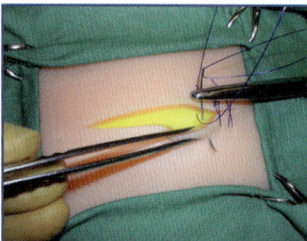

Release the needle from the needle holder (whilst still holding on to the near skin edge with your forceps).

Re-grasp the middle of the needle with your needle holder and pull the needle and suture material through the skin.
Once the needle is clear of the skin, release the skin from your forceps and palm them.
(Possibly once again using your fingers to hang on to the suture material to prevent it from becoming unthreaded.)

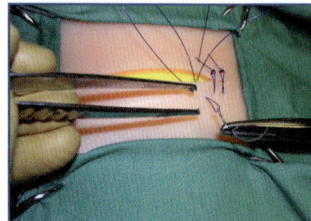

Square knot tying technique

Gather up the excess length of the suture material and the needle in the same hand that your 'palmed' forceps are in to have a working piece of suture material approx. 15 cm in length.

First throw

Place the needle holder (with jaws closed) in between the two strands of suture material over the wound, so that they are held *above and in line* with the incision.

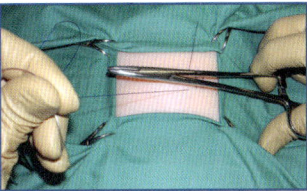

Wrap the long end of suture (that you are holding in your 'rat-tooth forceps hand' nearest you) *once* over the top and underneath the end of the needle holder, bringing your hand back towards your body.

NB: To perform a **surgeon's knot** – at this point you simply wrap the suture material *twice* around the end of the needle holder.

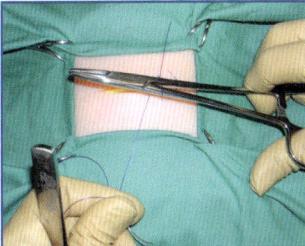

Open the jaws of the needle holder *slightly* and grasp the short free-end (or 'tail') of suture in the needle holder tips.

- Bring the short end *towards* you through the loop.
- At the same time move the hand holding the needle and forceps over the wound *away from* you, therefore both hands cross over the wound.

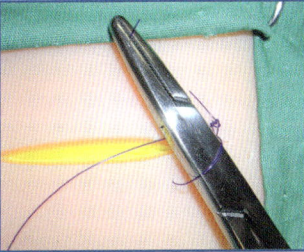

Tighten suture gently over the wound.

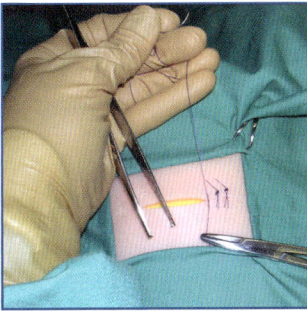

Square knot tying technique

Release suture material from the needle holder.

Second throw

Place the needle holder in between the two strands of suture material over the first knot as before.

- Wrap the long suture strand (furthest away from you) over the top of and around the end of the needle holder.
- Grasp and pass the short end through the loop *away* from you.
- Both hands cross over the wound.

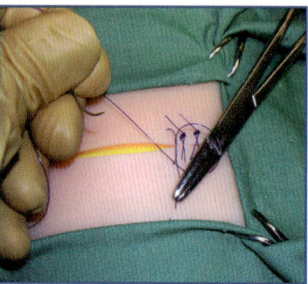

Tighten the knot down, keeping your hands low to ensure that a square knot is formed.

NB: Pulling on one strand more than the other will cause a slip knot to form.

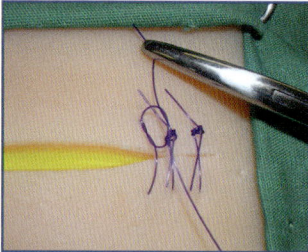

Third throw

Performed in the same way as the *first* throw with single wrap and tightened down to secure the knot.

You may put on another throw, or more, depending on circumstances. However, for most skin sutures, three knots are sufficient.

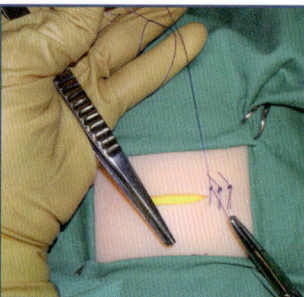

Square knot tying technique
Ensure even tension is applied when tightening sutures (to avoid half-hitch forming).
Cut suture, leaving approximately 1 cm.
The wound edge should be held together with even tension (i.e. not too tight or too loose, *apposing* edges just touching). • Knots are situated to *one side or the other* of the incision, not directly on top of it, which will prevent trauma to the healing wound on removal. 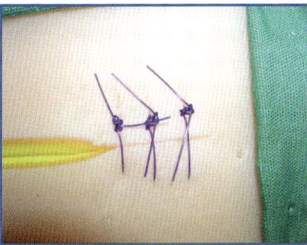

Footnote

It is 'good practice' to exit your needle through the centre of the incision; however, this depends on circumstances as to what/where anatomically you are suturing.

It also prevents you from accidentally picking up underlying structures and suturing these into the wound.

• This knot is also used to *start and finish continuous suture* patterns, though you will place more throws on to start and finish (depending on your choice of suture material).

© RVC

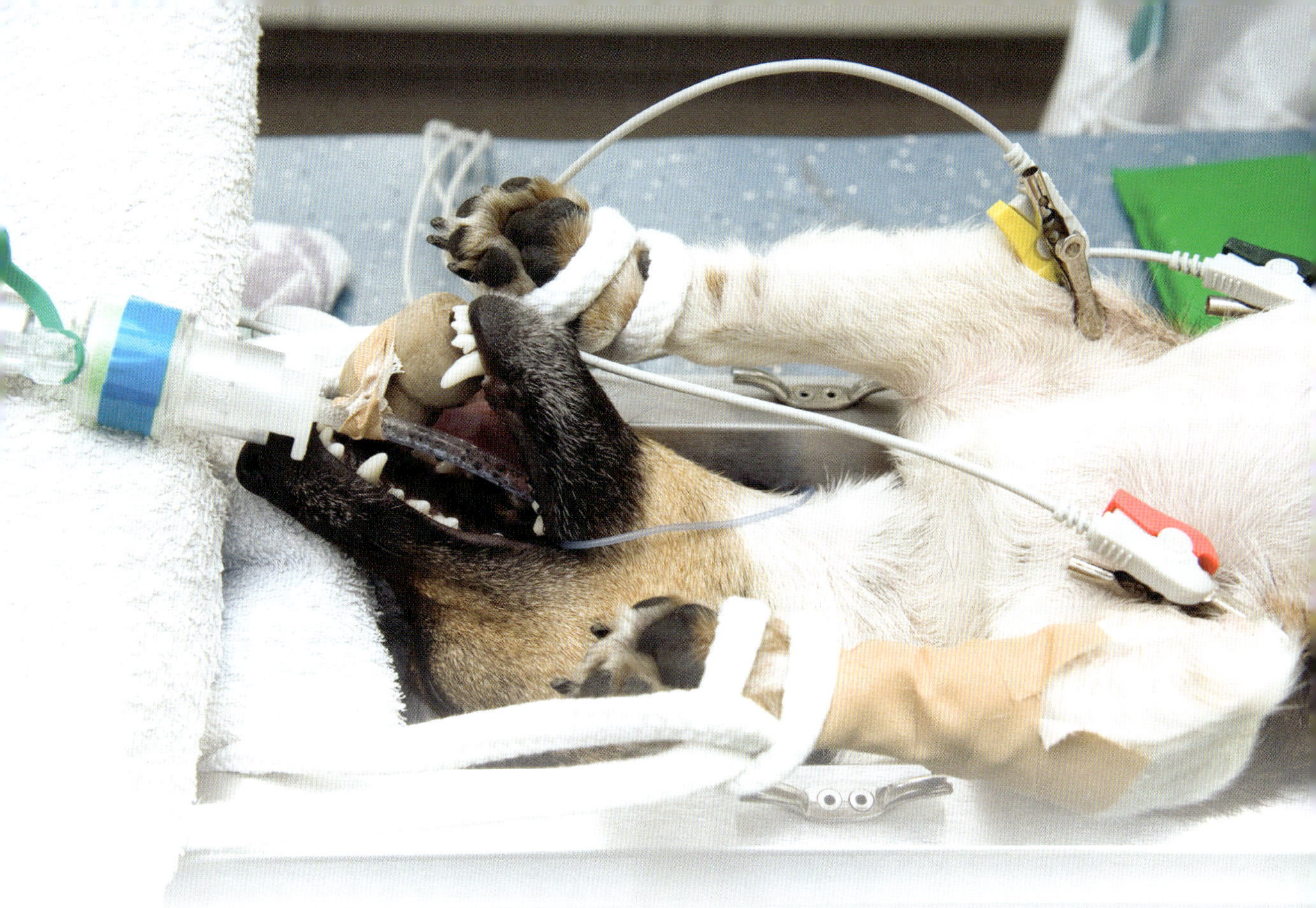

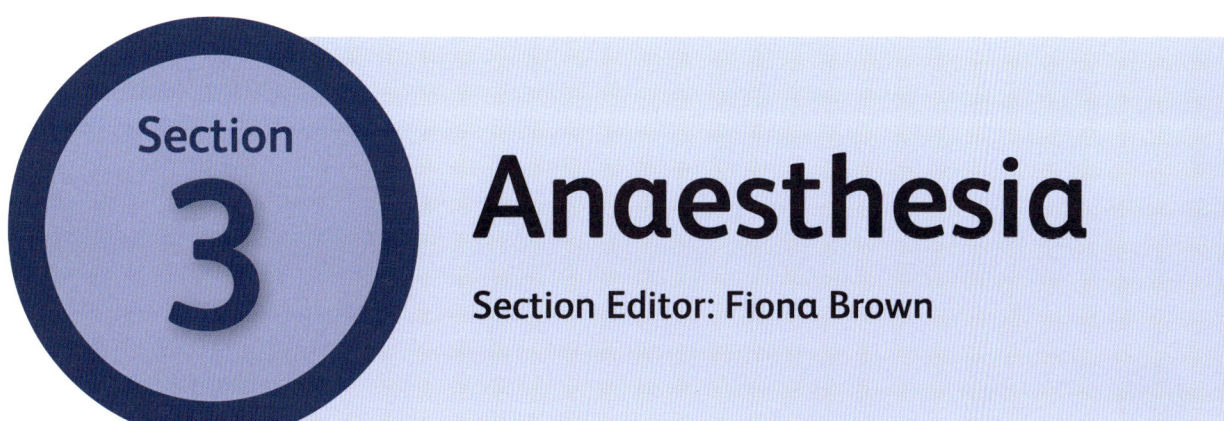

Section

3

Anaesthesia

Section Editor: Fiona Brown

Introduction

Anaesthesia is an essential skill in order to perform surgery. Setting up of the anaesthetic machine and checking that it is safe and fit for use is the first step in anaesthesia. How to manage the correct gases in the breathing mixture as well as which breathing system to use is an important decision to make. There are calculations that help to decide on anaesthetic gas flow and this depends on the size of the animal. Finally, intubation and monitoring the patient during anaesthesia while the surgery is being carried out is essential for patient safety and welfare.

Within this section there are two chapters:

Chapter 7: The Anaesthetic Machine

Chapter 8: Breathing Systems, Intubation and Monitoring Anaesthesia

Within each chapter you will find pictures and tips about how to practise relevant basic Day One skills. Each chapter will also detail key points for each set of skills and point out the health and safety considerations, which are critical to good practice.

An overview of all the learning outcomes is presented below and the more detailed learning outcomes are presented under each chapter.

Learning objectives

After studying this section, students should be able to:

- Identify and check the anaesthetic machine.
- Change an oxygen cylinder.

- Identify, select and check that a breathing system is safe and ready for use.
- Intubate and assess depth of anaesthesia of the patient.
- Monitor the patient using pulse oximeter, oesophageal stethoscope and Doppler.

What You Will Use

Clinical skills sheets (SS)

Six clinical skills sheets will be used in this section. Reference will be made to each skills sheet at the relevant point within the chapter. Clinical skills sheets for the following accompany this section:

SS 7.12 Anaesthetic machine set-up

SS 8.13 Parallel Lack breathing system

SS 8.14 Circle breathing system

SS 8.15 Bain breathing system

SS 8.16 Modified Ayres T-piece breathing system

SS 8.17 Anaesthesia help sheet: calculating fresh gas flow

Videos (V)

One video will be used in this section and reference will be made to it at the relevant point within the chapter. Videos will be hyperlinked and the following accompanies this section:

V 7.1 How to set up the anaesthetic machine

The Anaesthetic Machine

Fiona Brown[a] and Chris Seymour[b]

[a]The Royal Veterinary College, London; [b]Davies Veterinary Specialists, Hitchin, UK

Learning objectives

By the end of this chapter, students should be able to:

- Identify parts of the anaesthetic machine.
- Check that the anaesthetic machine is safe and ready for use.
- Change an oxygen cylinder.

Clinical skills sheet

One clinical skills sheet will be used in this chapter and this can be found at pages 102–104. Reference will be made to the skills sheet in the relevant section of the chapter. The details of the clinical skills sheet are as follows:

SS 7.12 Anaesthetic machine set-up

Video (V)

V 7.1 How to set up the anaesthetic machine

Health and safety!

Remember that gas cylinders are pressurized containers and should never be opened when not connected to an anaesthetic machine. The escaping gas can have dangerous consequences, either by causing damage in the form of cold burns to personnel or by propelling the cylinders forward like a rocket. They must be handled carefully and with respect.

- Larger cylinders need to be transported on appropriate trolleys and stored safely away from flammable material, with larger cylinders stored upright and secured with chains.
- They must never be greased or lubricated.
- Cylinders made from aluminium can be obtained for use adjacent to MRI scanners.

For piped gases there will be isolation switches in case of emergency.

Introduction

This chapter will begin by looking at the anaesthetic machine. All practices will have their own individual machinery that they use but the method employed to check that the equipment is safe and ready for use will follow a similar protocol. Plenty of textbooks feature a particular diagram showing the 'anatomy' of the anaesthetic machine; this is a very abstract concept away from the anaesthetic machine, but take that diagram and look at it next to an anaesthetic machine and the components become much easier to identify. A student should take every opportunity to view and explore the equipment away from the busy clinical environment either within the clinic out of hours or within a safe skills laboratory environment, providing the time to improve confidence.

7.1 The Anaesthetic Machine

Anaesthetic machines (Fig. 7.1) provide gases and a volatile agent in accurate concentrations, which improves safety.

© CAB International 2018. *Veterinary Clinical Skills Manual* (eds N. Coombes and A. Silva-Fletcher)

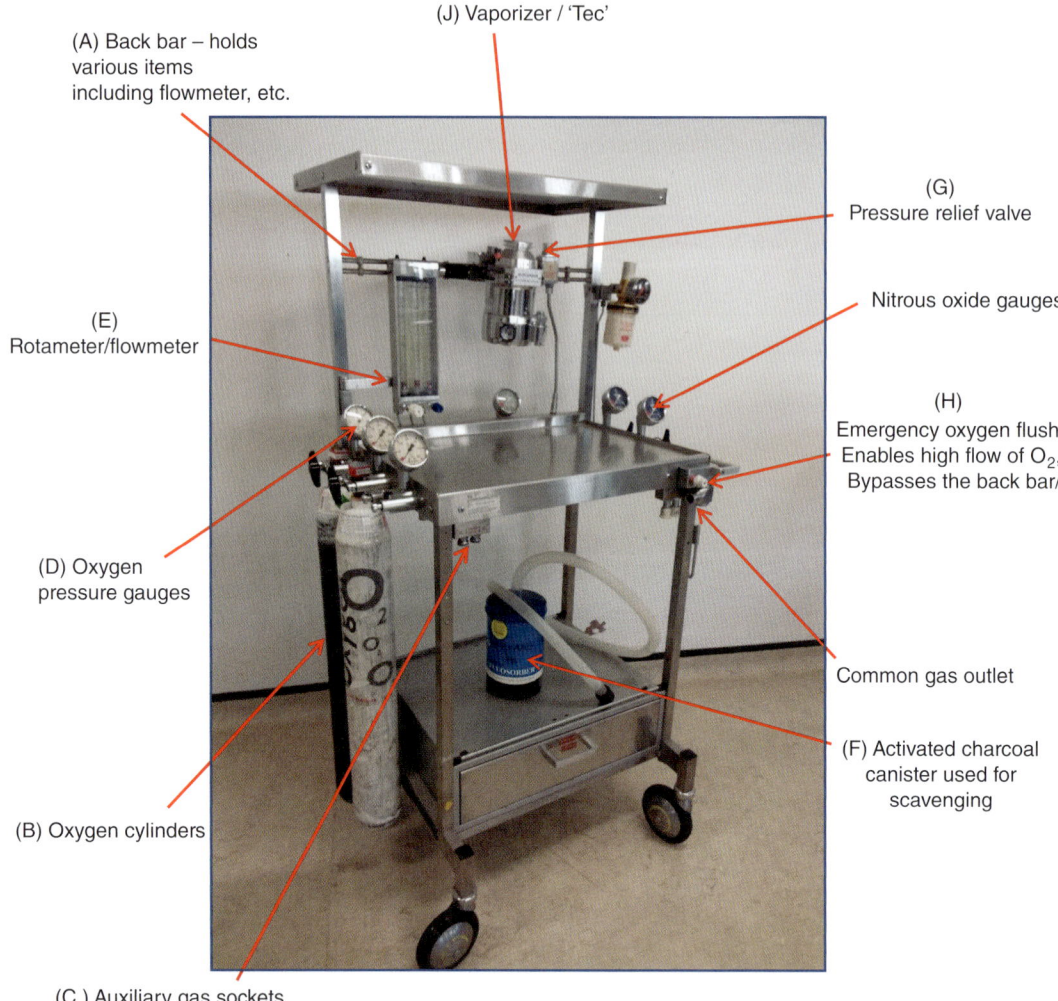

(A) Back bar – holds various items including flowmeter, etc.

(J) Vaporizer / 'Tec'

(G) Pressure relief valve

Nitrous oxide gauges

(E) Rotameter/flowmeter

(H) Emergency oxygen flush Enables high flow of O_2, Bypasses the back bar/

(D) Oxygen pressure gauges

Common gas outlet

(B) Oxygen cylinders

(F) Activated charcoal canister used for scavenging

(C) Auxiliary gas sockets

Fig. 7.1. The anatomy of an anaesthetic machine.

7.1.1   Stand/wall bracket

The anaesthetic stand is simply a structure that attaches all the separate components together, with all of the components integrated into the structure. If you look underneath you will see where all the tubes connect with each other.

This stand may be quite bulky, or lighter and mobile with wheels, or it may be attached to a wall in the practice. There will often be useful shelves, hooks or drawers integrated within the unit to make it user friendly.

7.1.2   Back bar

This holds the flowmeter(s) and vaporizer(s) (Fig. 7.1A).

7.1.3   Oxygen supply

To provide a volatile anaesthetic agent to your patient you need a carrier gas. Oxygen is usually supplied in pressurized cylinders (Fig. 7.1B) that are colour coded so you can ensure that you have correctly selected your chosen gas (Table 7.1). Cylinders are available in

Table 7.1. Colour codes of different gases.

Carrier gas	Colour (UK)
Oxygen	White (some older cylinders may still have a black body with a white neck)
Nitrous oxide	Blue

different sizes, from the smallest AA to J, with most mobile anaesthetic machines taking E-size cylinders. The largest cylinders are used when gases are piped.

Warning!

Medical air may be seen in practice to power equipment and must not be confused with oxygen (a medical air cylinder has a grey body with a black and white neck).

If a practice has piped gases, the primary source of oxygen is situated away from the anaesthetic machine and will be piped to areas of the building where it is required. There are wall-mounted sockets in the room, into which colour-coded pipes connect; they need to be pushed firmly into the socket until they lock into position. Turning on the flowmeter will confirm proper connection.

Many mobile machines may also have the facility for piped gases and will often use the smaller cylinders attached to the machine as a back-up if the pipeline supply fails.

The piped gas cylinders are very large and should be stored outside the practice building. There are commonly two banks of cylinders, with one in use and one as a reserve. When the in-use bank is running low, a loud audible alarm should sound so that staff can switch to the reserve bank. Although systems may be in place to change banks automatically, it is important for staff to replace the empty cylinders with full ones as soon as possible to ensure a back-up is always available. This system is very similar to the cylinders on the machine but on a much larger scale.

7.1.4 Alternative sources of oxygen

For very large veterinary practices it may be more economical to use liquid oxygen.

A vacuum-insulated evaporator (VIE) is needed to convert cryogenic liquid oxygen to gas form, which is then fed into the pipeline system.

7.1.5 Nitrous oxide

Nitrous oxide is an anaesthetic agent, supplied in cylinders, that can be used alongside oxygen as an additional carrier gas. Its anaesthetic properties are weak and it cannot be used to produce general anaesthesia alone, but has been found to provide a useful analgesic effect that helps to reduce the concentrations of volatile anaesthetic needed to maintain anaesthesia. These lower concentrations will have less profound cardiopulmonary side effects. The low blood solubility of nitrous oxide can cause diffusion hypoxia at the end of the anaesthesia. This is easily avoided by administering sufficient oxygen throughout the anaesthetic period and providing 100% oxygen for 10 min after the nitrous oxide has been turned off. If accidentally administered without oxygen, it will cause hypoxia and eventual death.

Although a useful anaesthetic drug, care must also be taken in any animals with suspected pneumothorax or gastric dilation/volvulus (GDV), as nitrous oxide can cause gas pockets to expand, which might be dangerous.

Nitrous oxide is usually administered at a concentration of between 50% and 70%, because it is not very potent. Care must be taken to ensure adequate scavenging systems are in place to prevent environmental exposure.

Having different gases available in a practice could lead to serious and potentially deadly errors. Steps have been taken to minimize the risk of accidental administration of the wrong gas.

7.1.6 Pin index

This system (Fig. 7.2) acts like a key: the cylinders have a specific keyhole pattern, which will only fix into the correct pins that are on the anaesthetic machine. Each gas has a unique pin index, which stops connection of the wrong cylinder to the wrong place on the anaesthetic machine, or to the wrong pipeline.

7.1.7 Pipeline connectors

Wall or ceiling-mounted hanging sockets for the pipes (Fig. 7.1C) will only allow the correct gas tube to connect.

7.1.8 Anti-hypoxic devices

Some modern anaesthetic machines provide a constant minimum amount of oxygen in order to prevent nitrous oxide being administered without adequate oxygen.

7.1.9   Checking the cylinder

To check if an oxygen cylinder attached to an anaesthetic machine is full, it needs to be opened. The cylinder can be opened using the ratchet key. Turn anti-clockwise to open or clockwise to close ('rightie tightie, leftie loosie'). Figure 7.3 shows how to open and close the cylinder.

The keys that have an integral ratchet are very user friendly as they are clearly labelled and will reposition/ratchet themselves into the correct position for use.

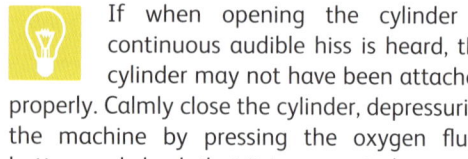

If when opening the cylinder a continuous audible hiss is heard, the cylinder may not have been attached properly. Calmly close the cylinder, depressurize the machine by pressing the oxygen flush button and check that it is connected correctly (see below).

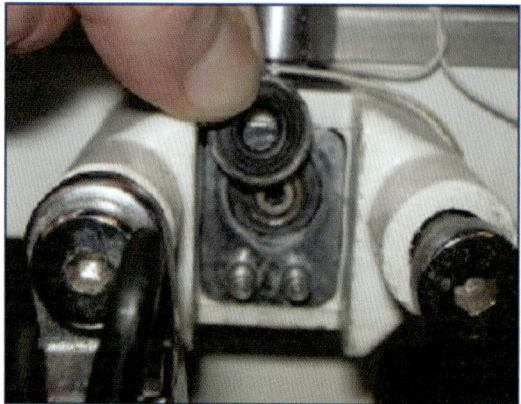
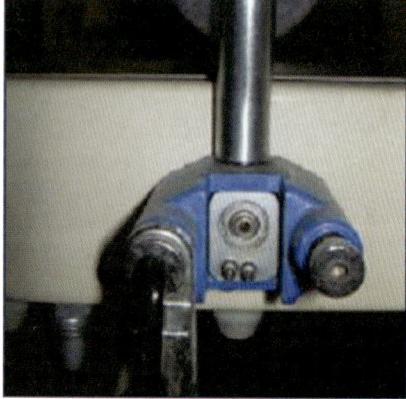

Fig. 7.2. Pin index showing the gas-specific arrangement of pins, which will only fit into the corresponding holes on the correct cylinder.

Turning on/opening the cylinder

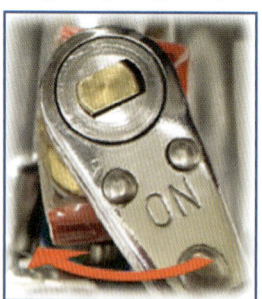

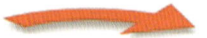

1. After putting the ratchet on the pressure gauge, make the first turn to the left. It should make a 'clicking' sound

2. Next, pull the ratchet handle to the right. You will not hear a clicking sound this time. Now your cylinder should be on and you should be able to get a pressure gauge reading

Turning off/closing the cylinder

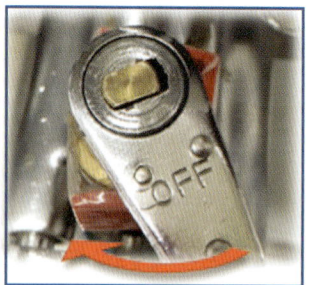

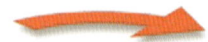

1. To turn off the tank, apply the ratchet to the cylinder in the off setting. Pull the handle to the left

2. Now pull the ratchet handle to the right. You should hear a 'clicking' sound. Push the emergency oxygen valve and you should hear the alarm whistle. The pressure gauge should drop to '0'

Fig. 7.3. How to use the ratchet key to open and close the cylinder.

7.1.10 Bodok seals

A small rubber ring called a Bodok seal prevents gas leaking between the cylinder and its mount on the anaesthetic machine. These rings are small but essential items and spares should always be kept. They may accidently stick to an empty cylinder when it is being removed from the machine, so that when a full replacement cylinder is attached and turned on, a sharp hissing sound is heard.

If this happens, do not panic. Turn the cylinder off and check that a Bodok seal is on the machine.

7.1.11 Pressure gauges

These show the pressure of the gas, in kilopascals (kPa) or bars, within the cylinder which, in the case of oxygen, is a direct indication of how much is remaining for use (Fig. 7.1D). A full oxygen cylinder will display 13,700 kPa, or 137 bar.

Because nitrous oxide is stored as a liquid and not as a gas, the pressure gauge cannot be used to calculate how much gas remains in the cylinder.

Both the in-use and reserve cylinder(s) should be checked before use to ensure adequate oxygen is available.

7.1.12 Pressure-reducing valves

These regulators reduce the pressure of gas coming from a cylinder to a safer, working value of around 400 kPa (4 bar) and also maintain it at a constant level.

7.1.13 Flowmeters (rotameters)

Flowmeters (Fig. 7.1E) control the flow of gases and are usually calibrated in ml/min or l/min. The flow is adjusted by turning a knob, which is colour-coded for each gas. As the gas flows, a bobbin or ball is seen to float in the gas stream: the height that it floats depends on the flow rate. A bobbin should also spin as the gas passes it, made easier to see by a white dot printed on the side of the bobbin. The actual gas flow is read from the top of a bobbin.

7.1.14 Oxygen alarm

This will sound when oxygen pressure in the cylinder drops below a certain level.

To check that the alarm is functioning, set an oxygen flow of at least 4 l/min and then close the cylinder or detach the pipeline supply from the anaesthetic machine. As the supply of oxygen decreases, the oxygen alarm should sound, usually as a high-pitched whistle.

7.1.15 Scavenging of waste anaesthetic gases

Properly functioning scavenging systems are essential to prevent waste gases from entering the room, to ensure a safe working environment for all staff.

- **Active scavenging** actively suctions waste gases away through a waste pipe (the most effective method).
- **Passive scavenging** (Fig. 7.1F) is not as effective as active scavenging: it simply allows a route for waste gases to be removed. This may be a tube connected to a hole in the wall or the ceiling, or to a canister containing activated charcoal (e.g. Fluosorber), which adsorbs waste volatile anaesthetics. Remember that charcoal does not adsorb nitrous oxide. Charcoal canisters must be weighed at least daily to ensure that they are not exhausted (usually they are discarded when their weight reaches 1400 g).

7.1.16 Pressure relief valve

If there is a build-up of pressure within the machine, such as caused by a blocked common gas outlet, this valve (Fig. 7.1G) will open to release the pressure. This is the valve that opens when the inner tube of a Bain breathing system is occluded when checking whether it is safe to use (see Bain skills sheet, SS 8.15).

7.1.17 Emergency oxygen flush

This bypasses the back bar (and so misses the rotameter and vaporizer) and supplies 100% oxygen via the common gas outlet (Fig. 7.1H). Oxygen from this source is supplied at a very high flow, so the patient should be disconnected from the breathing system first. It is used to clear the breathing system of anaesthetic gases at the end of anaesthesia.

7.1.18 Vaporizer

The agent used to maintain anaesthesia is a volatile liquid, which vaporizes when the carrier gas passes over it. There are various types of vaporizer and the most familiar type (plenum vaporizer) attaches to the back bar (Fig. 7.1J) and the gas passes through it from the adjacent flowmeter. The vaporizer, sometimes referred to as a 'tec', is a piece of equipment that holds the volatile agent in a reservoir and which is carefully calibrated to supply the anaesthetic agent at a desired percentage concentration. It is important that these pieces of equipment are treated with great care and are never dropped or tilted, to ensure that the careful calibration is maintained.

The dial: How much?

The concentration administered (as a percentage) is based on a number of considerations, including the minimum alveolar concentration (MAC) of the agent, which is the end-tidal concentration needed to provide surgical anaesthesia in at least 50 % of patients.

Examples:
Isoflurane MAC: dogs 1.3 % ; cats 1.6 %
Sevoflurane MAC: 2.5 %

This is a guide for maintenance. Actual required amounts may be influenced by other drugs administered and the animal's health status, age and body temperature.

7.1.19 Filling keys

Like the pin index safety system, there are key-filling systems for vaporizers that will only allow you to fill the vaporizer with the correct agent (Fig. 7.4).

 SS 7.12 gives step-by-step guidance on how to set up and check the anaesthetic machine

 V 7.1 on anaesthetic machine set-up demonstrates how this is done

V 7.1 video.cabi.org/dkwhy

7.2 Changing an Oxygen Cylinder on a Machine

7.2.1 When?

If it is a single cylinder with no reserve you will want to change the cylinder before it runs out completely. There is a red warning line on the pressure gauge and you may choose to change when this has been reached.

On machines where there is a reserve cylinder, you can wait for the cylinder to run out before turning on the reserve when the oxygen alarm sounds.

7.2.2 Removing

To remove the cylinder, ensure it is completely turned off using the ratchet key.

It is useful to position a foot under the cylinder to hold it steady whilst the clamp holding the cylinder in position is undone and the cylinder is lifted free and put into storage to await collection.

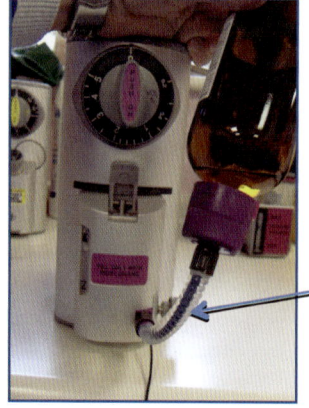

This is the filling key that prevents any spillage of the anaesthetic agent

Fig. 7.4. Filling key and bottle.

7.2.3 Replacing

Remove and discard the plastic wrapping on the cylinder neck and position the cylinder against the pins, checking that the Bodok seal is in position. Tightly close the cylinder clamp. Turn on the cylinder with the ratchet key.

> Having read this chapter and followed the skills sheet and video, you should feel more confident in your ability to safely use and set up an anaesthetic machine.

Further Reading: Alibhai, H.I.K. (2016) The anaesthetic machine and vaporizers. In: Duke-Navakovski, T., de Vries, M. and Seymour, C. (eds) *BSAVA Manual of Canine and Feline Anaesthesia and Analgesia*, 3rd edn. BSAVA Publications, Gloucester, UK.

Clinical Skills Sheet

7.12. Anaesthetic machine set-up

Note: this includes correctly attaching the breathing system provided.

Method
Generally check your machine first, making sure all oxygen cylinders are turned *off* and the pressure gauge dials are on 'red'.
Using the ratchet key provided, with the word 'on' facing uppermost, switch on the 'full' reserve oxygen cylinder. (The top key is showing 'On', the bottom key shows 'Off'.) 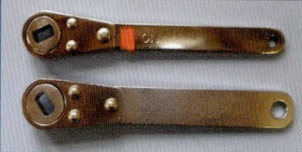
This key fits on to the *brass* fitting on top of the oxygen cylinder (When turning the cylinder *on*, you only need to make a half-turn with the ratchet key. *It makes no difference to the flow of oxygen if you turn the key any more than this.*) 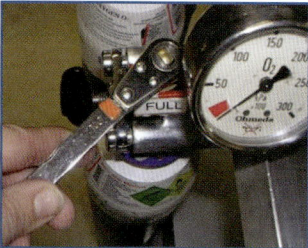
Check oxygen in the cylinder – state pressure. A full cylinder will read at 137 bar on the dial. 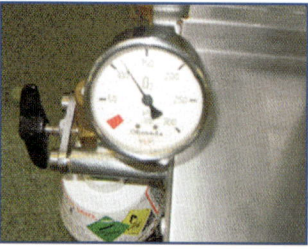
Check the O$_2$ emergency outlet button. Press it in and you should hear hissing of the O$_2$ 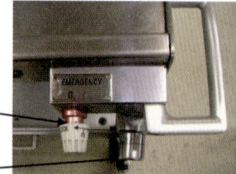 (O$_2$ outlet)

Method

Now check the flowmeter (rotameter):

Turn on the white knob (O_2) and check that the bobbin rises and returns to zero when turned down.

(The oxygen is read from the *top of the bobbin* in one type of flowmeter, but the *centre of a ballbearing* in another type of flowmeter.)

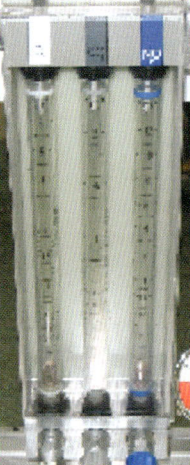

Turn the key over and turn off the 'full' reserve cylinder.

Now turn on the flowmeter, allowing the O_2 to empty from the machine, which checks the O_2 alarm (the alarm should sound – but only if fitted).

Now turn on the 'in use' cylinder.

State pressure in the cylinder (replace if empty). SEE WARNING BELOW.

If fitted – check contents of nitrous oxide cylinder by turning cylinder on.

Check the vaporizer (tec):
- Is it firmly attached to the back bar?
- If not, turn the switch to 'lock'.
- Check the fluid level in the window on the front.
- If it needs filling, this is done through the filling port – always with the correct anaesthetic agent as stated on the vaporizer.

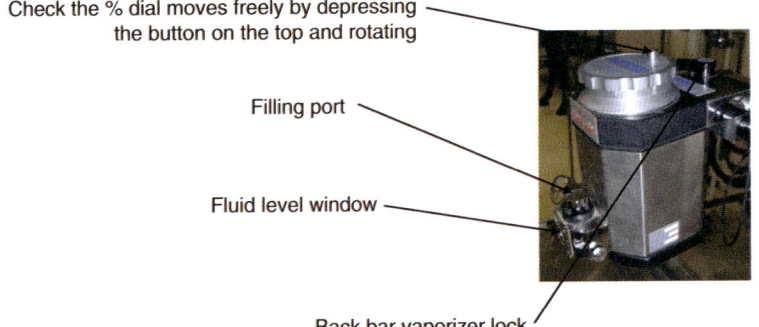

Check the % dial moves freely by depressing the button on the top and rotating

Filling port

Fluid level window

Back bar vaporizer lock

Attach the breathing system selected to the O₂ outlet

Now perform a circuit check for leaks:

1. Make sure the oxygen is on.
2. Attach the breathing system to the fresh gas outlet on the machine.
3. Close the APL Valve*.
4. Occlude the patient end of the breathing system with your thumb.
5. Turn the O_2 on at the flowmeter to approx. 4 litres.
6. The reservoir bag should fill; you can fill it quicker using the O_2 flush.
7. Once the bag is full, listen for any sounds of leaking gas.
8. The bag should stay inflated when you squeeze it.
9. Open the APL valve with your thumb still in place.
10. Squeeze the bag: the gas in the system should pass out through the scavenging system.

DO NOT ATTEMPT TO CHANGE AN OXYGEN CYLINDER UNLESS A MEMBER OF THE CSC STAFF IS PRESENT or you have been previously shown how to!

*APL valve

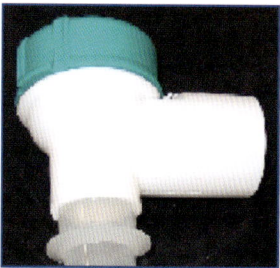

© RVC

Breathing Systems, Intubation and Monitoring

Fiona Brown[a], Chris Seymour[b] and Caroline Hoy[a]

[a]The Royal Veterinary College, London; [b]Davies Veterinary Specialists, Herts

Learning objectives

By the end of this chapter, students should be able to:

- Identify the common breathing systems.
- Select an appropriate breathing system for a patient.
- Check that a breathing system is safe and ready for use.
- Calculate oxygen flows required.
- Intubate the patient.
- Assess depth of anaesthesia.
- Monitor anaesthesia using:
  - Pulse palpation and pulse oximeter.
  - Heart rate using oesophageal stethoscope.
- Measure blood pressure using a Doppler.

Breathing Systems

Fiona Brown and Chris Seymour

8.1 Anaesthetic Breathing Systems

A breathing system is required to transport oxygen and the volatile anaesthetic agent from the anaesthetic machine to the patient, whilst also allowing the expired waste gases (including carbon dioxide) to be disposed of safely, through a scavenging system. The addition of a reservoir bag and adjustable pressure limiting (APL) valve facilitates controlled ventilation if required.

📗 Clinical skills sheets (SS)

Five clinical skills sheets will be used in this chapter and these can be found at pages 114–126. Reference will be made to each skills sheet at the relevant section within the chapter. The details of the clinical skills sheets used are as follows:

SS 8.13 Parallel Lack breathing system

SS 8.14 Circle breathing system

SS 8.15 Bain breathing system

SS 8.16 Modified Ayres T-piece breathing system

SS 8.17 Anaesthesia calculation help sheet

Danger of death!

APL Valve

It is vital that the APL valve is always kept open during anaesthesia. Remember that the animal is unable to exhale whilst this valve is closed.

The only time that this valve should be shut fully is when leak testing a breathing system before use (see later in chapter). When ventilating manually, this valve should be partially closed to provide enough resistance to give a breath (see section 8.15).

© CAB International 2018. *Veterinary Clinical Skills Manual* (eds N. Coombes and A. Silva-Fletcher)

8.2   Which Breathing System?

Several breathing systems are available and it can be confusing when deciding which one is the most suitable for your patient (Fig. 8.1). It is worth remembering that whilst most patients will breathe spontaneously during anaesthesia, sometimes controlled ventilation may be required.

 Controlled ventilation or intermittent positive pressure ventilation (IPPV) may occasionally be necessary during anaesthesia. This can be achieved either manually (by squeezing the reservoir bag) or with a mechanical ventilator. Indications include: hypoventilation; apnoea; and an open thorax, e.g. thoracotomy or diaphragmatic hernia. (See section 8.15 for how to ventilate safely.)

Some breathing systems work more efficiently when an animal is breathing spontaneously, whilst others are more efficient for controlled ventilation, so this is an important consideration when selecting which breathing system to use. The key point to remember is that there is not always a right or wrong choice – just maybe a better, more efficient one.

 What are rebreathing and non-rebreathing systems?

Rebreathing refers to the inhalation of some or all of the previously expired gases, including carbon dioxide and water vapour. If an animal rebreathes its exhaled carbon dioxide, it can cause a respiratory acidosis and have dangerous effects.

Breathing systems can be classified as either rebreathing or non-rebreathing systems:

- In rebreathing systems, carbon dioxide in expired gas is removed by chemical means (soda lime).

- In non-rebreathing systems, rebreathing is normally prevented by having enough oxygen flow into the system to wash away exhaled gas from the previous expiration. Because it is mainly the flushing effect of fresh gas that eliminates carbon dioxide,

these systems have the potential for rebreathing of carbon dioxide when oxygen flow is reduced.

Rebreathing systems include the circle and the to-and-fro, and both use soda lime to absorb carbon dioxide. If the circuit contains granules in a canister, then it is a rebreathing system. These systems can reuse exhaled gas and allow much lower oxygen flows to be used, with greater economy. Less volatile anaesthetic is used and the reaction of carbon dioxide with soda lime produces both heat and water, thus warming and humidifying inspired gases. It is important that you keep a close eye on the carbon dioxide absorber – as the soda lime becomes exhausted over time the animal will start to rebreathe carbon dioxide. As the soda lime becomes exhausted, it will change colour; it should be renewed when half of it has changed colour. (Note that if exhausted soda lime is left in the canister, the colour change can reverse, but this does not mean that it can be used again.)

Non-rebreathing systems are all named after their inventors: Magill, Lack, Bain, Ayre and Humphrey.

8.3   Rebreathing Systems

These are among the most efficient and economical of the breathing systems and are common in veterinary practices. They can be used on patients weighing over 10 kg. The circle system contains one-way valves, which direct the expired gases through the system so that carbon dioxide can be absorbed and reducing the oxygen flows needed. These systems can be used with relatively low oxygen flow rates in both spontaneously breathing and ventilated patients. There are many different designs of circle system.

 SS 8.14 for details of circle breathing system

8.4   Non-rebreathing Systems

There is no carbon dioxide absorber in these systems and elimination of carbon dioxide requires a high enough oxygen flow to flush away all the expired gases. Consequently, much higher flows are needed to prevent rebreathing. There are different systems based on the size of the animal. The Lack, Magill and Bain breathing systems are suitable in patients weighing over 10 kg, whilst the T-piece and mini-Lack breathing systems are suitable for those under 10 kg. The Humphrey system is suitable for all sizes. If a patient is close to 10 kg, it is helpful to consider their ideal weight and expected lung volume to decide which system to choose.

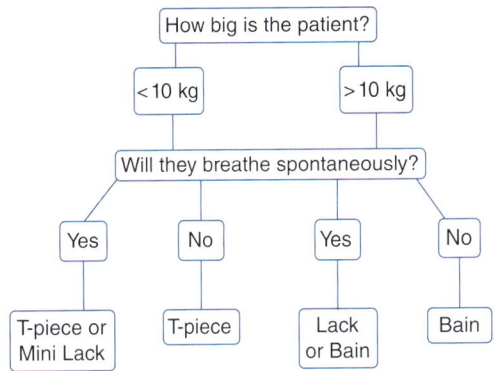

Fig. 8.1. Choosing a system relative to animal's body weight.

8.5 Mapleson Classification of Non-rebreathing Systems

Non-rebreathing systems were also classified by a physicist called Mapleson, based on theoretical considerations of exactly how much oxygen flow is needed to prevent rebreathing of previously exhaled gas (i.e. how efficient they are). This classification is from A to F. According to this system, the Magill and Lack are almost equally efficient and are classified as Mapleson A.

8.5.1 Mapleson A: the Lack and Magill breathing systems

These systems work very efficiently during spontaneous respiration and require a flow of at least the patient's minute volume. They are most suitable for spontaneous ventilation and short-term IPPV, though their efficiency decreases and the oxygen flow needs to be increased if controlled ventilation is required.

SS 8.13 for details of the parallel Lack breathing system. Note the patient end, tubing, machine end, valve, bag and the scavenge tube

8.5.2 Mapleson D/E/F: the T-piece and Bain

These classifications incorporate the Ayres T-piece, Jackson Rees modified and APL versions.

During spontaneous breathing, the T-piece and Bain systems are inefficient and wasteful as they need an oxygen flow of at least twice the patient's minute volume. They are, however, better systems for extended periods of controlled ventilation.

SS 8.15 for the Bain breathing system and **SS 8.16** for the T-Piece system. Please go through these and note the differences

8.5.3 Others

The Humphrey ADE is often called a hybrid system because it can work like either a Lack, or a T-piece, a Bain, or a circle system, depending on how it is set up and whether or not a soda lime canister is attached. In general practice, it is used mainly like a Lack or a circle. The T-piece configuration is used only in conjunction with a mechanical ventilator.

8.6 Checking the Systems

As with the anaesthetic machine (see Chapter 7), it is essential to check that breathing systems are safe and ready for use.

They should be visually inspected each day looking for signs of damage.

1. Attach the breathing system to the common gas outlet on the anaesthetic machine.
2. Close the APL valve.
3. Occlude the patient end with your thumb.
4. Fill the system with oxygen via the flowmeter or oxygen flush.
5. When the bag is inflated and tense, check for signs or sounds of leaking via tubing, connectors or bag.

6. Open the APL valve and check that gas can flow through it.
7. Remove your thumb from the end.

The Bain needs the inner coaxial tube checked in addition (see Bain skills sheet, SS 8.15.)

8.7 Oxygen: How Much?

Exact oxygen requirements are individual to each patient but calculations offer an estimate designed to prevent rebreathing of carbon dioxide.

What are we calculating?

- Respiration rate (RR) = the number of breaths in one minute.
- Minute volume (MV) = the amount (in ml) that an animal breathes in or out in 1 min.
- Tidal volume (TV) = the amount (in ml) that an animal breathes in or out in one breath (10–15 ml/kg).
- System factor = the multiple of the MV required to provide adequate oxygen flow to prevent rebreathing in a non-rebreathing system. Note that the system factor applies only to non-rebreathing systems and not to the circle.

SS 8.17 for an anaesthesia calculation help sheet with details of the two most commonly accepted suggested calculations

Calculating the minute volume

MV = TV (10–15ml/kg) × RR
Or:
MV = 200 ml/kg/min
For non-rebreathing systems, also take into account the system factor:
T-piece/Bain 2.5–3 × MV
Magill/Lack 1–1.5 × MV

If performed correctly, these calculations should ensure no rebreathing occurs. If a veterinary practice has access to capnography monitoring devices, then it may be possible to use lower flows, as these monitors will show if there is any carbon dioxide in the inspired gas.

Use capnography to ensure that no rebreathing is taking place (note wave returns to zero for each inhalation).

8.8 Conclusion

Not all veterinary practices will have every type of breathing system, but it is important that students and staff are confident with what they use most often, even if it is not the most economical. The student or staff member needs to select the most appropriate system for the patient's needs that hopefully is the most economic choice too. Care needs to be taken to ensure that breathing systems are safe and ready for use and that appropriate oxygen flows are selected.

Intubation and Monitoring Anaesthesia

Caroline Hoy, Chris Seymour and Fiona Brown

8.9 Before You Start

Detailed here are the questions you should ask yourself about your patient before you start the anaesthetic process. These will help you to focus on the essentials for safe anaesthesia.

- Look at the patient: what is normal for this dog/cat/rabbit?
- What is their demeanour? Quiet? Lively? Aggressive? Scared?
- Get a baseline set of observations: pulse and respiratory rate and temperature.
- What is their presenting problem? Are they receiving treatment?
- Do they have any other concurrent disease?

Will any of the above information affect your anaesthetic? Quiet patients may not need sedation, lively ones may need more. Your baseline observations are very important as they help you to decide whether the values during anaesthesia are appropriate or whether they are a cause for concern. Concurrent disease may mean that your normal preferred premedication is not appropriate or may even be contraindicated.

Always make a plan. You should take into account the worst-case scenario: it probably will not happen but if you expect the worst you will be prepared for it and you will only be pleased if it does not happen.

8.10 Intubation

An endotracheal (ET) tube delivers anaesthetic gases directly to the patient without contaminating the room and gives the anaesthetist control over respiration and the airway (Fig. 8.2).

The tube needs to be a good fit, but it is better to use a slightly too small tube than to place one that is too big and that could cause damage to the trachea (Table 8.1). Most tubes have a cuff that can be gently inflated to seal the tube against the trachea and prevent fluids from entering the lungs (Fig. 8.3).

The airway may be larger (sight hounds) or smaller (pugs, bulldogs) than you would expect for the size of the dog. Choose at least three sequentially sized tubes (e.g. 5.5 mm, 6 mm and 6.5 mm) and prepare more tubes if you suspect that the airway will be small. When selecting the ET tubes, it is important to check the length of tube is appropriate for the patient; the length should be no more than from the mouth to the point of the shoulder. If it is longer than this, there is a risk of intubating one bronchus only. If you are using cuffed tubes, inflate the cuff to check for leaks, and leave them inflated until you are ready to anaesthetize your patient. Deflate fully before induction. Once the patient is anaesthetized, get an assistant to hold the mouth open. It is easiest to intubate a patient in sternal recumbency.

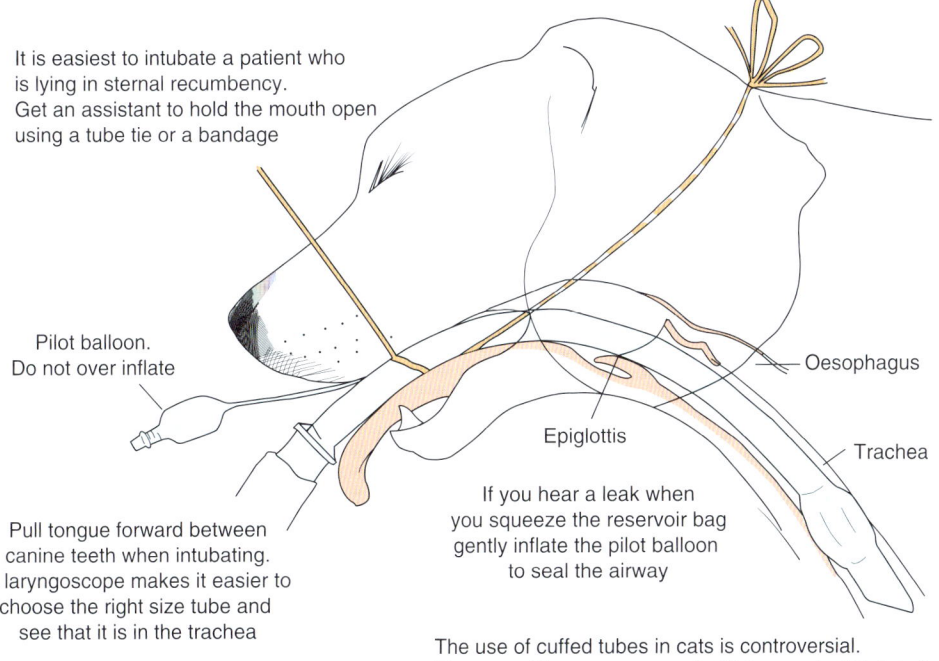

Use a tube tie or non-elastic bandage to secure the tube. Tie it firmly around the tube and then behind the ears or around the nose. Don't make it too tight

It is easiest to intubate a patient who is lying in sternal recumbency. Get an assistant to hold the mouth open using a tube tie or a bandage

Pilot balloon. Do not over inflate

Oesophagus

Epiglottis

Trachea

Pull tongue forward between canine teeth when intubating. A laryngoscope makes it easier to choose the right size tube and see that it is in the trachea

If you hear a leak when you squeeze the reservoir bag gently inflate the pilot balloon to seal the airway

The use of cuffed tubes in cats is controversial. Many practitioners use uncuffed tubes or don't inflate them

Fig. 8.2. Illustration of the position of endotracheal tube.

Table 8.1. How to select the size of the endotracheal tube based on weight of the animal.

Breed	Weight	Endotracheal tube size
Kittens and small cats	0.5–3 kg	2–3.5 mm
Cats	3–6 kg	4–5 mm
Small dogs	2–8 kg	4–7 mm
Medium dogs	8–20 kg	7–9.5 mm
Large dogs	20–40 kg	10–14 mm
Giant breed dogs	40 kg +	14–16 mm

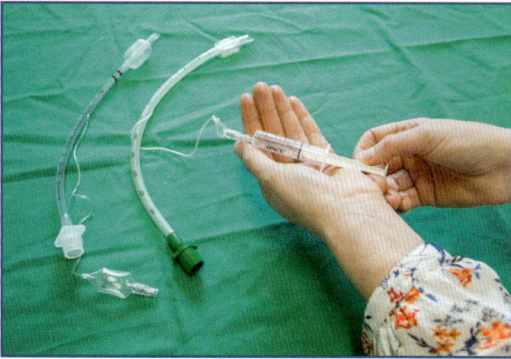

Fig. 8.3. Tube cuff inflated to seal the tube against the trachea.

A laryngoscope makes it easier to see the entrance to the trachea and choose the correctly sized tube. If you are intubating without a laryngoscope, slide the tube over the epiglottis and direct it ventrally towards the trachea, rotating it gently as it passes through the vocal cords. Connect it to the breathing system (oxygen turned on) and tie it in place.

Close the APL valve on the breathing system and squeeze the reservoir bag. The chest should rise with the breath – if you intubated 'blind' this is the easiest way to check that the tube is in the right place. A trace on a capnograph will also confirm correct placement. Make sure that the valve is opened when you have finished your checks.

Check your patient and their depth of anaesthesia and turn the vaporizer on.

 What if I can't intubate?

- Do not panic. Look at colour and respiration. If the patient is able to breathe spontaneously you have time.

- Check the depth of anaesthesia. If the patient is swallowing, they will deflect the tube down the oesophagus.
- Make sure that your assistant is holding the patient straight and at a comfortable height. Are they twisted or slumped? Reposition if necessary.
- Use a laryngoscope if one is available; if not a pen torch and a tongue depressor may help you to see if there are any obstructions or anatomical abnormalities.
- Can you pass a stylet or urinary catheter into the trachea? Slide it through an appropriately sized ET tube before you attempt to place it. You can then use the catheter as a guide and slide the ET tube down into the trachea. Remove the catheter or stylet once the tube is in the right place.
- You can also use a syringe and an ET tube adaptor to attach a urinary catheter to a breathing system and deliver oxygen while you look for a better solution.

8.11 Checking Depth of Anaesthesia

There are three tests you can perform to give a quick indication of the depth of anaesthesia:

- Gently brush the eyelashes from the corner of the eye outwards. Does this cause your patient to blink? Repeated checking will tire the reflex and it will stop.
- The eye should be rotated downwards if your patient is at the correct plane of anaesthesia when using a volatile anaesthetic (Fig. 8.4). A central eye means that the anaesthesia is either too deep or the patient may be about to wake up. A central eye may also be seen if ketamine is used as part of the anaesthetic protocol. Look at all the information you have available to you to decide whether you need to increase or decrease the depth of anaesthesia.
- It should be easy to open the jaw. If it is tense the patient may not be adequately anaesthetized. Some patients, such as Staffordshire Bull Terriers, never seem to relax their jaws fully, so you need to check the tone regularly to see what is normal for your patient and compare what you feel. If the

patient is lying in sternal recumbency, you will just feel the weight of the head.

It is not always possible to check these reflexes as you might not have access to the head. Some drugs, such as neuromuscular blocking agents, will suppress these reflexes, but you should get into the habit of checking them when you can.

8.11.1　What else can be done?

You need to monitor heart and respiratory rates in anaesthetized patients. If anaesthesia is too deep, the heart and respiratory rates may be decreased; if it is too light, the rates may increase.

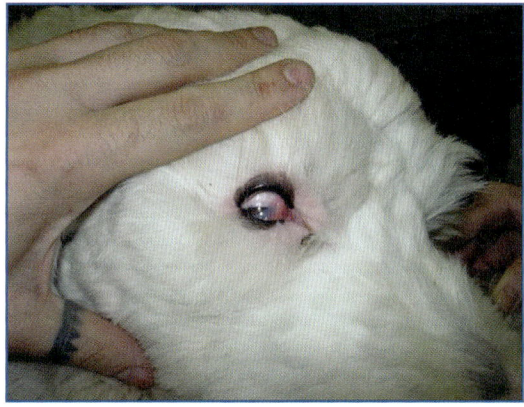

Fig. 8.4. Eye rotated down during anesthesia.

When the patient is intubated, the reservoir bag on the breathing system should expand and contract with each breath (note - it should not collapse completely), but beware that some surgical procedures may push on the diaphragm and also cause bag movement. You should look at the chest to see whether it too is moving. If your practice has a capnograph, you will see a trace that will most likely correspond to respiration, but this too can be affected by surgical activity.

8.11.2　Feeling a pulse

This is a skill that you will need to practise. You can listen to the heart with a stethoscope but it does not tell you whether the beats that you hear are causing blood to flow, or whether that flow is just confined to vital organs.

Figure 8.5 shows the sites that you can use. Get into the habit of feeling for a pulse. You always have your fingers with you and in a crash situation it is the pulse that you will want to feel to tell you whether your patient is alive.

You may not have high-tech monitoring but anyone can afford an oesophageal stethoscope (Fig. 8.6). It consists of a tube with a balloon at the end, which is passed down the oesophagus to the level of the heart; measure it against your patient before you pass it so that you have some idea of how deep it is going. Once it is in place, attach a stethoscope (you will need to remove the chest piece first) and move the tubing slowly within the oesophagus until you can hear the heart and respiratory sounds most clearly.

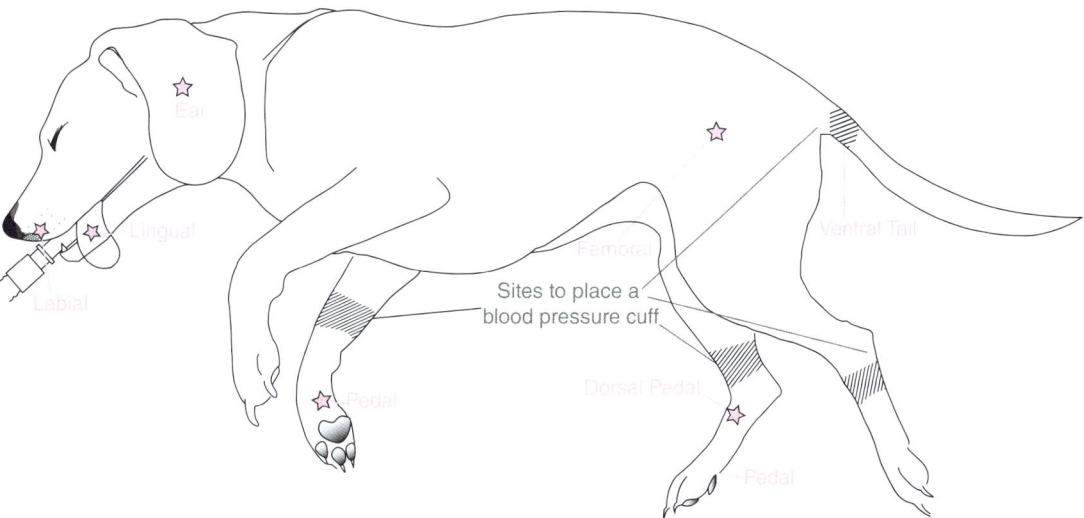

Fig. 8.5. Sites for feeling pulse.

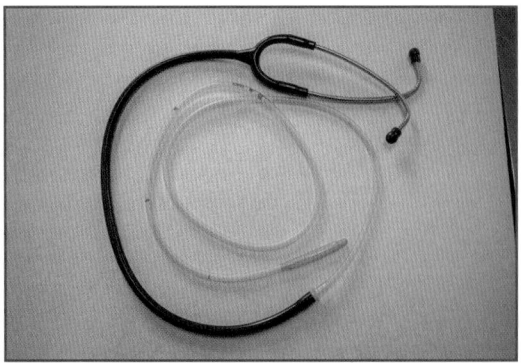

Fig. 8.6. Oesophageal stethoscope.

8.12 Using a Pulse Oximeter

If you shine light through blood, some of that light will be absorbed. A pulse oximeter measures this absorption and calculates the percentage of haemoglobin saturated with oxygen. Blood is there to carry oxygen to the tissues and haemoglobin should be 97–100% saturated.

The pulse oximeter has a probe that is clipped to the tongue or other pulsatile tissue, such as a toe or an ear. It may also work on the prepuce or vulva, or, if you are really struggling, you can try a fold of skin. The tissue should be well perfused and not too hairy or pigmented. Over time the clip can squeeze the blood out of the tissues, especially if blood pressure is low, and this would cause the displayed value to drop. If that does happen, try repositioning the probe; normally saturation will increase again afterwards.

If you have given a drug that causes peripheral vasoconstriction (e.g. medetomidine) you may not have enough perfusion for the pulse oximeter to work. Sometimes folding a moistened swab over the tongue before applying the clip improves the signal. A pulse oximeter also shows the pulse rate and in some a wave-like trace is displayed on a screen that can give some indication of pulse quality. Inaccuracies can arise from excessive ambient light, movement or poor perfusion, so try to look at both the trace and the displayed pulse rate when interpreting the information, rather than just writing the number down. If you are not sure about anything, count the pulse rate yourself.

If the pulse is irregular (for example, with a very pronounced respiratory sinus arrhythmia), the pulse oximeter will struggle to count accurately.

If the readings are worrying, always try repositioning the probe before deciding whether the values shown are real.

8.13 How to use a Doppler to Measure Blood Pressure

Clip the fur just above the main pad and feel for a pulse. Apply gel to the concave surface of the probe, place over the pulse and secure with tape. Turn the Doppler on with the sound volume at its lowest setting and slowly increase the volume, listening for pulse sounds. If you cannot hear anything, move the probe slightly under the tape and listen for a sound.

Select a blood pressure cuff of suitable size and wrap it snugly around the limb proximal to your probe, attach a sphygmomanometer and flick the rocker switch to the closed position.

With the Doppler switched on, inflate the cuff until the pulse sounds disappear. Open the rocker switch just enough to slowly let the air out of the cuff (this takes a bit of practice at first). Watch the sphygmomanometer needle as the cuff deflates and note the pressure at which the sounds reappear. This is generally close to systolic pressure, although in cats the value is thought to be between the systolic and mean pressures.

Common faults:

- Damaged probe.
- Turning the sound volume too high causes interference.
- Tape too loose or insufficient gel to get adequate contact between the probe and skin.
- Although you can check for pulse sounds without first taping the probe in place, it is likely to move when you tape it and the sounds may disturb your patient and other staff.

Too big a cuff will give you a falsely low pressure, too small a cuff a falsely high pressure.

8.14 What to Do if Blood Pressure is Low

Anaesthetic drugs are cardiovascular depressants. The commonest cause of low blood pressure (especially in an otherwise healthy patient) is too much anaesthetic agent. Check the depth and turn the vaporizer down if you can. If the blood pressure is low just after induction, it may improve once the effects of the induction agent have worn off.

It is difficult to tell if low blood pressure is caused by an inadequate circulating volume of fluids or by vasodilation, which will increase the space that the circulating fluids have to fill. If pressure does not improve, you can try giving a bolus of Hartmann's solution (5–10 ml/kg). If the patient has a history of heart disease, you must be careful not to overload with fluids. If the patient has a bradycardia, you may need to give drugs such as atropine to increase heart rate and therefore cardiac output.

8.15   Ventilating your Patient

During anaesthesia it is not a massive problem if the patient does not breathe spontaneously, as long as they are intubated and attached to a breathing system. Apnoea can be due to anaesthetic drugs or underlying disease. Make sure that the patient is not receiving too much anaesthetic agent and remember that positive pressure ventilation is more efficient in delivering anaesthetic gases to the lungs, so you might need to turn down the vaporizer if you need to ventilate for more than a few breaths. You will need a reliable assistant or a mechanical ventilator. Remember that respiration is triggered by the amount of carbon dioxide in the blood, so if you ventilate the patient too efficiently you will blow off more carbon dioxide and there is less chance that the patient will want to breathe spontaneously. If you are ventilating by hand, partly close the APL valve on the breathing system to stop too much gas escaping into the scavenging system. Do not close it fully; otherwise you might apply too much pressure to the lungs. Squeeze the reservoir bag and watch the chest, which should expand in a normal fashion. When you stop squeezing the bag, the lungs should empty due to the elastic recoil of the lungs and chest wall. You need to allow enough time for this to happen; otherwise the lungs will stay partially inflated. Aim for a rate that you would consider normal for the patient, and aim to keep the time of each expiration about two to three times as long as inspiration.

8.16   Pain: Detecting and Treating

Anything that a human would find painful will also be painful to an animal. There have been numerous studies that link good analgesia with better outcomes from surgery. It is considered unethical to perform surgical procedures without adequate analgesia.

If you are planning a painful procedure, give analgesia as part of your premedication plan. Pre-emptive analgesia is more successful than waiting for a pain response and trying to treat it.

How do you know if your patient is painful?

* Do you need high doses of anaesthetic agent to maintain anaesthesia? Common anaesthetic drugs such as propofol, alfaxalone, isoflurane and sevoflurane do not provide any analgesia. Increasing depth of anaesthesia will not treat pain.

* Have the heart rate and blood pressure increased from the baseline values you took before surgery? Has the respiratory rate increased? If the patient was painful before surgery, your baseline values may have already been raised. Would you expect a similar, non-painful patient to have the same heart/respiratory rate or blood pressure?

If you are not sure, it may be best to give a little extra analgesia and see if the values improve. Surgery on a patient with good analgesia on board is easier and smoother than on one that reacts to every stimulus. More advanced techniques such as nerve blocks with a local anaesthetic are worth doing for procedures such as dentals and limb surgery; with practice they take a few minutes more to perform at the start of anaesthesia but they can make everything run more smoothly.

Further Reading: Cooper, B., Mullineaux, E. and Turner, L. (eds) (2012) *BSAVA Textbook of Veterinary Nursing*, 5th edn. BSAVA, Gloucester, UK.

Hughes, L. (2016) Breathing systems and ancillary equipment. In: Duke-Novakovski, T., de Vries, M. and Seymour, C. (eds) *BSAVA Manual of Canine and Feline Anaesthesia and Analgesia*, 3rd edn. BSAVA, Gloucester, UK, pp. 45–64.

Schauvliege, S. (2016) Patient monitoring and monitoring equipment. In: Duke-Novakovski, T., de Vries, M. and Seymour, C. (eds) *BSAVA Manual of Canine and Feline Anaesthesia and Analgesia*, 3rd edn. BSAVA, Gloucester, UK, pp. 77–96.

Welsh, E. (2009) *Anaesthesia for Veterinary Nurses*, 2nd edn. Wiley-Blackwell, Chichester, UK.

Clinical Skills Sheet

8.13. Parallel Lack breathing system

General information:

- Non-rebreathing system.
- Classified as a 'Mapleson A'.
- Reservoir bag on the inspiratory limb.
- Inefficient for prolonged IPPV.
- Low system factor of 1–1.5 × minute volume.
- Use from 10 kg to 35 kg approx.

Task:

Assemble this system, perform a system check and calculate the fresh gas flow you would need for a 30 kg Doberman with a respiratory rate of 15 bpm.

Method
This is the main part of the Lack System.   The inspiratory (green) and expiratory (white) tubes used to come apart from the H connector, as did the APL valve, but it was often reassembled incorrectly and now comes 'glued' together.   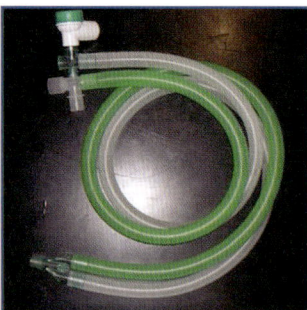
You will also need a 2 litre reservoir bag…   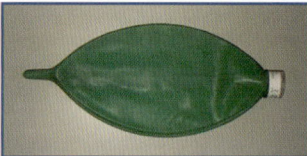

Method

…and scavenging.

This picture shows the scavenging tube with a black end connector that attaches to the APL valve.

The blue canister contains activated charcoal that scavenges waste anaesthetic agent. It does NOT remove nitrous oxide from the waste gases. This is a health hazard for you to breathe.

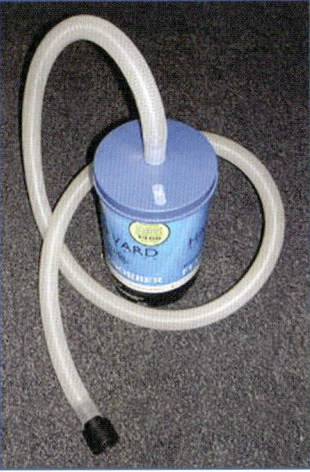

Attach the reservoir bag below the APL valve to the clear 'T'-connector.

The fresh gas enters through this part.

This part has a small rim on it that has the word 'bag' embossed on it.

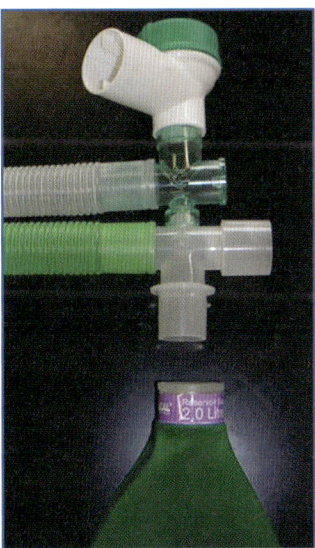

Method

It is very important that you know when an APL valve is OPEN or CLOSED.

The APL valve on the left is OPEN, the one on the right CLOSED.

You will need to know when a valve is OPEN or CLOSED to do a system check and if you need to perform IPPV (which cannot be done efficiently on this system).

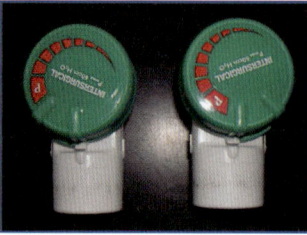

Attach the bag end to the anaesthetic machine and ensure scavenging is connected to the APL valve.

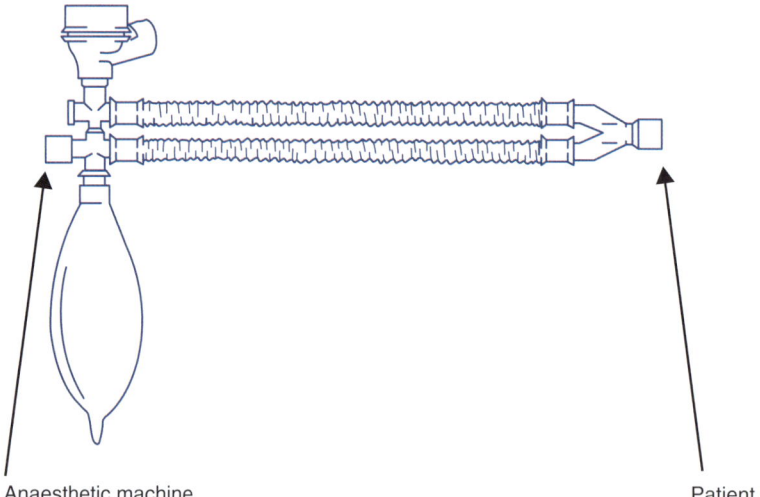

Anaesthetic machine   Patient

Now perform a system check (this method is the same with any system):

1. Make sure the oxygen is on.
2. Attach the system to the common gas outlet on the machine.
3. Close the APL valve.
4. Occlude the patient end of the system with your thumb.
5. Turn the O_2 on at the flowmeter to approx. 4 litres.
6. The reservoir bag should fill; you can fill it quicker using the O_2 flush.
7. Once the bag is full, listen for any sounds of leaking gas.
8. The bag should stay inflated when you squeeze it.
9. Open the APL valve with your thumb still in place.
10. Squeeze the bag: the gas in the system should pass out through the scavenging.

The system is ready for use – now work out your flow rate.

Calculation for use :

The formula for working out the flow rate for animals *over* 10 kg:

Tidal volume (body weight × 10 ml) × respiration rate (rr) × system factor (1 to 1.5)

30 kg Doberman × 10 ml × 15 rr × (1 to 1.5) = 4500–6750 ml or 4.5–6.75 l

© RVC

Clinical Skills Sheet

8.14. Circle breathing system

General information

- Rebreathing system.
- Can be used for IPPV.
- Very low flow rates can be used.
- Nitrous oxide can *only* be used safely if you are able to measure inspired oxygen concentrations.
- Use in patients with body weight of 10 kg and upwards.
- Has an absolute minimum flow rate of 10 ml/kg – *it does not have a system factor!*

Task:

Correctly assemble a circle system and do a system check.

Method
Collect the following items:
Soda-lime canister (sometimes looks like a hamster wheel).   This is filled with soda lime which absorbs CO_2 and changes colour when exhausted. At this point you would empty the exhausted soda lime and re-fill through the port on the back of the canister.   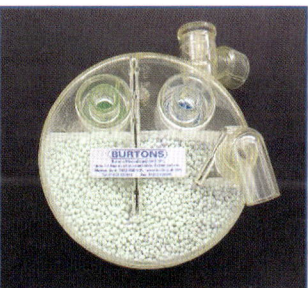
Fresh gas flow tubing, × 2 usually white tubes, open ended.   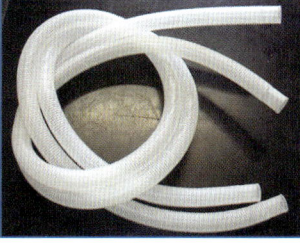   and a **Y-connector**.   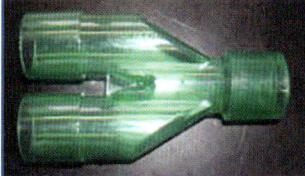

Method
Or you may have this type of tubing that has a 'built-in' Y-connector. 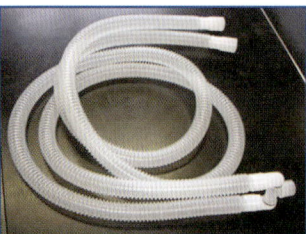
A 2 litre reservoir bag. (can be 5 l bag for large animal use). Check for holes or tears. 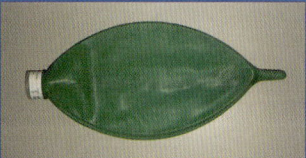
Scavenging tube with black connector. (The blue canister contains activated charcoal. This only removes waste anaesthetic agent, not nitrous oxide, which is a health hazard for you to breathe.) 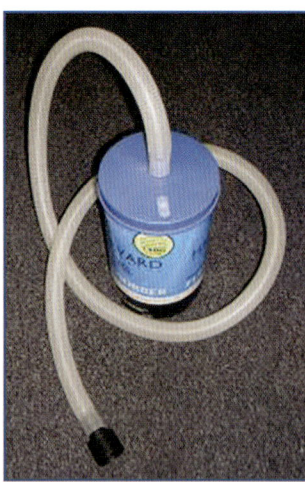

Method

This picture shows
- the green **oulet** one-way valve *(inspiratory)*.
- the blue **inlet** one-way valve *(expiratory)*.

These are built into the canister to ensure gases can only flow in one direction through the system.

(These valves mean the expired gas *has* to go through the CO_2 absorber.)

If you look closely underneath these valves you will see the words INHALE (green) and EXHALE (blue).

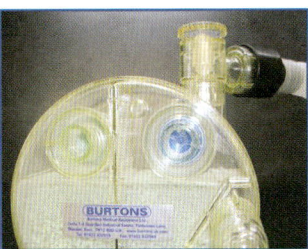

Put together as shown:

- The two breathing tubes attached to the inhale/exhale ports
- The scavenging tube attached to the outlet port on the APL valve
- The canister attached to the O_2 outlet on the anaesthetic machine. (You can see a small rigid plastic extender tube to keep the canister clear of the emergency O_2 outlet.)
- The reservoir bag hanging down attached to the elbow connector

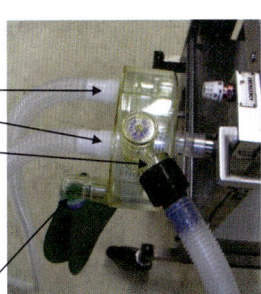

Now do a system check for leaks:
- Make sure the oxygen is on.
- Attach the system to the common gas outlet on the machine.
- Close the APL valve fully.
- Occlude the patient end (Y-connector) of the tubing with your thumb.
- Turn on the rotameter (flowmeter) to approx. 4 litres and allow the system to fill with O_2 until the reservoir bag is full.
- Listen for a sound of leaking gas/hissing.
- The reservoir bag should stay full when you squeeze it.
- Observe the bobbin on the rotameter – it should dip slightly.
- Open the APL valve fully and squeeze the bag: the gas should pass easily out of the system.

The system is now ready for use.

Work out your flow rate using the following calculation :

Minimum flow rate

10 ml/kg/min

For example, a 30 kg Doberman would need 30 × 10 = 300 ml *minimum*, though in reality it is unlikely that you will drop below 500 ml (0.5 l).

When using this system, you would generally start on about 4 l O_2 and gradually over a period of 20–30 min you would be reducing this amount to around 0.5 l. It depends on how your animal settles and how much you have the APL valve open.

© RVC

Clinical Skills Sheet

8.15. Bain breathing system

General information

- Non-rebreathing system.
- Classified as a 'Mapleson D'.
- Reservoir bag on expiratory limb.
- Can be used for IPPV.
- High system factor of 2.5 to 3 × minute volume.
- Used for patient weight between 10–20 kg.

Task:

Correctly assemble a Bain breathing system ready for use. Calculate the flow required for a 14 kg whippet breathing 18 times a minute.

Note: you have checked the anaesthetic machine and the oxygen supply is on.

Method
Collect the following items:
Anaesthetic tubing – wide corrugated tube with thin green inner tube.   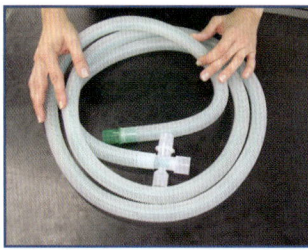
2 litre reservoir bag.   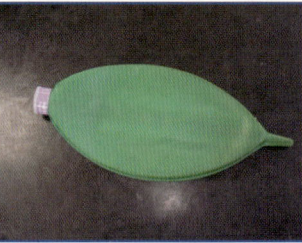
APL valve (adjustable pressure limiting).   Here shown *open*.   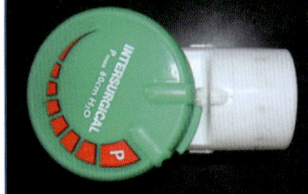

Method

Scavenging tube, with black end connector.

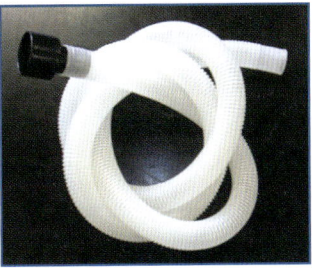

Put together as follows:

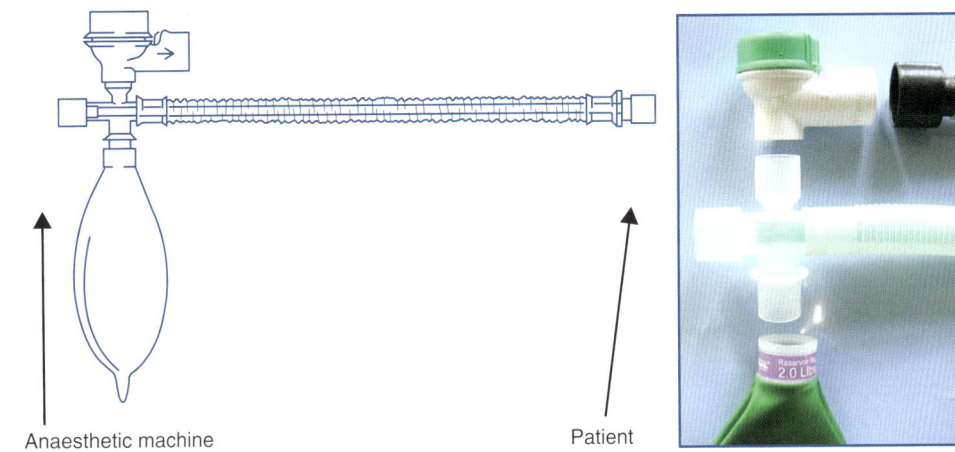

Anaesthetic machine   Patient

Connect the 'bag end' to the anaesthetic machine.

Ensure the scavenging tube is attached to the APL Value.

Ensure the scavenging is attached to a scavenging system.
(In this case a charcoal **Fluosorber**. This does not absorb nitrous oxide so should not be used with this gas.)

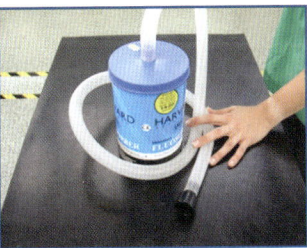

Method

Now perform a system check:

1. Make sure the oxygen is on.
2. Attach the system to the common gas outlet on the machine.
3. Close the APL valve.
4. Occlude the patient end of the system with your thumb.
5. Turn the O_2 on at the flowmeter to approx. 4 litres.
6. The reservoir bag should fill – you can fill it more quickly using the O_2 flush.
7. Once the bag is full, listen for any sounds of leaking gas.
8. The bag should stay inflated when you squeeze it.
9. Open the APL valve with your thumb still in place.
10. Squeeze the bag: the gas in the system should pass out through the scavenging.

You should also check the integrity of the green inner tube of the Bain. The details are at the end of this skills sheet.
The system is now ready for use.

Work out the flow rate for your 14 kg whippet with respiration rate of 18 bpm (breaths per minute) using the following calculation.

Calculation for use:
Tidal volume (body weight (kg) × 10 ml) × respiration rate × system factor (2.5 to 3)

$$14 \times 10 \text{ ml} \times 18 \times 2.5 \text{ to } 3$$
$$= 6300\text{–}7560 \text{ ml } (6.3\text{–}7.6 \text{ l})$$

So set your system to 6.3–7.6 l *before attaching to your patient.*

Question:
What are two main disadvantages of this system over a Magill or Lack?
Answer:
1. It has a high system factor of 2.5–3 times minute volume, therefore uses high fresh gas flow rates.
2. The inner tube may become disconnected.

Testing the integrity of a Bain system

The inner tube connections of the Bain can be tested as follows:

1. Attach the Bain to the common gas outlet on the anaesthetic machine and to the scavenging system.
2. Set the O_2 meter to approx. 4 l.
3. Using either a biro or the 'red tester' (ask CSC staff if not sure), occlude the INNER tube of the Bain.
4. If the inner tube (usually green) connections are patent, the O_2 flowmeter bobbin will dip briefly when blocked.
5. Stop occluding the inner tube and the flowmeter will return to normal.

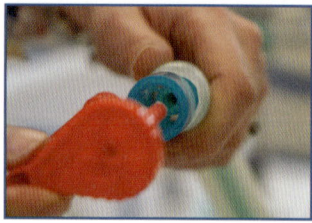

© RVC

Clinical Skills Sheet

8.16. Modified Ayres T-piece breathing system

General information

- Non-rebreathing system.
- Reservoir bag is on the *expiratory* limb.
- Can be used for IPPV (intermittent positive pressure ventilation).
- High system factor of 2.5 to 3 × minute volume.
- Use up to 10 kg patient weight.

Task: Correctly assemble a T-piece breathing system ready for use. Calculate the flow rate required for a 4 kg cat breathing 25 times a minute.

Note: you have checked the anaesthetic machine and the oxygen supply is on.

Method
Collect the following items:
Long fresh gas flow tube.   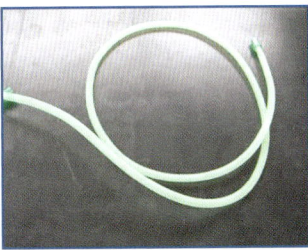
Short expiratory corrugated tube.   (These two tubes are usually permanently connected at the ET tube end.)   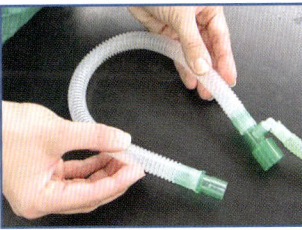
Blind-ended 0.5 litre reservoir bag.   (Can be blue or green.)   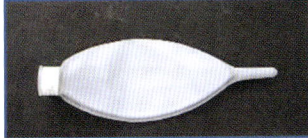

Method
T-connector. 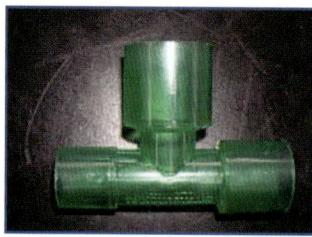
Scavenging tube. 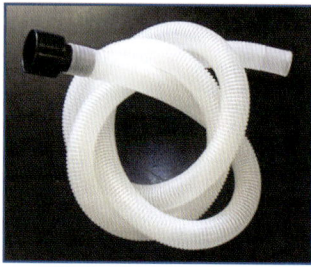
Blue low pressure APL valve (adjustable pressure limiting). (Here shown *open*.) 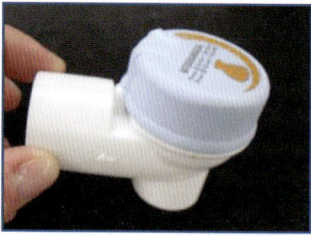
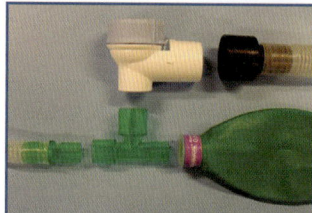
Put together: 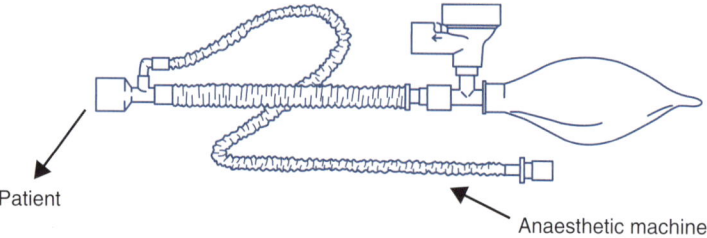

Method
Attach scavenging tube to APL valve, ensuring tube is attached to charcoal absorber or other scavenging outlet.
When attaching the green T-connector to the scavenging / APL valve / white tubing (as in the picture above), be aware that this will only fit together in one way so if you keep trying the different ends, it will eventually fit!
Connect fresh gas flow tube (the thin green tube) to the anaesthetic machine common gas outlet. 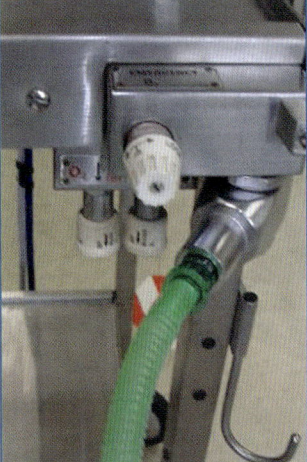
Now do a system check to check for leaks.

How to perform a system check (this method is the same with any system):

1. Make sure the oxygen is on.
2. Attach the system to the common gas outlet on the anaesthetic machine.
3. Close the APL valve.
4. Occlude the patient end of the system with your thumb.
5. Turn the O_2 on at the flowmeter to approx. 4 litres.
6. The reservoir bag should fill; you can fill it more quickly using the O_2 flush.
7. Once the bag is full, listen for any sounds of leaking gas.
8. The bag should stay inflated when you squeeze it.
9. Open the APL valve with your thumb still in place.
10. Squeeze the bag: the gas in the system should pass out through the scavenging.

The system is now ready for use.

Work out your flow rate using the following calculation.

Calculation for use:

The **formula** for working out the flow rate generally for animals *under* 10 kg body weight is :

Tidal volume (body weight × 15 ml) × respiration rate (rr) × system factor (2.5 to 3)

4 kg cat × 15 ml × 25 rr rate × 2.5 to 3

(4 × 15 ml × 25 × 2.5 to 3 = 3750 ml (3.8 l) or 4500 ml (4.5 l))

© RVC

Clinical Skills Sheet

8.17. Anaesthesia help sheet: calculating fresh gas flow

		Body weight	System factor (or circuit factor)	IPPV	Mapleson class
Non-rebreathing systems	T-piece	0–10 kg	2.5–3	Yes	F
	Mini-Lack	2–10 kg	1 litre under 5 kg, 200 ml/kg over 5 kg	No	A
	Bain	10–18 kg	2.5–3	Yes	D
	Lack	10–35 kg	1–1.5	No	A (very efficient)
	Magill	10–35 kg	1–1.5	No	A
Rebreathing system	Circle	10 kg + + +	Doesn't have one! _Minimum_ flow rate of 10 ml/kg. Start at 100 ml/kg then reduce to a maintenance setting of 50 ml/kg approx.	Yes	

Mapleson classification: named after a physicist, classed from A to F, relative to efficiency and how much fresh gas flow is required to prevent rebreathing.

The standard calculation is:

$$\textbf{Vt } (\text{weight} \times \textbf{10–15 ml}) \times \textbf{RR} \times \textbf{System Factor} = \textbf{FGF rate},$$

that is, the amount of gas the animal needs to have coming from the anaesthetic machine to enable safe anaesthesia without risking rebreathing of expired CO_2.

- **Vt** stands for **tidal volume** (weight (kg) × **10–15ml**).
- Why **10–15 ml**? It is the volume measured in millilitres that is allowed for each kilogram of body weight. If an animal weighs under 10 kg, its lung size in ratio to its body weight is _larger_, so you would use the **15 ml** part of the calculation here. If the animal is over 10 kg, its lungs are relatively _smaller_ in ratio to its body weight, so you use the **10 ml** part of the calculation.
- **Tidal Volume (Vt)** × **Respiration Rate (RR)** = **Minute Volume (MV)**.
- **MV** × **System Factor** = **Fresh Gas Flow Rate (FGF)**.

<u>An alternative and quicker method</u>

Assume the **MV** is 200 ml/kg, multiply this by the **System Factor (SF)**, so:

$$200 \text{ ml/kg} \times \textbf{SF} = \textbf{FGF rate}$$

<u>Example:</u>

25 kg dog, RR of 20, system = Lack **(SF of 1–1.5)**

Method 1:

25 kg × 10 ml (250 ml) × 20

= 5000 ml or 5 litres × 1–1.5

= 5–7.5 l

Method 2 (quicker):

25 kg × 200 ml

= 5 l × 1–1.5

= 5–7.5 l

© RVC

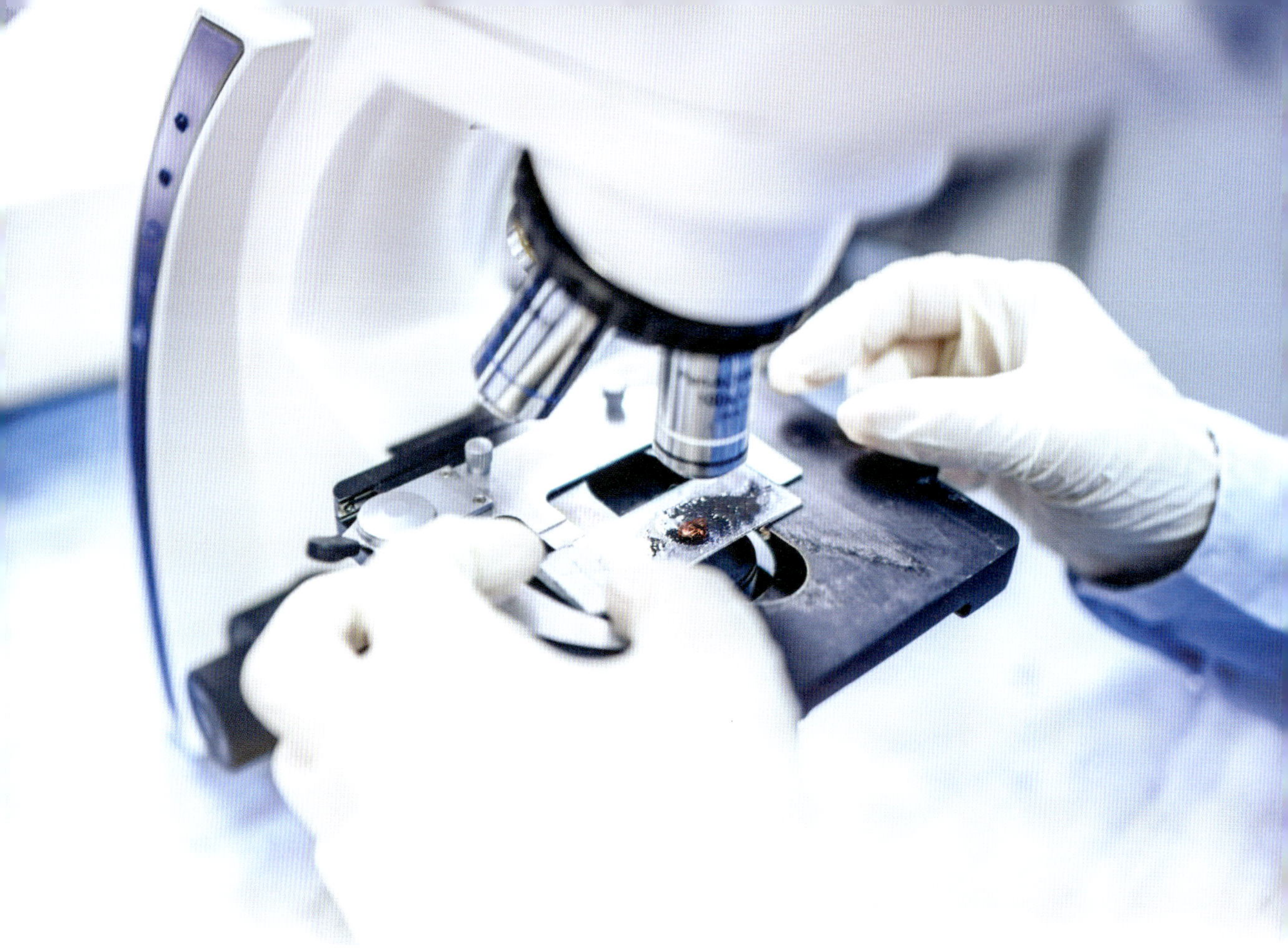

Section

4

Principles of Good Practice in the Laboratory

Section Editor: Alison Langridge

Introduction

All veterinary medicine and veterinary nursing graduates must be competent in basic laboratory skills. Using a microscope and preparing blood samples for initial screening tests are two of the most basic skills. The other important skills to practise are how to do initial tests on urine and faecal samples.

Within this section, there are three chapters:

Chapter 9: Laboratory Skills and Sample Collection

Chapter 10: Using a Microscope and Preparing Samples

Chapter 11: Urine and Faecal Analysis

Within each chapter you will find pictures and tips about how to practise relevant basic Day One skills. Each chapter will also detail key points for each set of skills and point out the health and safety considerations, which are critical to good practice.

An overview of all the learning outcomes is presented below, with more detailed learning outcomes presented under each chapter.

Learning objectives

After studying this chapter, students should be able to:

- Identify the principles of good laboratory practice, including relevant legislation relating to Health and Safety in the laboratory.
- Demonstrate understanding and safe use of laboratory equipment.
- Demonstrate the safe and appropriate collection, preservation, legal packaging and transport of laboratory samples.
- Dispose of all materials and tissue safely and appropriately.
- Safely and effectively use a binocular microscope and apply the principles of maintaining the microscope in good working order.
- Prepare a blood smear and stain and conduct a packed cell volume measurement.
- Perform urinalysis and faecal analysis.

What You Will Use

Clinical skills sheets (SS)

Ten clinical skills sheets will be used in this section. Reference will be made to each skill sheet at the relevant point within the chapter. Clinical skills sheets for the following accompany this section:

SS 9.18 Venepuncture techniques: blood collection by Vacutainer

SS 9.19 Venepuncture techniques: blood collection by syringe + needle

SS 9.20 Fine-needle aspirate biopsy (FNAB) and smear

SS 9.21 Packing a laboratory sample

SS 10.22 Microscope set-up

SS 10.23 Preparing and examining blood smear and stain

SS 10.24 Packed cell volume (PCV)

SS 11.25 Obtaining a urine specific gravity reading and a dipstick reading

SS 11.26 Preparing a urine sample for microscope analysis

SS 11.27 McMaster faecal egg count technique

Videos (V)

Four videos will be used in this section and reference will be made to each video at the relevant point within the chapter. Videos will be hyperlinked and the following accompany this section:

V 10.1 Microscope set-up (shorter video)

V 10.2 Blood smear and stain

V 10.3 Packed cell volume (PCV)

V 11.1 Urine SG

Laboratory Skills and Sample Collection

9

Kate English and Alison Langridge
The Royal Veterinary College, London

Learning objectives

By the end of this chapter, students should be able to:

- Identify the principles of good laboratory practice in a working veterinary environment.
- Identify relevant legislation relating to Health and Safety in the laboratory.
- Demonstrate understanding and safe use of laboratory equipment.
- Dispose of all materials and tissue safely and appropriately.
- Demonstrate the safe and appropriate collection and preservation of laboratory samples taken from animals.
- Demonstrate and describe safe and legal packaging and transport of laboratory samples.

Clinical skills sheets (SS)

Four clinical skills sheets will be used in this chapter and these can be found at pages 135–144. Reference will be made to each skills sheet at the relevant section within the chapter. The details of the clinical skills sheets used are as follows:

SS 9.18 Venepuncture techniques: blood collection by Vacutainer

SS 9.19 Venepuncture techniques: blood collection by syringe + needle

SS 9.20 Fine-needle aspirate biopsy (FNAB) and smear

SS 9.21 Packing a laboratory sample

Introduction to Laboratory Skills

Kate English and Alison Langridge

Most veterinary practices are now equipped with in-house laboratory equipment. The main advantage of this is that they can obtain diagnoses quickly and accurately. Many laboratories in veterinary practices are manned by a Registered Veterinary Nurse (RVN) but the accuracy of the diagnostic results is reliant on more than equipment or an RVN; it is multifactorial and is wholly dependent on all staff being able to work safely and effectively within the veterinary practice laboratory environment. This includes ensuring that all equipment is correctly maintained and calibrated every day.

9.1 Health and Safety

Aside from the potential to obtain inaccurate results through poor maintenance or protocol, the veterinary laboratory harbours many potential hazards. These include:

- Zoonotic diseases and other biological agents.
- Equipment.
- Biological waste, including sharps and glassware.
- Fumes and/or aerosols.
- Chemicals.
- Fire or explosion.
- Slip or trip injuries.

All veterinary laboratories should have a laboratory Code of Conduct, within which there should be strict

© CAB International 2018. *Veterinary Clinical Skills Manual* (eds N. Coombes and A. Silva-Fletcher)

Standard Operating Procedures (SOPs). The practice management will have developed these SOPs following a risk assessment of the laboratory area. The SOPs should be clearly displayed and should specify not only how to stay safe in the laboratory, but also what course of remedial action to take if there is an accident or incident, or if a member of staff is unwell or becomes pregnant.

9.2 Laboratory Basics: Before You Begin

9.2.1 Appropriate attire for laboratory work

In-house veterinary laboratories can be as hazardous as any other laboratory and it is imperative that personnel are appropriately attired.

Laboratory coats should be worn, but in practice it is rarely practical to do this. It is advisable therefore for any staff conducting lab work to wear a disposable plastic apron to protect themselves.

Footwear should not be open-toed and should ideally have a non-slip pattern on the sole.

9.2.2 Appropriate conduct in the laboratory area

General laboratory rules should apply to the in-house laboratory area so there should be no eating or drinking by any personnel in this area.

There should be a clinical waste bin in the laboratory and all attire should be removed and a clinical hand wash performed before moving to another area of the building.

9.2.3 Personal protective equipment (PPE)

PPE is equipment that will protect the user against health or safety risks at work. This includes an array of equipment, but in an in-house veterinary practice laboratory this list needs to include sterile and non-sterile non-latex gloves, eye protection (such as goggles), plastic disposable aprons, caps, masks, gauntlets and radiography PPE.

Radiography PPE should include at least one gown with a lead equivalence throughout of not less than 0.25 mm, at least one lead thyroid protector, lead gauntlets and lead forearm protectors with a lead equivalence of not less than 0.5mm.

Further guidance on general PPE can be found at http://www.hse.gov.uk/toolbox/ppe.htm. Further advice on radiography PPE can be found at http://www.rcvs.org.uk/document-library/pss-review-2015-small-animal-draft-modules/, Module 5, pp. 36–40.

9.3 Disposal of Laboratory Consumables

In a veterinary laboratory, it is important to ensure that all disposable items are in the correct receptacle. There are usually four receptacles in the veterinary laboratory.

9.3.1 Sharps bin

This is a bright yellow, hard plastic bin with a yellow fixed lid. The lid will almost always have a push-down flap and a niche whereby syringes can be safely removed from the needle hubs.

Items for the sharps bin should include only those items which can puncture the skin and cause harm (apart from those sharps used with cytotoxic drugs) (Fig. 9.1).

9.3.2 Pharmaceutical bin

This is a bright yellow, hard plastic bin with a blue fixed lid.

This bin must only contain:

* Glass injection or medication bottles.
* Vaccination bottles.
* Expired medication (both loose and blister-packed).
* Returned medication (both loose and blister-packed).

9.3.3 Clinical waste

Clinical waste will be recognizable by a bright yellow bin liner. Items for this bin should include only those items that are detailed below:

* Any bodily waste (blood, vomit, urine, faeces, bodily tissue, saliva, pus, body parts, teeth).

- Anything that has touched any of these bodily fluids (tissue paper, swabs, gloves, aprons).
- Disposable surgical items that are not sharp (drape, suture material, cap, mask).
- Any soft consumables that are not sharp (giving set minus spike, angiocath minus stylet, Pasteur pipette, urinary or blood dipsticks, transport swabs.
- Blood tubes (unless glass).
- Any disposable item from an isolated patient that would normally be in general waste (food, equipment wrappers, empty hand rub bottles etc.)

Clinical waste items do not include:

- Anything that is sharp.
- Anything that is cytotoxic or has been in contact with cytotoxic medication or patients receiving cytotoxic medication.
- Any general waste (for example, blood slide wrappers, bandaging wrappers, food wrappers) unless it is contaminated by a bodily fluid.

9.3.4 Cytotoxic bin

This is a bright yellow, hard plastic bin with a purple fixed lid.

This bin must only contain:

- Cytotoxic drugs.
- Cytotoxic sharps.
- Any materials that have come into contact with cytotoxic drugs or patients receiving cytotoxic medication.

9.4 General Waste

General waste bins will be recognizable by a black bin liner. They are for general domestic waste and all packaging that is not contaminated by bodily fluids or chemicals.

General waste items must not include:

- Any items listed in the sharps, pharmaceutical or clinical waste sections.
- Medications.
- Vaccination bottles.

✔	✘
Scalpel blades	Syringes (unless not detachable, e.g. insulin syringe)
Stitch cutters	Disposable scalpel handles
Hypodermic needles	Suture material
Suture needles	Blood tubes
Giving set spikes	Paper tissue
Any stylets	Swabs
Glassware (e.g. microscope slides/ampoules)	Organic matter
Capillary tubes	Urinary dipsticks
Lancets	Pasteur pipettes
Autoinjectors (e.g. Epipen)	Eppendorfs
Broken rigid plastic (e.g. gutter splint off-cut)	General waste and packaging
Sharp orthopaedic or dental disposables (e.g. mandible wire)	Urinary dipsticks

Fig. 9.1. Items that should and should not be put in the sharps bin.

Further details on waste disposal are available from http://www.bsava.com/Resources/BSAVAMedicinesGuide/Medicinewastedisposal.aspx

Principles in Sample Collection

Kate English

Samples may be taken from living patients or deceased patients. If samples are being taken from a living patient, then considerations as to whether this may be performed under manual restraint or require sedation or anaesthesia may be considered. If obtaining samples from a deceased patient it is preferable to take samples as soon as possible after death. If immediate sampling is not possible, then refrigeration or freezing may be considered. Where feasible, refrigeration is preferred, as freezing and then thawing will create changes in the tissue that may obscure or alter pathological findings. If submitting the patient for a pathologist post mortem, it is preferable to discuss the optimal way to submit with the pathologist as early as possible.

9.5   Blood Sampling

When obtaining a blood sample, consideration should be given to the safe amount of blood that can be obtained from the patient. For small animals, particularly 'pocket pets' or similar, the amount of blood that can safely be taken should be calculated before sampling. When the volume of whole blood that can be obtained is known, the available plasma or serum (approximately one-half to one-third of the whole blood) can be estimated. This will be the amount available to run laboratory tests. The tubes that are used will depend on what laboratory tests are required (Fig. 9.2). Colours of tubes referred to here are applicable to the UK, but in other countries the colours of the tubes may vary and examination of the label to determine the content (or otherwise) of the tube is always recommended. When filling the tube always make sure that you only fill it to the level of the arrow indicated on the label. This may be halfway up the label or at the top of the label.

A smear made from blood or fluid at time of sampling is recommended to be additionally submitted in all instances.

See section below on packaging and sending samples on for further details on appropriate labelling.

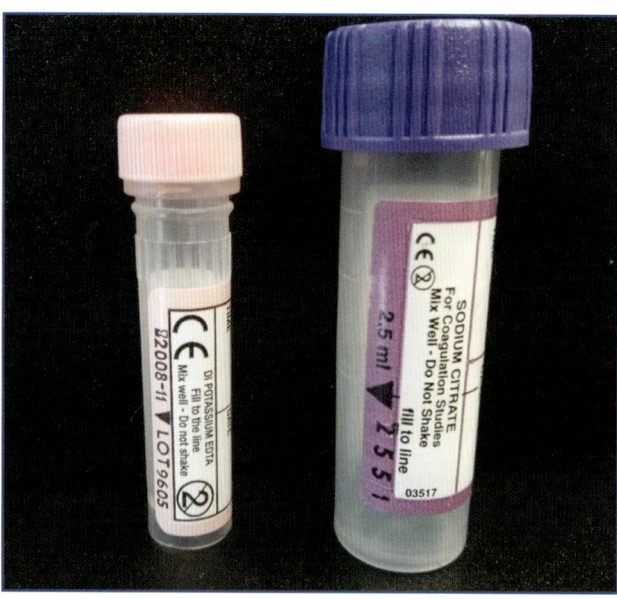

Fig. 9.2. Two types of blood collection tube (note the arrows that indicate how much blood to collect).

9.5.1 Blood tube selection

Species and test will influence the tube selection.

- For reptiles and the majority of avian species, heparin (usually lithium heparin) is the tube of choice.
- For mammalian haematology and for fluid cytology submissions, EDTA is preferred.
- For biochemistry serum, clotted blood with no anticoagulant or heparin is preferred. EDTA will interfere with many of the biochemistry assays.
- For PCR testing, EDTA or heparin is usually preferred.

It is important when sending the sample to an external laboratory to check what the laboratory recommends as the optimum sample. If the volume they request cannot be safely collected from the patient, then contact them to discuss before sampling.

For biochemistry tests it is better to separate the serum or plasma before submission. Samples may become haemolysed if in contact with the cell clot and this will interfere with the assay.

SS 9.18 for detailed guidance on venepuncture techniques, blood collection using Vacutainer

SS 9.19 for detailed guidance on venepuncture techniques, blood collection using syringe + needle

9.6 Cytology Collection

Cytology is used to evaluate cell types in a fluid, effusion, or solid mass or organ. The cells are assessed to determine if they are cells that would be expected to be sampled from that area. Also assessed are whether the numbers of cells are as expected or higher.

Samples may be obtained by direct palpation and visualization, as for a skin mass; or by 'blind' sampling, as for peritoneal tap, or non-endoscopic bronchoalveolar lavage; or under ultrasound or endoscopic guidance.

9.6.1 Equipment needed

- Fine-gauge needle, usually a 22G or 23G.
- Syringe for aspiration and expiration, usually a 2.5 ml, 5 ml or 10 ml.
- Sample pots, EDTA for cytology, plain for microbial culture.
- Glass slides for smear preparation, for aspirates and to make smears from fresh fluid.
- Other equipment as appropriate for site.

9.6.2 Site preparation

- If appropriate (e.g. joint fluid), sterile surgical preparation is required.
- Some sites (e.g. respiratory flush samples) would not be appropriate for this.
- If sampling an ulcerated surface for evidence of infection, then cleaning of the site may not be very helpful.

The technique on aspiration of a lymph node would apply to aspiration of other peripheral sites, such as skin masses. For internal organs, other more specific considerations would apply and there would be additional concerns when aspirating structures within the thoracic cavity and the abdominal cavity, as aspiration of the thoracic cavity contains a risk of a pneumothorax being introduced, which can result in severe complications.

SS 9.20 for detailed guidance on fine-needle aspirate biopsy (FNAB) and smear

9.6.3 Biopsy

- Techniques available for skin or externally accessible structures include punch biopsies, Tru-cut biopsies, incisional biopsies and excisional biopsies.
- For deep or internal structures or organs, punch biopsies would be unrealistic. Tru-cut biopsies may be achieved transcutaneously; and grab, incisional or excisional biopsies may be achieved with visualization of the organs, either endoscopically or via exposure through surgical incisions.
- Surgical aseptic site preparation is required for this type of sampling.
- Place tissues into formalin fixative as soon as possible. The ×10 rule works well: 10% formalin saline solution, 1:10 ratio of tissue to formalin (if you are squashing the tissue into the pot you need a bigger pot).

9.7 Post-mortem

A standard approach to a post-mortem, as you would have to a physical examination, is recommended, because if you go through a step-by-step process you are more likely to identify something abnormal and less likely to miss something out.

- External examination.
- Assess skin and subcutis.
- Evaluate the abdominal cavity.
- Evaluate the thoracic cavity.
- Remove the pluck.
- Examine the abdominal organs *in situ*, include checking the patency of the gall bladder and the urinary bladder.
- Remove the organs, including the intestine, and place on the table for a full evaluation, and before excising.
- Examination of the pluck: open the trachea and bronchi and slice through the lung parenchyma.
- Examination of the heart: ensure that you have evaluated all chambers and valves, as well as observing the thickness of the walls.
- If appropriate, examine the brain: place immediately without incising into formalin. Fix for 5 days before making incisions.
- If concerned over microbes and requiring culture: tissues should be swabbed or placed on saline-moistened surgical swabs in plain containers for submission for culture.
- For architectural examination of the tissue, to identify inflammatory lesions, or neoplasms: fixation in formalin saline, as for biopsies, is required.

9.8 Packing and Posting

Local mail guidelines may be variable and checking that you are adhering to legal requirements is your responsibility.

- It is usually acceptable to mail samples within your own country; however, mailing samples in general post across country borders may not be permissible.
- Mailing of known infectious material, particularly if it is a notifiable disease, or zoonotic hazard (i.e. in-contact humans could become infected), is also not permitted.

For packing samples:

- The sample container should be leakproof.
- It should be labelled with patient name, species and date of collection.
- It should be wrapped within sufficient absorbent material to 'mop up' if the container does leak in transit.
- The container and absorbent material should be placed within a second leakproof container and placed within a rigid leakproof structure.
- A laboratory form with patient details, submitted sample details and laboratory requests should be included.
- Samples in formalin should be submitted separately from unstained smears and fluids (formalin fumes change the staining properties of cells and may make them unrecognizable).
- The envelope should be clearly labelled with the delivery address and the address of the sender.
- The envelope should also be clearly labelled with 'pathological sample' and 'fragile with care' or similar.
- Samples should be sent to have as short a time in the post as possible, i.e. first class and not over a weekend.

 SS 9.21 for detailed guidance on packing a laboratory sample

Clinical Skills Sheet

9.18. Venepuncture techniques: blood collection by Vacutainer

Method
This collection method is preferably for personnel who are already confident in taking venous blood samples.
Please also see Help Sheet on blood sampling from bovine coccygeal vein (Ref: A Sykes BVM4 RP2 Project 2016).
Vacutainers are designed to exert a strong negative pressure and are used on larger-bore veins to avoid venous collapse (thus rarely used for small animals). They also facilitate multiple blood tube collection with a good degree of biosafety.
There are three parts to the collection system: a double-ended needle, a holder and a Vacutainer. 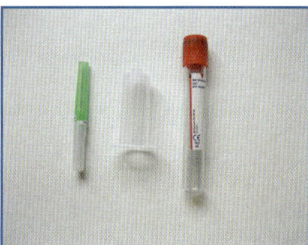
There are many types of needle (the green sheathed shown is 21G (gauge) × 1.5″) …
… and many types of Vacutainer (the tube pictured is for serum analysis). (http://www.bd.com/vacutainer/pdfs/plus_plastic_tubes_wallchart_tubeguide_VS5229.pdf)
Remove white top of double needle and screw grey rubber-covered needle into the holder. 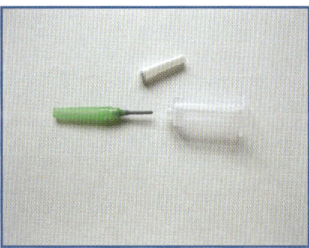
Slide the Vacutainer part way into the end of the holder, resting the lid against the grey covered needle. *Do not push home* as the vacuum will be lost! 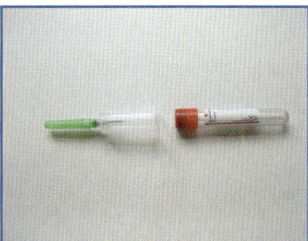

Method
Unsheath the second needle and hold Vacutainer and holder as shown below. 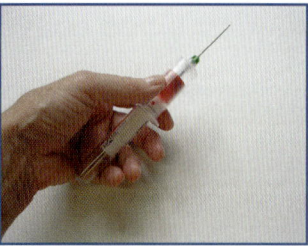

Sample collection
Slowly advance the needle into the already occluded (raised) vein, taking care not to insert too far (thus puncturing the far wall of the vein). For details, see SS 9.19: Blood collection by syringe + needle.
• Once the needle is in the vein, rest the tube against your palm, securing with both ring and little fingers. • Steady the holder with your index finger, brace the holder wings with thumb and middle finger, push the tube fully against the 'grey' needle. • The vacuum seal will be punctured and the tube should begin filling immediately.
When the tube is filled, slide it back down the holder. If more samples are required immediately insert the next tube for blood collection.
When sampling is complete, stop vein occlusion and remove the needle from the vein.
As the needle is withdrawn, apply pressure (with your thumb) over the puncture site for a few seconds to reduce the likelihood of a haematoma forming.
Dispose of the needle and sheath into a sharps clinical waste bin.

Clinical Skills Sheet

9.19. Venepuncture techniques: blood collection by syringe + needle

Method
There are many sizes and types of syringe: 1, 2, 5, 10, 12 and 20 ml pictured.

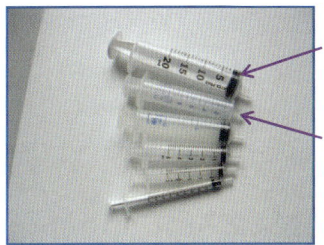

Three-part syringe, has black rubber inside which gives better suction for blood sampling

Two-part syringe, used for repeat injections where suction is not important

There are also many sizes and types of needle, e.g. 16G (gauge) × 1″ (A) and 25G × 5/8″ (B). Unsheathed pictures: A above, B below.

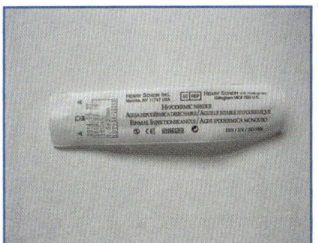

A

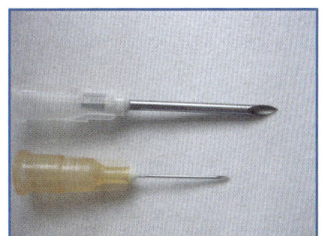

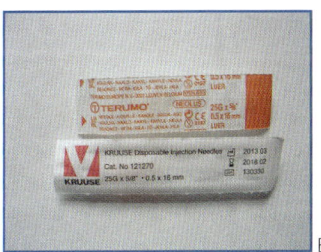

B

Blood can be collected from a number of venous sites, such as the cephalic, saphenous or jugular. It is easier to collect large samples from the jugular vein.
The size of the animal and the chosen vein will determine the needle gauge (G) and length. For example, 24–26G × 5/8″ is suitable for a rabbit ear vein; 19G × 1″ is suitable for a sheep jugular vein.
The amount of blood required for analysis will determine the syringe size.
Snap the protective shield off the end of the needle sheath and attach the needle hub firmly to the syringe.
The collection site should ideally be shaved or clipped free of hair or fur before sampling.
It is essential that an assistant correctly restrains the animal for blood sampling (see picture examples below). The animal should be as still as possible so as not to damage the vein or haemolyse the sample.
The sample vein must be occluded *proximally* by thumb to 'raise' it for easier needle insertion and subsequent blood collection. It takes a few seconds for the vein to become 'visible'.

Method

Canine right forelimb, cephalic vein raised by the assistant (note needle pointed cranially).

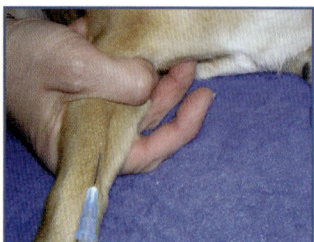

Please note: The dog in the picture is a model only, so the hair on the leg is not clipped. In a real patient, the fur would be clipped and the skin prepared with a spirit swab.

Ovine left jugular occluded.

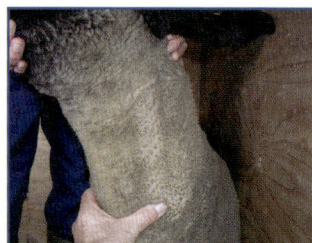

NB: the *sampler* occludes this vein

Sample collection

Unsheath the needle and place it *bevel edge facing upwards* at a shallow angle (5–10 degrees) against the vein.

Picture shows inserting the needle into sheep's raised jugular vein (note needle pointed cranially).

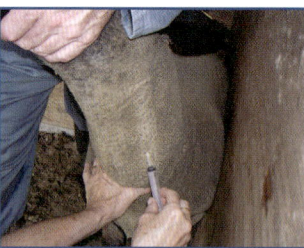

Slowly advance the needle into the vein, taking care not to insert too far (thus puncturing the far wall of the vein).

Start to retract * the syringe plunger using thumb and middle finger. The forefinger acts as a brace against the wings of the syringe.
(You may prefer a different method, e.g. thumb and ring finger on the plunger and fore and middle fingers as a brace on each wing.)
* If no blood appears in the syringe, **stop immediately**, pull the needle back a little subcutaneously and reattempt at a slightly different angle.

Slowly draw up the required volume of blood into the syringe.

When sampling is complete, stop occluding the vein. As the needle is withdrawn, apply pressure (with your thumb) over the puncture site for a few seconds to reduce the likelihood of a haematoma forming.

Dispose of the needle and sheath into a sharps clinical waste bin (picture shows four types of port for bracing the needle hub so the needle safely drops into the bin).

Method
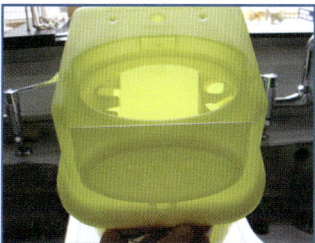
It is no longer considered safe practice to re-sheath a needle. However, in circumstances where there may not be a clinical waste bin (maybe on-farm, for example), it is better to re-sheath than leave an exposed needle to endanger others.
Blood may now be expelled into one or more storage tubes for later analysis.

© RVC

Clinical Skills Sheet

9.20. Fine-needle aspirate biopsy (FNAB) and smear

Task:

Obtain a fine-needle aspirate biopsy (FNAB) from the left popliteal lymph node and make a 'squash' smear preparation on the slide.

Gloves are not necessary but your hands should be clean.

Method
Equipment: • Hand rub. • 5 ml or 10 ml syringe. • 21G or 23G needle. • 2 clean microscope slides. • Pen. 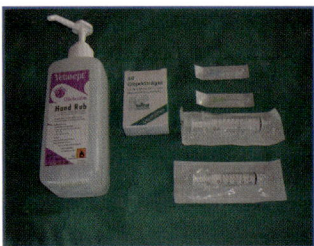
Prepare two slides on the bench.
Open the syringe packaging taking care not to contaminate the syringe; draw back on the plunger to ¾ the volume of the syringe, then place back on the sterile packaging.
Open the needle packaging in the same way and leave *in situ*. 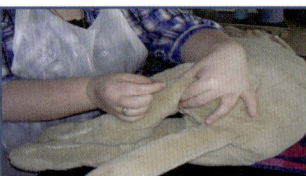
Stabilize the biopsy site firmly between your thumb and index finger.

Method

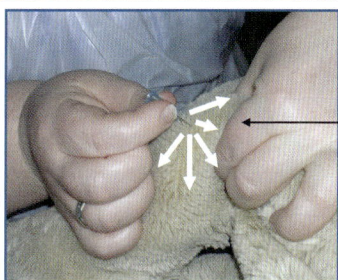

Insert the needle through the skin perpendicular to the skin surface.
Redirect the needle tip forwards and backwards a few times in a fan shape within the mass.
Do not remove the needle tip from the mass during this procedure.

Ensure that the needle has been handled aseptically throughout.

The correct way to hold the needle during sample harvesting is by the hub only (see picture above). Do not cover or contaminate the end of the hub during the procedure.

Withdraw the needle from the lesion.

Attach the needle to the prepared air-filled syringe.

Smear preparation

Position the tip of the needle closely over the microscope slide.

Rapidly depress the plunger and express the sample on to the slide.

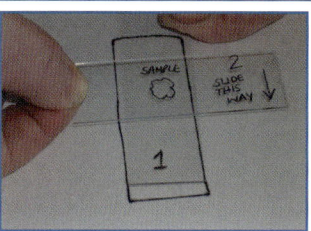

Place a second clean slide on top of the first slide at right angles to it.
Squash the sample gently between the two slides.
Smoothly slide the top slide away from you.

Turn the top slide over so that you have two smeared samples.

Air dry and label both slides.

© RVC

Clinical Skills Sheet

9.21. Packing a laboratory sample

Task:

Complete the lab form and package the sample for postage as described below.

Method
Wear disposable examination gloves.
Assume the tubes contain a blood sample sufficient to reach the fill line (marked by an arrow). Also assume the fluoride oxalate and EDTA samples have already been gently inverted to mix blood with anticoagulant.
Select the following tubes: Plain (for general biochemistry*) 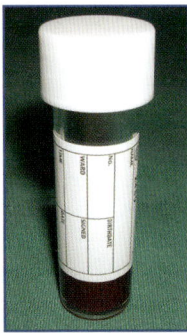
Fluoride oxalate (for glucose*) 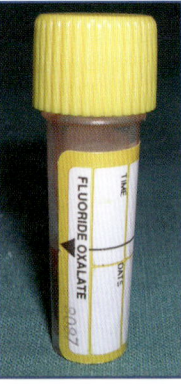

Method
EDTA (for general haematology**) 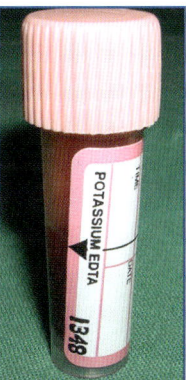
Label each tube with reference number/owner name and date.
Complete laboratory form: • Sender's details. • Patient and client details. • Required tests. • Brief clinical history.
Wrap each sample in sufficient cotton wool to absorb contents should breakage occur. 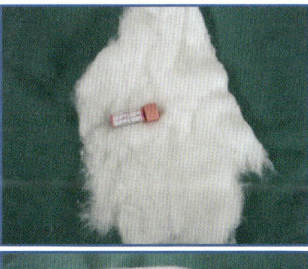 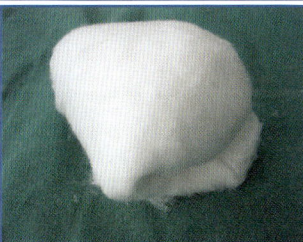
Place each sample into a sealable plastic bag.
Place all of these into a rigid outer container (a hard 60 ml syringe case or similar may be used if approved container not available).
The container should then be sealed with Sellotape. (In the CSC we provide a less adhesive alternative, so these samples can be reused.)
Place the lab form into a separate sealable plastic bag.

Method
Label the envelope conspicuously with the words: **'Pathological Sample'**   **'Fragile – with care'**   (or similar).   Write the laboratory address.   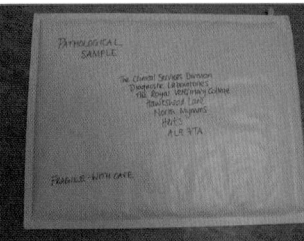
Write the sender's address on the reverse of the envelope.   
Place the lab forms and sealed samples into the envelope.
Seal the envelope (either using self-adhesive strip or adhesive tape such as Sellotape).

*Please note that ideally:
- **Plain** samples should be centrifuged after the blood sample has been allowed to clot at room temperature for 20–30 min. The serum can then be separated and placed into another plain tube and posted.
- **Fluoride oxalate** tubes should also be centrifuged and the plasma transferred into a plain tube before posting.

However, the method stated in this skills sheet is a quicker but still acceptable method.

Ideally, you should make a **fresh smear and send this with the EDTA sample for haematology. The laboratory will make smears from EDTA sent samples, but cell morphology changes can occur even overnight.

© RVC

Using a Microscope and Preparing Samples

10

Kate English and Alison Langridge

The Royal Veterinary College, London

Learning objectives

By the end of this chapter, students should be able to:

- Safely and effectively use a binocular microscope.
- Effectively view a microscope slide.
- Safely and effectively use oil immersion technique.
- Effectively use a Vernier scale.
- Understand and apply the principles of maintaining the microscope in good working order.
- Prepare a blood smear and stain the slide for viewing under the microscope.
- Conduct a packed cell volume measurement.

 Clinical skills sheets (SS)

Three clinical skills sheets will be used in this chapter and these can be found at pages 149–158. Reference will be made to each skills sheet at the relevant section within the chapter. The details of the clinical skills sheets used are as follows:

SS 10.22 Microscope set-up

SS 10.23 Preparing and examining blood smear and stain

SS 10.24 Packed cell volume (PCV)

 Videos (V)

Three videos will be used in this chapter to demonstrate how to perform the clinical skill and these are:

V 10.1 Microscope set-up

V 10.2 Blood smear and stain

V 10.3 Packed cell volume (PCV)

Introduction

Microscopes are an essential piece of equipment within veterinary practices and are likely to be used most days by veterinary surgeons, RVNs and students as part of a clinical work-up. Therefore, it is essential that all members of the team understand how to operate them safely and effectively in order for the diagnostic processes to continue uninterrupted. It is also vital that all staff employ good standards of clinical responsibility and make it their duty to ensure that the microscope is handled, cleaned, used and stored correctly.

Although different microscopes are constructed in slightly different ways, it is important that students recognize the common features and are able to apply this knowledge. The common features of a microscope are shown in Table 10.1. The item numbering in the column on 'During set-up' denotes the order in which these should be adjusted during set-up.

 SS 10.22 for a detailed procedure in setting up the microscope

 V 10.1 for a demonstration of microscope set-up

V 10.1 video.cabi.org/owjba

10.1 Viewing the Slide

Once the slide has been secured on the stage, the student needs to learn how to scan the slide in a methodical way. The most common method is the 'battlement technique' whereby the stage control is used to

© CAB International 2018. *Veterinary Clinical Skills Manual* (eds N. Coombes and A. Silva-Fletcher)

Table 10.1. Component functional parts of a microscope and how to use these during set-up. (Adapted from Irvin-Porter, 2011)

Common feature	Function	During set-up
Stage	A flat, slitted platform which securely holds the microscope slide. Can be moved laterally, forwards and backwards using stage control knobs	1. Move the stage to its lowest position using the coarse focus knob
Sub-stage condenser	Condenses light from the light source on to the specimen on the slide	2. Adjust the condenser so that it is just a few millimetres below the stage
Rheostat	A dial, usually on the side of the microscope. Alters the level of light produced by the light source	3. Turn the rheostat to its lowest setting *before* switching on the microscope
Objective lenses	Four lenses (×4, ×10, ×40, ×100) which sit on a rotating nosepiece above the stage	4. Move the lowest objective lens to the ×4 position. Ensure that it clicks into place
On/off switch	Usually located on the side of the microscope. This should be switched OFF after use	5. Switch to the ON position *only after* adjusting the rheostat to its lowest position
Eyepiece (two if binocular)	Contains ocular lenses which magnify the primary image formed by the objective lens	6. Look down the eyepieces and adjust the distance between them so that the view is whole
Focus knobs (for fine or coarse focus)	These two knobs operate on the same dial to move the stage up and down and to focus	7. The coarse focus knob is used during the first step of set-up to lower the stage to its lowest position
Light source	A flat disc on the base of the microscope underneath the sub-stage condenser. This contains a light bulb providing a light, which can be altered by the rheostat, condenser and iris diaphragm	
Iris diaphragm	This can be adjusted to let more or less light through the condenser	
Vernier scale	Horizontal and vertical scales allow points of interest on a slide to be accurately recorded and easily located by others	No set-up required.

move the stage in a shape that resembles the top of a battlement (Fig. 10.1).

Once the microscope has been set up as above, follow the steps below.

1. Place the microscope slide on to the stage, using the metal spring clips to hold it in place. Be careful to ensure that the clips are placed in position carefully and that they do not snap. This can break the slide.
2. Move the lowest objective lens (×4) into place, ensuring that it clicks into position.
3. Without looking down the eyepiece, move the stage up until it almost touches the objective lens. Ensure that the lens does not touch the slide.
4. Look down the eyepiece and slowly move the stage downwards using the coarse focus knob until the image comes into view.
5. If you cannot see the image and need to move up a magnification, lower the stage and repeat steps 2–4. Do this for each objective lens shift until you have found your image.
6. Once you have found the image, use the fine focus control to sharpen the image.

10.2 Using oil immersion

Once the slide has been viewed in a methodical way and you have secured your image, you may want to use oil immersion as below:

1. First, complete steps 1–6 as above.
2. Fully dilate the iris diaphragm.
3. Move the stage down and place a drop of oil on to the specimen.
4. Rotate the nosepiece until the objective lens ×100 has clicked into place.

Fig. 10.1. Diagram illustrating the 'battlement technique' for viewing specimens on glass slides. (Author's own diagram.)

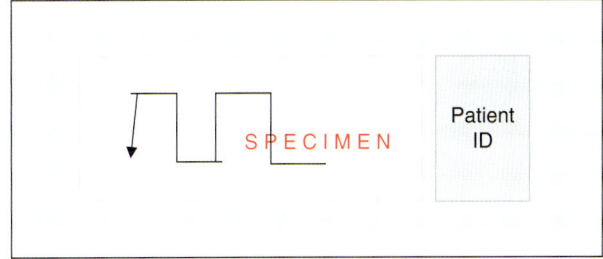

5. Without looking down the eyepiece, move the stage upwards slowly until the objective lens comes in contact with the oil on the slide.
6. Look down the eyepiece and slowly focus the image using the fine focus control.

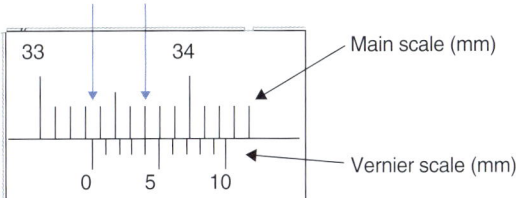

Fig. 10.2. Details of Vernier scale. (Author's own diagram)

10.3 Vernier scale

The Vernier scales are located on the horizontal and vertical aspects of the stage (commonly referred to as the x and y axis) and are always adjacent to each other (Fig. 10.2). They are useful for recording specific locations of points of interest on a slide; for example, an unusual blood cell or parasite.

Using a Vernier scale

- Lower the stage if required, in order to see the scales clearly, but *do not adjust the slide*.
- On each axis, there is a large (or main) scale and smaller (Vernier) scale located next to it.
- The main scale reading is taken first from where the Vernier scale matches it. If the Vernier scale '0' is between numbers, read the one it has just left.
- On the scale in Fig. 10.2, the '0' is between 33 and 34 mm therefore the first reading is **33 mm**.
- Then look down the Vernier scale and see where the Vernier scale and the main scale are most closely in alignment.
- On the scale in Fig. 10.2, this occurs at **4** on the Vernier scale.
- Therefore, the reading on this x axis should be recorded as **x = 33.4 mm**.

10.4 After viewing the specimen

1. Turn down the rheostat to its lowest position.
2. Lower the stage to its lowest position.
3. Remove the slide and either store or dispose of appropriately.
4. Rotate the nosepiece to its lowest objective lens (×4).
5. Switch off the light.
6. Remove the plug from the mains socket.
7. Clean the microscope lenses using lens tissue.
8. Replace the dust cover.

Care of your microscope

- The microscope must be stored in an upright position, in a clean, dry, cool area.
- The base must be supported at all times during lifting of the microscope.
- The microscope should never be pushed or pulled along a surface.
- The microscope should be cleaned regularly using an appropriate disinfectant. *It should never be sprayed with any fluid.*
- The light must not be left switched on.
- Electrical safety checks must be carried out regularly by an approved engineer.

10.5 Preparing a blood smear and stain

This is one of the basic Day One skills and all students should be able to prepare a blood smear and stain the slide for microscope viewing. Take care not to contaminate the slide with your own fingers prior to staining. You should, of course, be wearing gloves, but slides do get handled occasionally prior to this.

 SS 10.23 for a detailed procedure in preparing a blood smear and staining

 V 10.2 for a demonstration on how to perform a blood smear and stain

V 10.2 video.cabi.org/atcyd

 Stain use and maintenance

1. In-house stains will usually be a Romanowsky type – a variant of a Wrights–Giemsa, or Giemsa–Wright which stains samples blue or red, unless the substances are metachromatic, or have an intrinsically pigmented nature, so they do not stain.
2. Other stains that are sometimes used include supravital stains such as New Methylene Blue or May–Grunwald–Giemsa.
3. It is important to get to know your own stain and to know whether it is staining well or not, as this will mean that you will know when it needs changing more reliably.
4. Stains dislike water. Avoid getting water in the stain pots, and make sure your samples are thoroughly dry before starting the staining process.
5. Solution 1 is usually pale blue and is the fixative step. Although most manufacturers recommend the same amount of time in each stain pot, longer time in the fixative will often result in better staining, particularly if your sample is quite thick. The exception is aspiration from adipose tissue as fat will dissolve in the fixative.

6. Solution 2 is usually the red stain and requires the standard staining time. Blotting off the excessive fixative by dabbing the end of the smear on absorbent paper before placing it in the stain pot will not hurt.
7. Solution 3 is the blue stain and will often 'go off' quicker than the other stains.
8. General maintenance requires covering the stain with airtight lids in between use.
9. If a scum forms on the top of the jar, it can be removed with a little bit of tissue paper or blotting paper.
10. If there is a large amount of stain precipitate (this may be worse in some preparations if the stain became cold – it is best to keep your stain at room temperature), then filtering through blotting paper or a coffee filter can help.
11. When changing stains, thoroughly rinse and then dry the stain jars before refilling.
12. It is best to have a set of stains just for use in ear swabs or skin scrapes, as bacterial growth will often be high.

10.6 Packed cell volume (PCV) measurement

This is another basic skill that must be practised. Packed cell volume in blood is an important measurement to screen for most clinical conditions and to ascertain the hydration status of the animal.

 SS 10.24 for a detailed procedure in preparing a blood for PCV measurement

 V 10.3 for a demonstration of the technique to perform a PCV

V 10.3 video.cabi.org/yvslj

Further Reading: Davis, J. (2008) Diagnostic laboratory techniques. In: Aspinall, V. (ed.) *Clinical Procedures in Veterinary Nursing*, 2nd edn. Butterworth-Heinemann, Oxford, pp. 243–276.
Irvin-Porter, G. (2011) Laboratory diagnostic aids. In: Cooper, B., Mullineaux, E. and Turner, L. (eds) *BSAVA Textbook of Veterinary Nursing*. BSAVA, Gloucester, UK, pp. 538–546.

Clinical Skills Sheet

10.22. Microscope set-up

Method
This is an expensive and sensitive piece of equipment.   It should *only* be moved by gripping the main vertical frame and with your other hand under the microscope foot.   *Always* switch off the light bulb after use, and switch off at the mains.   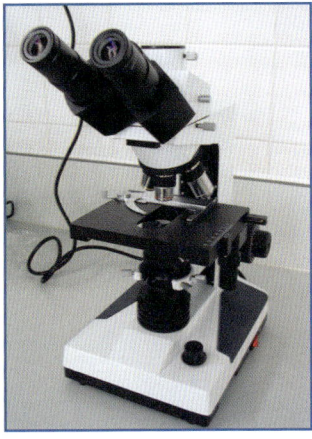
Check microscope is plugged in and switched on at the mains supply.
Ensure that the rheostat (light intensity dial) is turned to the lowest setting (to avoid damaging the bulb and your eyes). 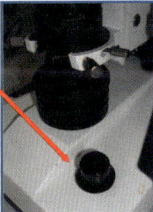
Turn the microscope on.   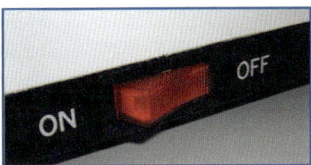
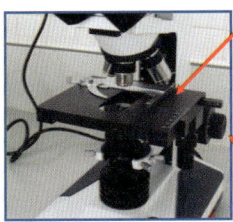 Rack down the mechanical stage as low as possible   (using the coarse focus dial)

Method

Select the lowest power objective lens (×4 or ×10 depending on machine), rotate and 'click' into position.

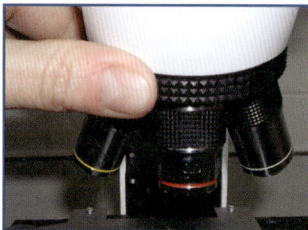

Place the microscope slide on to the stage (ensuring it is the right way up and label to the right).

The slide is held in position using the specimen holder shown here →

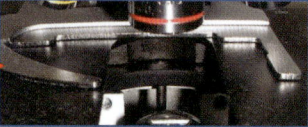

Look at the stage directly, rack it up using the coarse focus so that the slide is positioned just below the objective lens.

Adjust the rheostat as necessary (usually to a medium light intensity).

Adjust the binocular eyepieces to fit your eyes – and to ensure that only one image is seen.
If you find this difficult, look up and focus into middle distance then look through the eyepieces again.

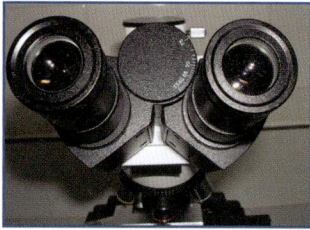

Check the position of the substage condenser and adjust to give the best possible image (usually racked up to just a few millimetres below the stage)

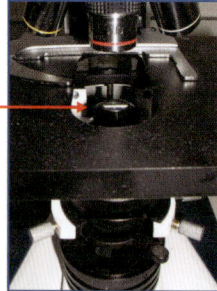

Substage condenser dial

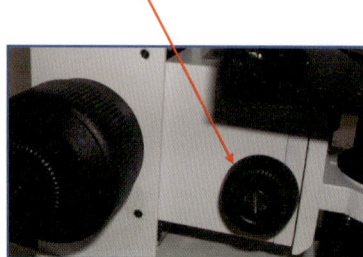

Method
Move the slide using the position adjustment knobs so that the area of interest is under the lens.
Rack the stage down using the coarse focus to focus the slide.
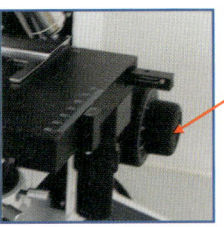 Adjust the fine focus
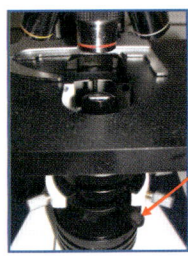 If necessary, adjust the iris diaphragm to provide optimal lighting
Scan the slide methodically, using the 'battlement' technique (up–along–down–along–up, etc.) to locate the object of interest. 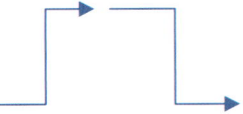
Once object is located, position in the middle of the field and adjust fine focus if necessary.
Reading the **Vernier Scale**: think of it as reading the coordinates of a point on an x–y graph. 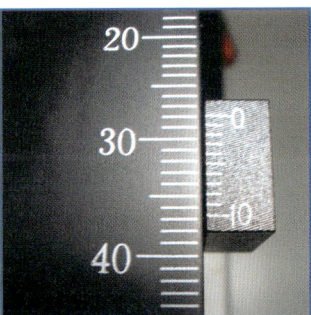
Read the horizontal (x) scale first, followed by the vertical (y) scale.
Method: Read off the larger Vernier scale and note where the '0' of the smaller scale lines up. In the above photo of a vertical scale it is at 28, so the coordinate will be '28 point something'.
For the decimal point, read where the lines of both scales match up **exactly**, and use the number from the small scale. In the above photo it is at '7'.
The reading (coordinate) for the above vertical scale is therefore 28.7

© RVC

Clinical Skills Sheet

10.23. Preparing and examining blood smear and stain

Method
1. Blood smear technique:
Always wear gloves.
An EDTA blood sample is provided (pink sample pot). •   Check that this is not clotted or overfilled.
Mix the sample gently, by rotating the pot end to end (up to a dozen times).
Remove a capillary (microhaematocrit) tube from container.
Remove the lid from the selected blood sample pot.
Holding the sample tube at an angle, insert the capillary tube completely into it to enhance the flow of blood up the capillary tube. If there is only a small amount of blood, tipping the tube *almost horizontal* will ensure enough blood enters the capillary tube. 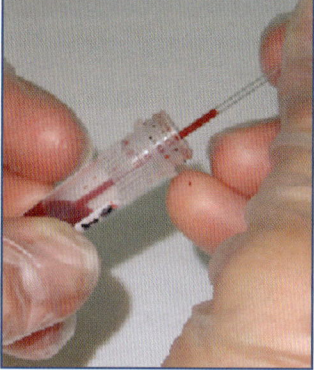
Fill capillary tube with blood to at least 1 cm.
Place a finger gently over the top end of the tube, which will create a vacuum and thus hold the sample in the tube.
Put a dot of blood (by releasing finger vacuum briefly) near one end of the slide. Dispose of the tube in a sharps bin.
Replace the lid on the blood sample to prevent spillage.
Place the spreader (another slide) on to the main slide – approximately in the middle.
At a 30–45 degree angle, pull the spreader towards the dot of blood. 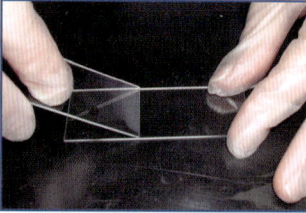

Method
Allow the dot of blood to *seep along* the edge of the spreader, by capillary action. 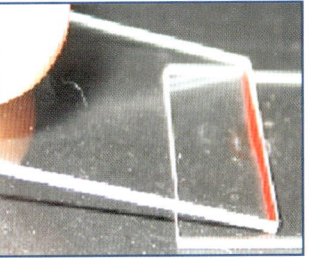
Push spreader smoothly *away* from the sample, along the slide. Do *not* drag the spreader *over* the blood dot, as the cells will be damaged (haemolysed) 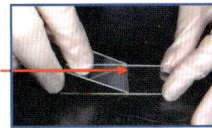
Air dry the slide by standing it upright against a coplin jar, or in a glass cradle.
(In a clinical set-up the sample would be labelled by indelible pen and usually on the right-hand side with the patient's identity and date.)

2. Staining technique:

Dip slide into coplin jar containing pale blue solution (fixative = methanol).
- Dip slowly five times, or hold in fluid for 5 sec.
- Allow excess fluid to drip back into the jar.

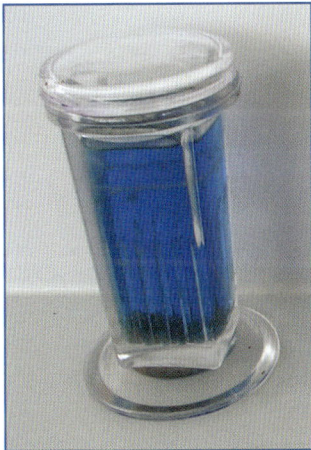

Method

Dip slide into coplin jar containing red solution (solution 1 = acid dye: eosin).
- Dip slowly five times, or hold in fluid for 5 secs.
- Allow excess fluid to drip back into the jar.

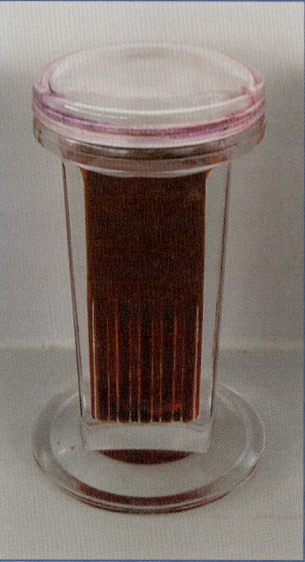

Dip slide into coplin jar containing purple solution (solution 2 = basic dye: methylene blue).
- Dip slowly five times, or hold in fluid for 5 sec.
- Allow excess fluid to drip back into the jar.

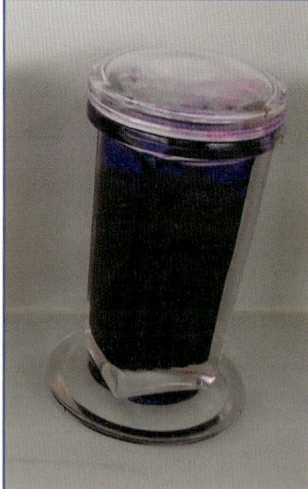

Rinse the slide with distilled water from squeezy bottle or dip into 4th coplin jar containing distilled water.

Wipe underside of slide and allow to air dry upright.

The slide is now ready to look at under the microscope (refer to SS 10.22 (Microscope set-up)).

Method

Common faults with smear technique:
- too thick – use smaller drop of blood.
- too thin – use larger drop of blood or faster spreading motion.
- banding – use smoother spreading motion.
- streaking – dirty spreader slide.
- holes in smear – dirty/greasy slide).
- narrow smear – allow blood to spread across spreader slide.

© RVC

Clinical Skills Sheet

10.24. Packed cell volume (PCV)

Method
Always wear gloves.
Select EDTA (pink) or heparin (orange) sample pot.
Make sure the sample is not clotted or overfilled.
Mix the sample gently, by rocking the pot (up to a dozen times).
Remove two capillary (microhaematocrit) tubes from container.
Remove the lid from the selected blood sample tube.
Holding the sample pot at an angle, insert the capillary tube completely into it to enhance the flow of blood up the capillary tube. If there is only a small amount of blood, tipping the tube *almost horizontal* will ensure enough blood enters the capillary tube. 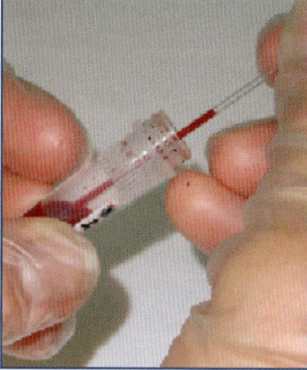
Fill the capillary tube with blood *at least* ¾ full.
Place a finger gently over the top end of the tube, which will create a vacuum and thus hold the sample in the tube.
Wipe the outside of the capillary tube with a tissue.

Method
Plug one end of the tube with soft-clay sealant, holding the tube at an angle whilst pushing *gently* into the clay. The plug should be about 3 mm depth. (Don't push too hard or you'll shatter the tube, and possibly have shards of glass in your finger!) 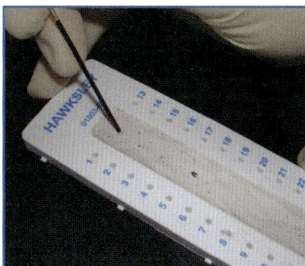 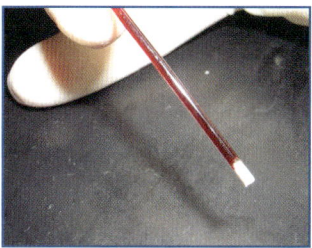
Place tube into a microhaematocrit centrifuge.
Clay plug facing outwards against outer rim. 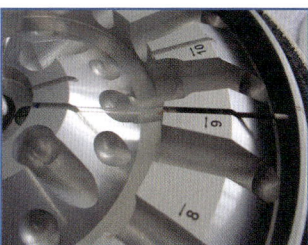
Repeat the procedure to fill another capillary tube.
Replace the lid of the blood sample tube.
Place the second tube into the centrifuge (plug facing outwards) – *always* opposite the first tube for balance. (There must be an even number of tubes in the centrifuge placed opposite each other or the machine will spin out of balance.) 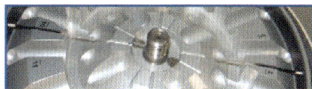
Important: screw inner safety lid (just hand tight) down over samples. If you forget, the samples will not be secured and will shatter as the centrifuge begins to spin – dangerous and messy to clear up.
Close *and* lock the main lid.
Set at 10,000 rpm for 5 min or 'fast' setting.

Method

Correctly read prepared sample if available; if not, read the sample you have done.

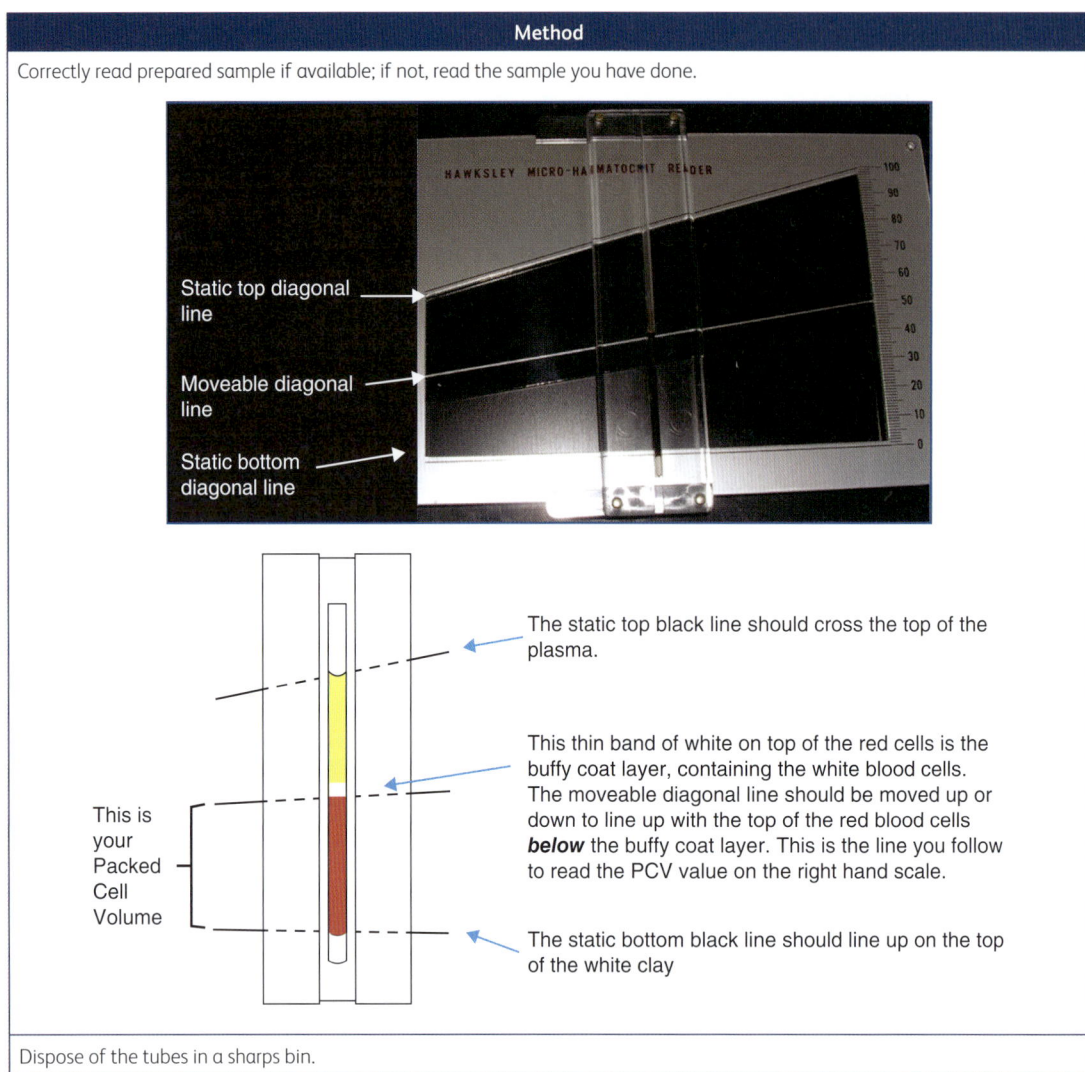

Static top diagonal line

Moveable diagonal line

Static bottom diagonal line

The static top black line should cross the top of the plasma.

This thin band of white on top of the red cells is the buffy coat layer, containing the white blood cells. The moveable diagonal line should be moved up or down to line up with the top of the red blood cells **below** the buffy coat layer. This is the line you follow to read the PCV value on the right hand scale.

This is your Packed Cell Volume

The static bottom black line should line up on the top of the white clay

Dispose of the tubes in a sharps bin.

© RVC

11 Urine and Faecal Analysis

Alison Langridge and Kate English

The Royal Veterinary College, London

Learning objectives

By the end of this chapter, students should be able to:

- Perform urinalysis for initial screening using specific gravity measurement and dipstick.
- Prepare a urine sample for examination under the microscope.
- Perform McMaster faecal egg count technique for gastrointestinal parasites.

Clinical skills sheets (SS)

Three clinical skills sheets will be used in this chapter and these can be found at pages 163–168. Reference will be made to each skills sheet at the relevant section within the chapter. The details of the clinical skills sheets used are as follows:

SS 11.25 Obtaining a urine specific gravity reading and a dipstick reading

SS 11.26 Preparing a urine sample for microscope analysis

SS 11.27 McMaster faecal egg count technique

Video (V)

One video will be used in this chapter to demonstrate how to perform the clinical skill:

V 11.1 Urine SG

Introduction

Urine and faecal analyses are extremely valuable to understand the health status of an animal. Some analysis can be done quickly for initial screening and further analysis can be undertaken based on initial results.

11.1   Urinalysis

Urinalysis is a cheap and easy laboratory procedure that can provide valuable information very quickly. A complete urine analysis comprising urine dipstick, specific gravity (SG) and sediment examination should be performed, even if one component part shows no abnormalities. To gain maximum benefit from urine analysis, concurrent serum or plasma biochemical analysis is often required. Terms used in urinalysis are defined in Table 11.1.

11.1.1   Gross appearance

When the urine sample is first presented, it should be appraised for colour and turbidity before any tests are performed (Table 11.2). Odour is also a good parameter to record.

11.1.2   Specific gravity

The specific gravity (commonly referred to as SG or USG) of urine is a key indicator of the patient's ability to concentrate their urine. This can be easily obtained by measuring the refractive index (RI) on a calibrated refractometer.

Reminder

The refractive index (RI) is dependent on the amount and type of solute in the liquid that is placed on it. Thus, the SG of a solution depends on the number and molecular weight of particles in the solution.

As distilled water has an SG of 1.000, the concentration of urine as a comparison is recorded as a percentage.

© CAB International 2018. *Veterinary Clinical Skills Manual* (eds N. Coombes and A. Silva-Fletcher)

Table 11.1. Key terminology used in urinalysis. (Adapted from Villiers and Blackwood, 2005.)

Word	Meaning
Osmolality	The concentration of a solution expressed as the total number of solute particles per kilogram
Specific gravity (SG) (also referred to by the abbreviation USG or SpGr)	Refers to the concentration of the urine compared with the concentration of distilled water. SG is not expressed in units
Isosthenuria	Refers to the maintenance of a constant osmolality of the urine, regardless of changes in osmotic pressure of the blood
Refractive index (RI)	The ratio of the velocity of light in a vacuum to its velocity in a specified medium
Refractometer	An instrument for measuring a refractive index and ascertaining results for specific gravity, total proteins of urine

Table 11.2. Sample appearance and possible causes (adapted from Villiers and Blackwood, 2005).

Appearance	Cause
Clear, very pale straw colour	Low SG (dilute urine)
Clear to slightly turbid, deep yellow	High SG (concentrated urine)
Bright red	Fresh blood (un-oxidized)
Red	Free haemoglobin/lysed RBC
Red-brown	Older (oxidized), haemoglobin/lysed RBC
Dark red-brown	Myoglobin Transfusion of haemoglobin-based oxygen-carrying solution (oxyglobin)
Red-pink	Consumption of beetroot or red food dyes
Dark yellow/ greenish	Bilirubin
Orange/yellow	Tetracyclines
Cloudy	Increases in any constituents: Cells WBC RBC Epithelial cells Casts Mucus Bacteria Amorphous material/crystals

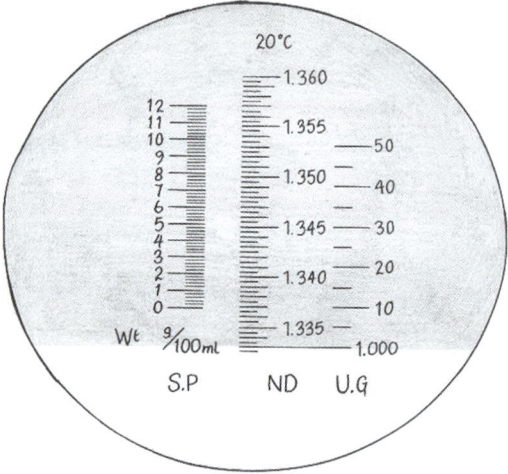

Fig. 11.1. The scale in a refractometer. The blue area (represented here in grey) ends precisely on the line reading 1.000. This means that it is calibrated and ready to use. (Courtesy of RVC Clinical Skills Centre.)

shaded area (which is normally blue in refractometers) is sitting on the 1.000 line at the bottom of the scale. This occurs after a drop of water has been placed on the prism and the refractometer has been manually calibrated to bring the blue area down on to that 1.000 line.

Once the refractometer has been calibrated to 1.000 with distilled water, the water needs to be wiped off the prism and the cover with a tissue. A drop of the urine should then be placed on the prism and the cover closed.

11.1.3 Refractometer

Figure 11.1 is a diagram depicting the scale in a refractometer and what it looks like when it is calibrated, before the urine is placed on the prism. You can see that the

 You must wipe off the water to prevent dilution of the sample, which could result in an incorrect diagnosis.

The light through the prism will now refract relative to the 'weight' of the urine, so when you look down the refractometer, the blue area will have moved up. Where the blue and white areas meet is where you record the patient's urinary SG (Fig. 11.2).

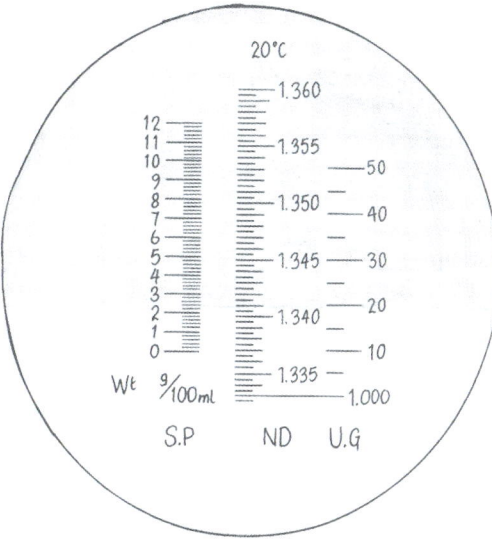

Fig. 11.2. An example of a reading from a urine sample on the refractometer. In this diagram, the blue area (represented here in grey) has moved away from the baseline 1.000 and is now sitting at 19. This means that the SG for this patient is 1.019. For efficient communication, this representation is often verbally conveyed as 'ten' followed by the number given on the scale. In this case, we would simply say this result is 'ten nineteen'.

11.1.4 Urinary dipstick

For a general investigative urinalysis, a combination dipstick provides the most holistic overview of clinical wellness. Table 11.3 outlines the different types of dipsticks that are available.

Before you start the test:

- Observe appearance and record colour, turbidity and odour.
- Record the time the sample was collected and what time it was dropped off at the surgery.
- Ensure that the sample is in an appropriate receptacle (for example, not in a boric acid tube or a jam jar which may have residual glucose present).

Materials required for basic urinalysis:

- Non-sterile gloves.
- Pasteur pipette.
- Kidney bowl.
- Timer or clock.
- Tissue.
- Distilled water.
- Combination dipsticks.
- Refractometer.
- Clinical and domestic waste bins.
- Sharps bin.

 SS 11.25 for a detailed procedure in how to do urinalysis using the refractometer and/or dipstick

 V 11.1 for a USG measurement demonstration

V 11.1 video.cabi.org/qzsgj

Table 11.3. List of dipsticks available and the components measured by each stick. (Adapted from Cooper *et al.*, 2011)

Type of stick	What it measures
Combination	pH, protein, glucose, ketones, urobilinogen, bilirubin, haemoglobin, myoglobin. They also measure leucocytes, though a positive urinary leucocyte reading is widely accepted as being unreliable
Diastix	Glucose
Keto-diastix	Ketones, glucose
Uristix	Protein, glucose
Ketostix	Ketones

11.1.5 Prepare a urine sample for microscope analysis

If the urine is cloudy and/or if a sediment is suspected, it is necessary to examine urine under the microscope.

 SS 11.26 for a detailed procedure in how to prepare urine sample for microscope examination, with examples of some urine crystals

References and Further Reading: Cooper, B., Mullineaux, E. and Turner, L. (2011) *BSAVA Textbook of Veterinary Nursing*, 5th edition. BSAVA, Gloucester, UK.

Irwin-Porter, G. (2011) Laboratory Diagnostic Aids. In: Cooper, B., Mullineaux, E. and Turner, L. (eds) *BSAVA Textbook of Veterinary Nursing*, 5th edition. BSAVA, Gloucester, UK.

Osborne, C.A. and Stevens, J.B.(1999) *Urinalysis: A Clinical Guide to Compassionate Patient Care*. Bayer Corporation and Bayer AG Leverkusen, Kansas, USA.

Villiers, E. and Blackwood, L. (eds) (2005) *BSAVA Manual of Canine and Feline Clinical Pathology*, 2nd edn. BSAVA, Gloucester, UK.

11.2 Faecal Analysis

If gastrointestinal parasites are suspected, it is necessary to examine faeces for parasite eggs. This is conducted using the McMaster technique. A special microscope slide is available for counting eggs (if they are present) and this is called a McMaster chamber, as shown in Fig. 11.3.

You need to take suitable PPE precautions as with handling any sample, as detailed in Chapter 9.

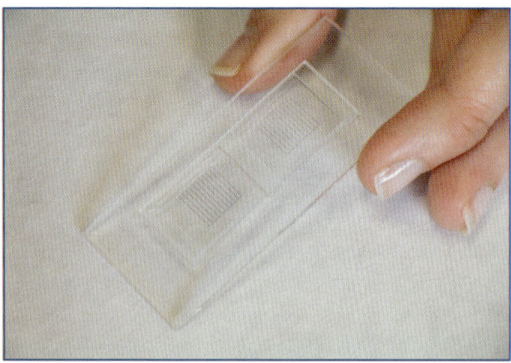

Fig. 11.3. The McMaster chamber.

 SS 11.27 For a detailed procedure in how to check for parasite eggs and how to count these

Clinical Skills Sheet

11.25. Obtaining a urine specific gravity reading and a dipstick reading

Method
Specific gravity (SG) measurement:
Calibrate refractometer – lift the cover plate and place 2–3 drops of distilled water on the prism surface.
Hold refractometer up to a light source and read the scale – calibrate to 1.000 if necessary (there is usually a screw on top of the refractometer for this purpose, which may be adjusted by hand or by mini screwdriver, depending on the model – please do not do this unless you have been previously shown)
Lift the cover plate and dry the prism surface with a tissue.
Wear gloves.
Gently mix the urine sample.
Pipette the urine and place 2–3 drops on the prism surface.
Replace the cover.
Hold the refractometer up to the light source.
Read the scale correctly (from the right-hand scale) *For example, the reading in this diagram is 1.019*
Rinse the prism with distilled water (over a sink) and wipe dry with a tissue.
Dipstick analysis:
Select the appropriate dipstick test strips.
Ensure the test strips are in date.
Remove one stick and place the reagent side up on the Benchkote.
Immediately replace the lid.
Gently mix the urine sample.
Pipette approximately 1ml of urine.
Drop one drop of urine on each of the reagent pads of the urine dipstick.
Note the time.
Leave for the recommended time/s as identified on the dipstick container.

Method
Hold the stick the correct way up against the dipstick container and compare. 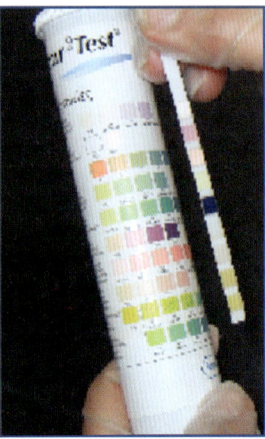
Read and record the results correctly.
Dispose of the stick correctly into clinical waste.

© RVC

Clinical Skills Sheet

11.26. Preparing a urine sample for microscope analysis

Method
Wear gloves.
Remove supernatant (the fluid above the sediment) with a disposable pipette, being careful not to disturb the sediment. Leave a drop of supernatant in the tube with the sediment. *Do not suck it dry.* 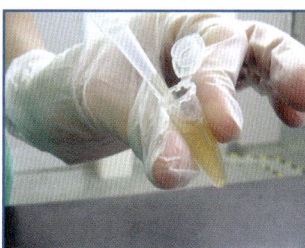
Discard supernatant into a kidney dish.
Flick the sample tube to re-suspend the remainder of the sediment.
Add one drop of 'Sedistain' and mix. (*The sample does not have to be stained to see urinary crystals; the staining is optional and situation dependent.*)
Pipette up some of the sample and place one drop on to a microscope slide.
Apply cover slip • Lower slowly over the sample. • Avoid air bubbles.
This station does not use a real sample (in fact it is cider and bicarbonate of soda). With a true sample, at this stage you would check under a microscope at ×4 or ×10 magnification.
Identify photographs of urine crystals (see images below).
Question: At what speed and for how long would you centrifuge this sample?
Answer: 1–2000 rpm for 2–5 min.

Method

Urine Crystals

A. Cystine

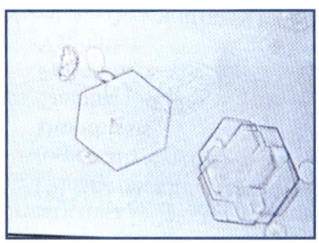

B. Calcium oxalate

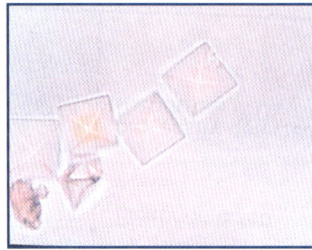

C. Struvite (triple phosphate)

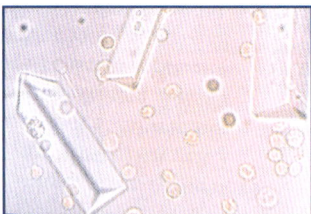

D. Ammonium urate

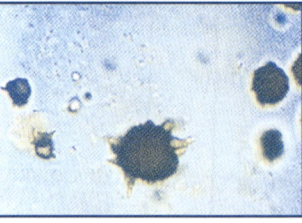

© RVC

Clinical Skills Sheet

11.27. McMaster faecal egg count technique

Method
Wear gloves.
Prepare all the equipment you will need: • 2 glass beakers. • 100 ml measuring cylinder. • faecal sample. • spatula. • scales. • fine sieve. • flotation fluid – 400 g sodium chloride (NaCl) in 1000 ml water, this is a general-purpose flotation fluid. • plastic pipette. • lab tissues. • McMaster slide. • microscope.
Place a glass beaker on the scales and calibrate the scales to 0.
Using the spatula, measure out 4 g of faeces into the glass beaker.
Pour 56 ml of flotation fluid into the 100 ml measuring cylinder. *Make sure the fluid is thoroughly mixed as it tends to separate.*
Pour the measured flotation fluid into the container with 4 g of faeces. Mix well with the spatula.
Select a second container and the sieve.
Filter the faecal solution through the sieve into the second container, pressing the retained solid material to force through as much liquid as possible.
Stir the filtrate in container 2 with a plastic pipette.
Using the pipette, withdraw a sub-sample of the filtrate as you are stirring.
Fill the first compartment of the McMaster counting chamber with the sub-sample of the filtrate, taking care not to introduce any air bubbles.
Stir the filtrate again with the pipette and take a second sub-sample.
Fill the second compartment of the McMaster counting chamber.
Wipe off any excess fluid from the underside of the slide.
Allow the counting chamber to stand for 5 minutes – this allows the eggs to float to the surface and the debris to sink to the bottom of the chamber.
Microscope examination of slide:
Examine the sample under the microscope at 10 x 10 magnification. DO NOT USE HIGH POWER as you will break the slide.
Starting in the top left corner of the grid, scan vertically between the 'tram-lines' within the engraved areas of the two chambers.
Count and identify any eggs seen within the engraved area of chambers (using the 'tram-lines' for guidance), ignoring those outside the squares.
To estimate the number of eggs per gram of faeces (epg) use the following calculation: • Number of eggs seen in chamber 1 + number of eggs seen in chamber 2. • Then multiply the total number of eggs seen by 50. e.g. (12 + 15) × 50 = 1350 epg.

Method
Question: Are the number of eggs found always an indication of the number of worms present? Suggest reasons for your answer.
Answer: No. While the number of eggs per gram usually gives an indication of the worm burden, there are exceptions. Reasons include: • Eggs are only produced by fertile adult females – therefore, immature or single sex male infections will be missed. • Output of eggs is influenced by host physiological factors (e.g. increased during stress, lactation; decreased with immunity). • Chemotherapy – corticosteroids increase egg production; sub-lethal anthelmintic doses will decrease egg production. • Concentration of eggs influenced by volume of faeces produced; rate of passage through intestine; distribution of eggs throughout faecal mass. • Some types of eggs are heavier than others and thus may not float in the chosen flotation fluid.

NB: All excess faeces and faecal fluid mix should be flushed down a toilet or otherwise suitably disposed of.

© RVC

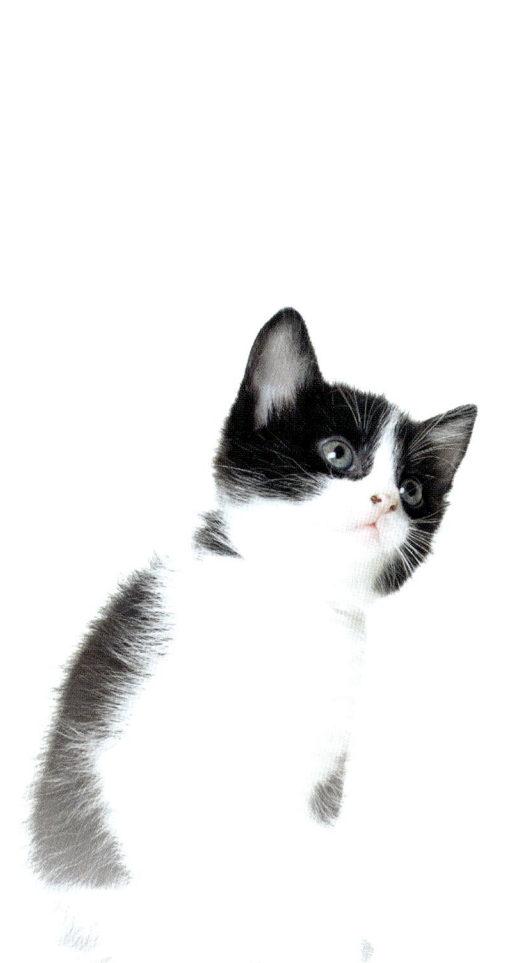
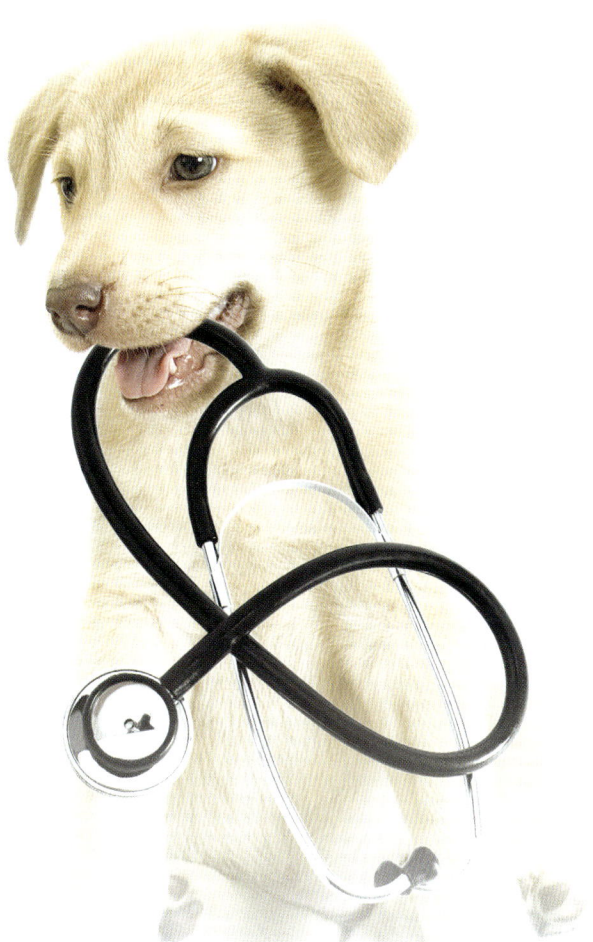

Section 5

General Clinical Skills

Section Editor: Alison Langridge

Introduction

A high level of competence in general clinical skills is fundamental to the process of disease diagnosis and treatment. The three chapters in this section are based on the skills required to perform a basic clinical examination and initial treatments. An underlying knowledge of pharmacy underpins all treatments and therefore this section on first contact with the patient will explore the principles in pharmacy.

The aim of this section is to provide that basic knowledge to start diagnosis and treatment. Within this section there are three chapters:

Chapter 12: Physical Examination, Fluid Therapy, Tube and Drain Management

Chapter 13: Principles of Small Animal Bandaging

Chapter 14: Pharmacy

Within each chapter you will find pictures and tips about how to conduct relevant basic Day One skills. Each chapter will also detail key points for each set of skills and point out the health and safety considerations, which are critical to good practice.

An overview of all the learning outcomes is presented below and the more detailed learning outcomes are presented under each chapter.

Learning objectives

After studying this section, students should be able to:

- Conduct a physical examination including triage, cranial nerve and ophthalmic examination.
- Maintain a urethral catheter, thoracostomy tube, abdominal drain and tracheostomy tube.
- Obtain samples and aseptically handle these tubes/catheters.
- Identify different layers of a bandage and different types of dressings.
- Identify risk factors for iatrogenic injuries.
- Apply a safe, effective bandage to a small animal.

- Identify and utilize the relevant legislation and guidelines associated with storage, dispensing and disposal of veterinary medication.
- Interpret written prescriptions or drug orders and calculate the required doses.
- Dispose of equipment used in the administration of medication according to relevant legislation and guidelines.

What You Will Need

Clinical skills sheets (SS)

Nine clinical skills sheets will be used in this section. Reference will be made to each skills sheet at the relevant point within the chapter. Clinical skills sheets for the following accompany this section:

SS 12.28 Cranial nerve examination.

SS 12.29 Ophthalmology practical: eye examination.

SS 12.30 Assessing urinary output in a catheterized patient.

SS 12.31 Catheterizing a limb.

SS 12.32 Setting up intravenous fluids.

SS 13.33 Applying a canine forelimb bandage.

SS 13.34 Applying a canine chest drain bandage.

SS 13.35 Applying an ear bandage.

SS 15.40 Applying a lower-limb protective bandage on a horse.

Videos (V)

Four videos will be used in this section and reference will be made to each video at the relevant point within the chapter. Videos will be hyperlinked and the following accompany this section:

V 12.1 Ophthalmic examination.

V 12.2 Place an intravenous catheter in a dog.

V 12.3 Prepare and set up fluid admin (small animal).

V 13.1 Ear bandage.

Physical Examination, Fluid Therapy, Tube and Drain Management

Karen Humm

The Royal Veterinary College, London

Learning objectives

By the end of this chapter, students should be able to:

- Understand the importance of appropriate animal handling when performing a physical examination.
- Perform a triage examination.
- Perform a cranial nerve examination.
- Peform an ophthalmic examination.
- Understand the reasons for placement of a urethral catheter, thoracostomy tube, abdominal drain and tracheostomy tube.
- Maintain these tubes/catheters appropriately.
- Quantitatively assess fluid obtained from these tubes/catheters.
- Obtain samples from these tubes/catheters.
- Understand the importance of aseptic handling of these tubes/catheters.

 Clinical skills sheets (SS)

Five clinical skills sheets will be used in this chapter and these can be found at pages 177–189. Reference will be made to each skills sheet at the relevant section within the chapter. The details of the clinical skills sheets used are as follows:

SS 12.28 Cranial nerve examination
SS 12.29 Ophthalmology practical: examination
SS 12.30 Assessing urinary output in a catheterized patient
SS 12.31 Catheterizing a limb
SS 12.32 Setting up intravenous fluids

 Videos (V)

Three videos will be used in this chapter:

V 12.1 Ophthalmic examination
V 12.2 Place an intravenous catheter in a dog
V 12.3 Prepare and set up fluid admin (small animal)

Introduction

Physical examination of the patient is essential to allow accurate patient assessment. Without this, further diagnostic tests cannot be decided upon and treatments cannot be administered. Essentially, a diagnosis cannot be made with confidence. Depending on the patient's presentation, detailed specific examinations may be required, such as a cranial nerve or ophthalmic examination. This chapter describes how to perform these examinations. It also describes common procedures performed when caring for hospitalized patients, once they have undergone initial evaluation.

12.1 Safe Handling and Patient Welfare

A physical examination should cause minimal stress to the animal involved. All efforts should be made to maximize the safety of the person performing the examination, any bystanders (including owners and other members of staff) and the animal itself.

171

Stress can be difficult to assess in some species, so knowledge of how this may be displayed by the animal involved is important. Appropriate personal protective equipment is generally required when performing a physical examination, which again varies depending on the species involved.

12.2 Physical Examination

A physical examination is required prior to making a diagnosis or prescribing drugs and is also necessary to monitor hospitalized patients and disease progression. The results of every physical examination should be noted in patient records and in some cases may need to be supplemented with photographs or diagrams for particular disease processes. As experience grows, each individual will develop their own technique for physical examination, in terms of order and style, but all points must be covered.

Physical examination can be distressing for a patient, particularly if they are painful, so appropriate handling, empathy and a careful technique are required. It is often best to leave examination of any suspected painful area until the end of the examination.

12.2.1 Triage examination

A triage examination involves assessing a patient for stability of the three major body systems (Table 12.1):

- Cardiovascular system.
- Respiratory system.
- Neurological system.

Major dysfunction in any of these systems can be life-threatening, with total loss of function rapidly leading to death.

 If a patient is showing signs of major body system dysfunction, stress must be minimized and very careful handling is required to prevent further decompensation.

 Remember that dysfunction in one major body system can lead to changes in other body systems. For example, cardiovascular dysfunction can lead to weakness, meaning the patient may not be ambulatory. When performing a triage examination, try to consider what the primary problem is.

 Once the major body systems have been assessed, abdominal palpation and body temperature measurement should be performed. Altogether, this information allows recognition of an unstable patient that requires immediate therapy.

Table 12.1. Major body systems and how they are assessed in a triage examination.

Major body system	Assessment methods
Cardiovascular	Cardiac auscultation (murmur or gallop) Pulse palpation (central and peripheral) Heart rate and pulse rate calculation Heart rhythm and pulse rhythm assessment (regular, irregular, sinus arrhythmia) Mucous membrane assessment (colour and capillary refill time)
Respiratory	Orthopnoea assessment Respiratory effort (inspiratory or expiratory, paradoxical) Respiratory rate Audible noise assessment (suggesting upper respiratory tract pathology) Lung field auscultation (crackles, harshness, wheezes) Mucous membrane assessment (colour)
Neurological	Mentation (normal, quiet, obtunded, stuporous, comatose) Ambulatory

12.2.2 Cranial nerve examination

A cranial nerve examination is an important part of a full neurological examination, allowing assessment of neurological function. If cranial nerve abnormalities are noted, this could be due to pathology in the brainstem, cerebellum, forebrain, eye, middle ear or the C1–C5 spinal cord segment, or a peripheral neuropathy or myopathy may be present. Abnormal findings in a cranial nerve examination should be interpreted alongside a full neurological examination and physical examination, as well as patient history, to allow understanding of the likely cause.

Tools required:

- Pen torch.
- Cotton buds.
- Cotton wool balls.
- A secure room with 'obstacles' (e.g. chairs).
- Food with a strong odour.

 Many animals resent cranial nerve examination. Having a colleague present to help with handling and recording of results may be very helpful in making the process smoother.

 SS 12.28 for a detailed examination follow the steps for cranial nerve examination

12.3 Ophthalmic Examination

A full ophthalmic examination is not necessary in every patient, but is required if there are historical or physical examination findings that suggest ocular disease.

 There are many pieces of equipment which aid ophthalmic examination, but the essential items are:

- A strong light source.
- Schirmer tear test strips.
- Fluoroscein dye.
- Indirect ophthalmoscope.
- 20D (dioptre) lens.

 SS 12.29 For a detailed examination, follow the steps for a practical ophthalmology exam

 V 12.1 Ophthalmic examination

V 12.1 video.cabi.org/jknha

12.4 Principles of Tube and Catheter Insertion and Care

Tubes and catheters can be placed to improve patient comfort, to obtain a diagnosis, or to treat a disease process. Patients with these tubes and catheters need to be hosptialized and carefully nursed while they are *in situ* to decrease the risk of complications. The reasons for placing a tube, precautions to observe during the procedure and the maintenance of the tubes are outlined under each subheading below.

12.4.1 Urethral catheter

Urethral catheters are placed for many reasons, including:

- Obtaining a urine sample.
- Accurate measurement of urine output.
- De-obstruction of the urethra.
- Aiding management of the recumbent patient (preventing urine scald).
- Aiding management of patients with neurological bladder dysfunction.

Urethral catheters can be placed for a short period (minutes) or for days. They can be made of many different materials and in differing designs. Ease of placement varies between patient species and sex. However, it is always imperative that they are placed in an aseptic manner. They also need to be managed in a sterile fashion to decrease the risk of hospital-acquired infection.

If a urethral catheter is going to be left *in situ* in a patient, it must not be left open as this will lead to urine scalding and will greatly increase the risk of catheter-associated urinary tract infection, which will cause increased morbidity and mortality. Urine collection systems should therefore be used which are cheap to purchase or can be made in-house.

 Many patients will require a buster collar when they have a urethral catheter in place as they may interfere with the catheter, leading to possible damage or dislodgement.

 SS 12.30 for details regarding using a urethral catheter for assessing urine output

12.4.2 Thoracostomy tube

Thoracostomy tubes (often referred to as 'chest drains') are placed in patients to allow drainage of pathological fluid and/or air from the pleural space. There are two main types of thoracostomy tube: wider-bore tubes placed with a trochar; and much narrower tubes that are placed via a Seldinger technique. Both types can be used in surgical (thoracotomy) or non-surgical patients. In all cases, however, they are placed aseptically and aseptic handling is required at all times to minimize the risk of hospital-acquired infection.

 Patients with thoracostomy tubes may have undergone surgery or trauma and so may be in some discomfort. It is important, therefore, to be careful and empathetic when handling these patients. Thoracostomy tube use itself, however, is not painful.

When using a thoracostomy tube to drain the pleural space, the volume of fluid and/or air should be accurately recorded and samples of fluid taken as appropriate.

12.4.3 Abdominal drain

Abdominal drains are generally placed in patients with abdominal pathology where continued fluid production is anticipated. This is most commonly in post-surgical patients. The drains vary in style and material, but all must be placed and managed in an aseptic fashion to minimize the risk of hospital-acquired infection.

 Patients with abdominal drains may have undergone surgery or trauma and so may be in some discomfort. It is important, therefore, to be careful and empathetic when handling these patients. Abdominal drain use itself, however, is not painful.

12.4.4 Tracheostomy tube

Tracheostomy tubes are placed in patients with upper respiratory tract pathology that impairs effective respiration. They are placed aseptically under general anaesthesia, allowing bypass of the upper respiratory tract.

 The upper respiratory tract allows humidification, filtering and warming of inhaled air, but the use of a tracheostomy tube prevents this from occurring. These patients are therefore at risk of inhaling foreign bodies and drying of the trachea and lower airways resulting in 'thicker' respiratory secretions. To minimize these adverse effects, inhalational risks, such as cat litter, must be avoided and regular nebulization over the tracheostomy tube entrance is required.

 Patients with a tracheostomy tube must be monitored constantly, as dislodgement or obstruction of the tube can rapidly lead to severe respiratory distress and death. If dislodgement does occur, on placement, two stay sutures will have been placed in the tracheal rings cranial and caudal to the tracheostomy site labelled 'up' and 'down', respectively. When these are gently pulled, this will reveal the tracheal opening and the tracheostomy tube can be replaced.

A spare tracheostomy tube should be available by the patient's cage at all times in case of tube blockage, allowing rapid replacement.

 Never insert the obturator of the tracheostomy tube into the tube while it is *in situ* in the patient. It is designed to aid insertion and not to assess how the patient can cope without the tracheostomy tube. Use of the obturator in this way causes almost complete obstruction of the patient's airway.

12.5   Intravenous (IV) Catheter Placement

Placing an intravenous catheter is an essential skill. This allows:

- Repeated intravenous administration of drugs without the risk of extravascular administration or venous damage (e.g. haematoma).
- Intravenous fluid therapy.
- Continuous-rate infusion of drugs.
- Intravenous access for emergency administration of drugs in unstable cases at risk of cardiopulmonary arrest.

Selecting the appropriate vein is the first step (Table 12.2). This depends upon the species, breed, demeanour and underlying disease process (e.g. hind limb veins are to be avoided in patients with diarrhoea, but may be preferred in an aggressive patient).

Once the vein has been selected, the site must be prepared by clipping the fur; the skin must be thoroughly

cleansed to remove any dirt and then aseptically prepared to ensure sterility before the catheter is placed. The person placing the catheter should carefully wash their hands prior to the procedure to minimize the risk of catheter site contamination.

 SS 12.31 offers detailed guidance regarding the materials required and the steps to follow for insert an IV catheter successfully

 V 12.2 Place an intravenous catheter in a dog

V 12.2 video.cabi.org/yfjvn

12.6   Fluid set-up

Crystalloid fluid therapy is required for:
- Correcting hydration deficits.
- Treating hypovolaemia.
- Correcting electrolyte abnormalities.
- Maintenance of volume status in patients under general anaesthesia.

 Great care should be taken when selecting the fluid to be administered to a patient, as the packaging of most isotonic crystalloid solutions looks very similar although their components can vary markedly.

 SS 12.32 offers detailed guidance regarding the materials required and the steps to follow for successful fluid set-up

 V 12.3 Prepare and set up fluid admin (small animal)

V 12.3 video.cabi.org/kzpgr

Table 12.2. Veins used for intravenous catheter placement in different species.

Species	Veins most commonly chosen for IV catheter placement
Dog	Cephalic or lateral saphenous
Cat	Cephalic or medial saphenous
Rabbit	Marginal ear vein
Horse	Jugular
Cow	Jugular

Further Reading: Brown, A.J. and Drobatz, K.J. (2007) Triage of the emergency patient. In: King, L.G. and Boag, A.K. (eds) *BSAVA Manual of Canine and Feline Emergency and Critical Care*, 2nd edn. BSAVA, Gloucester, UK.

Garosi, L. and Lowrie, M. (2013) The neurological examination. In: Platt, S. and Olby, N. (eds) *BSAVA Manual of Canine and Feline Neurology*, 4th edn. BSAVA, Gloucester, UK.

Heinrich, C. (2014) Ophthalmic examination In: Gould, D. and McLellan, G. (eds) *BSAVA Manual of Canine and Feline Ophthalmology*, 3rd edn. BSAVA, Gloucester, UK.

Clinical Skills Sheet

12.28. Cranial nerves examination

	Method
1	**Pick up a form** • Good clinical practice.

2	**Observe**
	• Facial symmetry, CN **Facial (VII)**
	   ○ Observe for any droopy eyelid, ear, lips and nostrils size.
	• Head tilt, **Vestibular (VIII)**
	   ○ Observe for rotation of the head on its axis.

3	**Olfaction**
	CN **Olfactory (I)**
	• Test ability of the animal to smell, using food.
	   ○ Should cover the eyes.
	   ○ Do not use irritants (i.e. alcohol); these will stimulate the sensory receptor of the trigeminal nerve.

4	**Vision** CN **Optic (II)** • Dropping cotton balls (tests eye movements as well, see below). ○ Normal reaction expected is eye and head will follow the cotton ball.

5	**Menace**
	CN **Optic (II)** and **Facial (VII)**
	• Gently move the hand towards the eye.
	   ○ Normal reaction is blinking, present in animals over 4 months of age.
	   ○ It is possible to test medial lateral visual fields by covering one eye.

6	**Check pupil size** CN **Oculomotor (III)** and **Sympathetic (Horner's)** • In a dark room, at arm's distance with the pen light behind your eyes, shine in both the animal's eyes and look at both pupils 'retro-illuminated' by the reflection of the tapetum. ○ Do not use a strong light, to avoid pupil contraction.
7	**Pupillary light reflex (PLR)** CN **Optic (II)** and **Oculomotor (III)** • Shine the pen light in one eye. • Repeat on the opposite side. ○ Normal response is brisk contraction of the pupil.
8	**Consensual** PLR CN **Optic (II)** and **Oculomotor (III)** • While performing the direct PLR, look at the contra-lateral eye. ○ Normal response will be contraction of the pupil.
9	**Check strabismus** CN **Oculomotor (III), Troclear (IV)** and **Abducent (VI)** ± **Vestibular (VIII)** • Observe the eye position in normal horizontal position of the head. • Then move the head upwards (vestibular stimulation VIII). ○ Check if both eyes are in the same position.

Method

10	**Positional nystagmus**
	CN **Oculomotor (III), Troclear (IV) Abducent (VI)** and **Vestibular (VIII)**
	• Move the head upwards.
	  ○ This will stimulate the vestibular system.
	  ○ Normally the eye should follow the head; and once the head has stopped, the eye movements should stop too.

11	**Oculovestibular (oculocephalic) response** CN **Oculomotor (III), Troclear (IV) Abducent (VI)** and **Vestibular (VIII)** • Move the head side to side and observe the eyes' movements. ○ The eyes should follow the head with a jerky movement similar to the nystagmus.

12	**Facial sensation**
	CN **Trigeminal (V)**
	• Ophthalmic branches
	  ○ Touch the nasal septum with forceps as a test of sensory awareness
	• Maxillary branch
	  ○ Pinch the upper lip.
	• Mandibular branch
	  ○ Pinch lower lip.
	  ○ The reaction expected is the animal moving the head away from the stimulus.

13	**Palpebral reflex** CN **Trigeminal (V)** ophthalmic/maxillary branches and **Facial (VII)** • Tap the medial (ophthalmic) and lateral (maxillary) cantus. ○ Observe the blinking.
14	**Corneal reflex** CN **Trigeminal (V)** (ophthalmic branch) and **Abducent (VI)** ± **Facial (VII)** • Touch the cornea with a clean and moist cotton bud. ○ The reaction expected is retraction of the eye bulb, the third eyelid comes across and in some cases the animal blinks.
15	**Temporal muscle mass** CN **Trigeminal (V)** • Palpate the muscle of the head. ○ Check for asymmetry and muscle wastage.
	The following three tests can be performed in one action:
16	**Jaw tone** CN **Trigeminal (V)** Mandibular branch • Open the jaw. ○ Test for the resistance.

17	**Swallowing gag reflex**
	CN **Glossopharyngeal (IX)** and **Vagus (X)**
	• Stimulates the pharyngeal mucosa.
	  ○ Look for gag action (elevation of the palate and contraction of the pharyngeal muscles).
	  ○ Ideally test right and left.
	• Alternatively, in case of aggressive animals the pharyngeal region dorsal to the pharynx can be palpated externally.

18	**Tongue**
	CN **Hypoglossal XII**
	• Observe for:
	  ○ Symmetry, atrophy, deviations and movements.
	  ○ In some cases the tongue can be pulled out (more in large animals).

© RVC

Clinical Skills Sheet

12.29. Ophthalmology practical: eye examination

Method

During this ophthalmology practice, you will perform a complete eye exam on your dog. *You are responsible for the welfare of your dog.* Therefore, do not place it on the table unless one person acts as a 'back-stop' and another is suitably restraining the dog. If unsure or you have any concerns, please ask a member of staff present.

Please perform each test/examination in the order set out below.

You should have:
- a light source (pen torch).
- a dioptic lens.
- an ophthalmoscope.
- an examination sheet and pen.

Complete the examination sheet provided where possible to indicate test results or abnormal findings.

---

1. Examine both eyes from a distance *first* and consider the following (2 minutes)
- Pupil size and symmetry – be aware of the shape, size.
- Relationship of the globe to the orbit and eyelids and its relationship to the other globe:
  - Is the eye small, normal, or enlarged?
  - Is the eye protruding (exophthalmos) or sunken (enophthalmos)?
  - Can you see the eyelid margin? Are the lids turned in towards globe (entropion), or turned out away from globe (ectropion)?
- Periorbital swelling?
- Squinting/blinking? May indicate evidence of pain or discomfort.
- Ocular discharge? Note presence and nature.

---

2. Record each of the following four ocular reflexes (5 minutes)

(1) Pupillary light reflex *(tests: CN II and III)*

Direct

Shine a bright light into the eye. Pupil constriction indicates a normal response.

Indirect

Shine the light in the right eye. When the pupil constricts, *quickly* swing the light to the left eye. If the left pupil is in a constricted state, this is a normal response; the left pupil may constrict more in response to the direct light.

(2) Menace response *(tests: CN II and VII, visual cortex)*

Make a menacing gesture with the hand towards the eye, taking care not to touch the vibrissae or cause excessive facial currents, which may induce a false positive result. Blinking or moving the head away indicates a normal response.

(3) Dazzle reflex *(tests: CN II and VII (rostral colliculus and orbicularis oculi muscle) – subcortical reflex)*

Shine bright focal light source into each eye. Blinking or squinting indicates a normal response.

(4) Palpebral reflex *(tests: CN V and VII)*

Gently touch medial then lateral canthus. A blink reflex is a normal response.

---

3. Examine each of the following structures (10 minutes)

Complete the exam in one eye before moving on to the other eye. Note any abnormalities on exam sheet.
- Eyelids.
- Nictitating membrane/third eyelid – gently depress the globe with your index finger to see the third eyelid.
- Conjunctiva – bulbar and palpebral.
- Cornea.
- Anterior chamber – shine light from the front but look into chamber from the side.
- Iris.

Method

4. Examine the lens (2 minutes)

To examine right eye:

- Hold penlight at arm's length in right hand.
- Shine through dilated pupil in order to elicit a bright tapetal reflection.
- Use your left hand to hold upper eyelid open.
- Note any opacities in what should otherwise be a clear lens.

5. Fundic exam (any remaining time)

Indirect ophthalmoscopy with pen torch + indirect (dioptic) lens

To examine right eye:

With penlight in your **right** hand, illuminate tapetum (as for lens exam above).

- Hold the indirect lens in your left hand between thumb and forefinger and rest the remaining fingers of the left hand on superior orbital rim.
- Maintaining contact with the dog, turn left wrist to bring lens into the path of light approximately 5 cm in front of the cornea.
- Maintain lens in an upright position.
- If light and lens are in the correct position, you will see the fundus.

If time allows:

Direct ophthalmoscopy, with pen torch or ophthalmoscope

To examine the right eye:

- Turn dial to 0.
- Select large circle of white light.
- Hold ophthalmoscope up to your right eye, arm's length away from animal.
- Shine light to see a good tapetal reflection.
- Whilst maintaining a good fundic reflection, move to within 2–3 cm of the animal's right eye.

© RVC

Clinical Skills Sheet

12.30. Assessing urinary output in a catheterized patient

Task:

Aseptically drain a urinary bag, calculate the output and assess whether it is low, normal or high.

Method
Equipment: • Hand rub. • Gloves. • Spirit swab. • Measuring receptacle.
Wash hands or use hand rub.
Wear gloves.
Swab end of urine bag drain and tap with spirit swab. 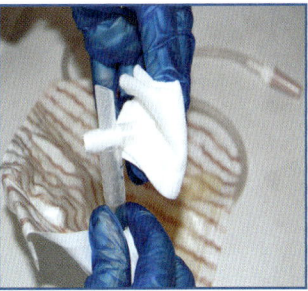
Slide the white tap sideways and empty contents of bag into appropriately sized measuring jug. Measurement should be as precise as possible, so this urine may be condensed into a smaller receptacle for accuracy. 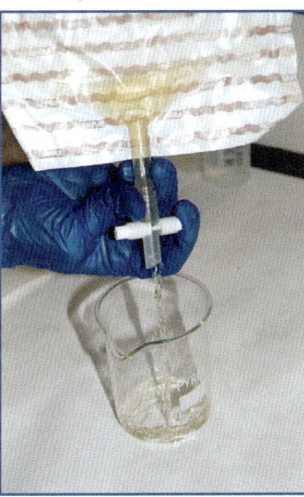 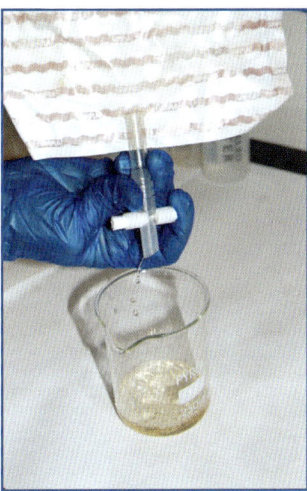

Method
Swab end of urine bag drain again and close the tap. 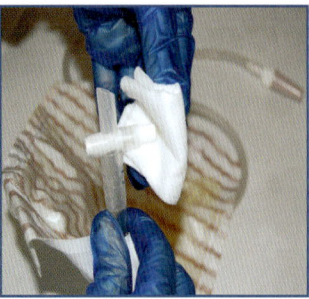
Calculate urine output.
Normal urinary output for well hydrated cats and dogs (including those on intravenous fluid therapy) is **1–2 ml/kg/h**[*]. Normal urinary output for rabbits ranges from **0.8 to 10.4 ml /kg /h**. However, **the average is around 5.5 ml/kg/h**[**].   [*]Cooper, B., Mullineaux, E. and Turner, L. (eds) *BSAVA Textbook of Veterinary Nursing*, 5th edition. BSAVA, Gloucester, UK.   [**]Harcourt-Brown, F.M. (2002) *Textbook of Rabbit Medicine*. Butterworth-Heinemann, Oxford, UK.

© RVC

Clinical Skills Sheet

12.31. Catheterizing a limb

Task:

Select the equipment and catheterize the dog's cephalic vein in preparation for administering intravenous fluids. Note: you can assume that the area over the vein has already been clipped to remove the fur and cleansed.

Method
Select and collect all of the following equipment *before* continuing: • Scissors.   • 3 strips of 2.5 cm wide × 40 cm long elastoplast-type securing tape, e.g. eband.   • Bandaging material – 5 cm wide Orthoband and a conforming bandage (e.g. Knit-fix or *red* cohesive bandage).   • T-connector – flushed with hep-saline.   • 5 ml syringe filled with hep-saline.   • Intravenous catheter – size 18/20 gauge.
Wash your hands.
Open the catheter packet but leave the catheter inside at this stage.
Ask your assistant to restrain the patient and raise the vein.
Remove the catheter from the packet (do not touch any part of the needle).
Using your left hand, immobilize the vein by stretching the skin between the thumb and fingers.
Position your thumb so that it is just lateral to the vein to help stabilize the vein.   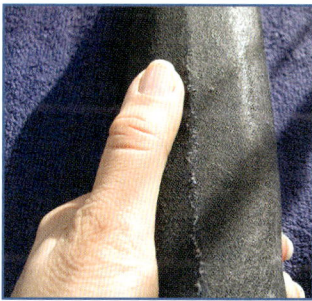
Holding the catheter in right your hand, insert the needle through the skin at a 20–30° angle, bevel facing upwards.   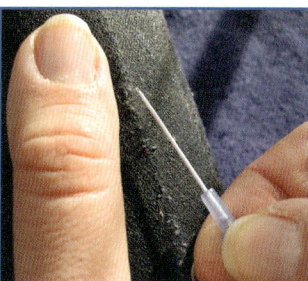

Method
Advance the catheter one-third way into the vein – blood should appear in the hub when it enters the vein. 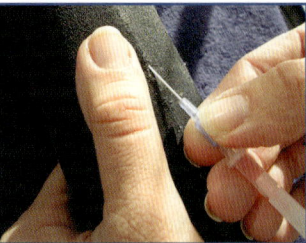
Stabilize the stylet hub with your left hand. 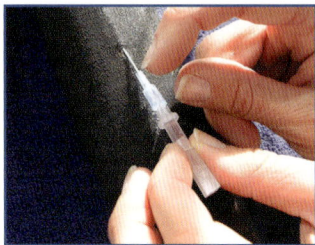
With your right hand, gently slide and advance the catheter into the vein.
Observe to ensure blood is still flowing freely from the catheter hub.
Continue holding the catheter in place to prevent dislodgement.
Ask your assistant to stop raising the vein and move your thumb over the skin over the catheter to help reduce blood flow.
Remove the catheter stylet.
Attach pre-filled T-connector.
Secure the catheter with tape appropriately:
1st strip placed *underneath* the catheter and then wrapped over the skin insertion site and the catheter hub.
2nd strip placed under the T-connector and wrapped around the limb and over the T-connector.
Loop made in the T-connector tubing and a 3rd strip placed to secure the loop in place. 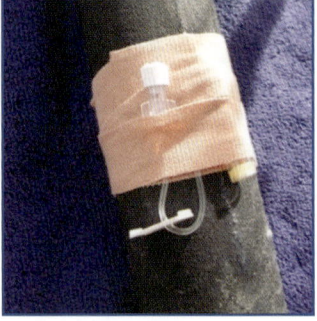
Flush catheter with a small quantity of hep-saline through the injection port – drawing back first to make sure blood appears in the needle.
Apply a final bandage layer over the catheter and connector (if available, use *red* cohesive).

Method
Question: For up to how many days may this catheter be left in if there are no problems?
Answer: 3 days.

Please note:

- When you are subsequently connecting your fluid line to the T-connector, *do not* swab the connection point of the T-connector; this would, in effect, break sterility.

- You should only swab – with a sterile swab (or swab and surgical spirit) – the injection port when using it to administer drugs or check for patency.

© RVC

Clinical Skills Sheet

12.32. Setting up intravenous fluids

Task:

Using the most appropriate equipment available, collect and set up all the equipment/materials required to administer intravenous fluids to an acidotic 24 kg dog.

Method
Select and collect all of the following equipment *before* continuing:
Gauze swabs (cotton wool if swabs unavailable). Or alternative sterile swabs, e.g. 'sterettes'. 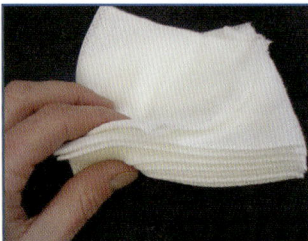
Scrub solution and isopropyl alcohol.
Scissors.
3 strips of 2.5 cm securing tape × 30–40 cm long. 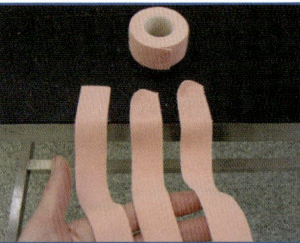
Bandaging material, e.g. 'Soffban' and a conforming bandage. The conforming bandage may be replaced with a light cohesive-type bandage, e.g. 'Vetrap'. *This is usually red if the catheter is completely bandaged over as a warning that there is an in-dwelling catheter in place.* 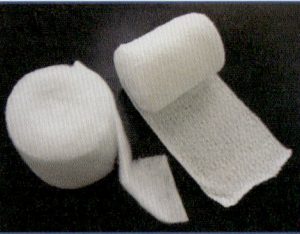

Method
T-connector flushed with hep-saline. 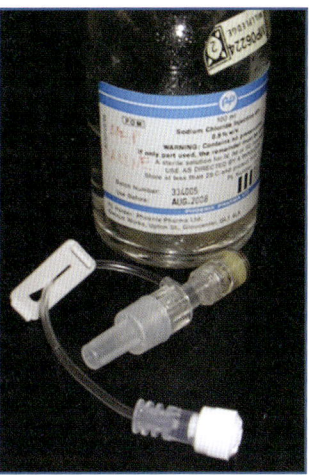
5 ml syringe hep-saline.
Intravenous catheter – 18 (green) or 20 (pink) gauge (for this size of dog). 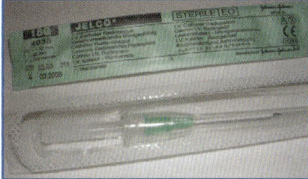
Administration set – 20 drops/ml.
1 l compound sodium lactate 'Hartmann's'. 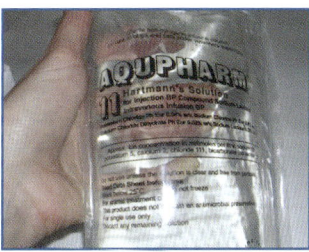
Wash hands – or use hand rub.
Check date and contents of the bag of fluids (for leakage, particles, cloudiness). Work out your drip rate (see CSC sheet on this).
Remove the outer bag. 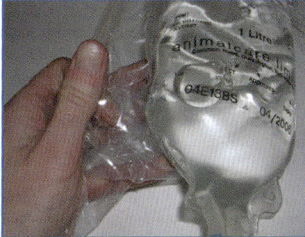
Hook the bag on to the drip stand.

Method

Remove the tag over the administration port.

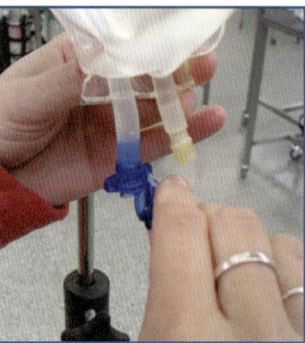

Remove the administration set from the outer packaging.

Close the flow control clamp fully.

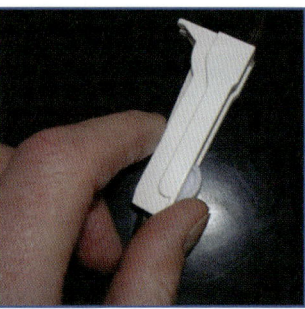

Remove the protective cover from the spike of the administration set.

Taking great care not to touch the spike of the administration set, insert it into the bag of fluids by pushing and twisting until it is fully inserted.

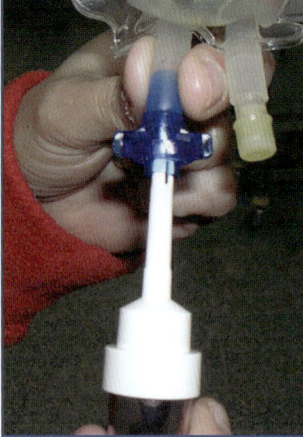

Method
Squeeze drip chamber and allow to half fill. 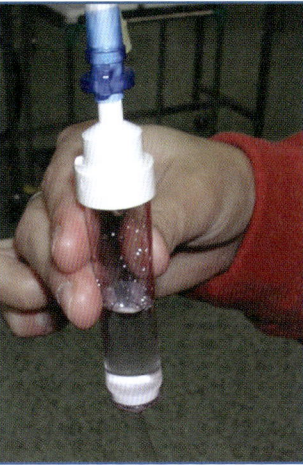
Partially open the flow control clamp and fill the drip line – *in a controlled manner without spilling any fluid*. (Have a kidney dish to hand in case you do have to run any fluids through; it is more important that you make sure there aren't any *air bubbles* in the line. You can then draw up the spilt fluids into a syringe and take them out of the calculation.) 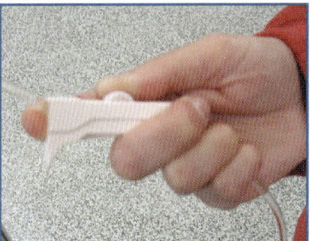
Ensure there are no air bubbles in the line – this cannot be stressed enough!
Close the flow control clamp and hook the line over the drip stand.
Maintain sterility of the administration set throughout.
Question: What are the main electrolytes in this solution? **Answer:** Sodium, chloride, bicarbonate and potassium.
Question: Give four common causes for the flow of fluids to stop unexpectedly. **Answer:** • Patient flexing elbow. • Tubes kinking. • Blood clot in catheter. • Empty bag.

Very important note:
When connecting the drip line to the catheter/T-connector you have placed (see SS 12.31, Catheterizing a limb), you should *only* sterilely swab the *injection port* of the T-connector *before* you flush it through with hep-saline solution.
You do *not* need to swab the T-connector port before you attach the drip line. *To do so would break sterility*.

© RVC

Principles of Small Animal Bandaging

13

Alison Langridge
The Royal Veterinary College, London

Learning objectives

By the end of this chapter, students should be able to:

- Identify different layers of a bandage.
- Understand the principles of safe practice whilst applying dressings or bandages.
- Identify different types of dressings and their use.
- Identify risk factors for iatrogenic injuries.
- Apply a safe, effective bandage to a small animal.

Clinical skills sheets (SS)

Four clinical skills sheets will be used in this chapter and these can be found at pages 194–202 and 241–245. Reference will be made to each skills sheet at the relevant section within the chapter. The details of the clinical skills sheets used are as follows:

SS 13.33 Applying a canine forelimb bandage
SS 13.34 Applying a canine chest drain bandage
SS 13.35 Applying an ear bandage
SS 15.40 Applying a lower-limb protective bandage on a horse

Videos (V)

One video will be used in this chapter to demonstrate how to perform the clinical skill:

V 13.1 Ear bandage

Health and Safety key points

Good hygiene and common sense are essential when applying dressings and bandaging. You must ensure that:

- The patient is safely, comfortably and appropriately restrained. Remember that the patient may be in pain, so be mindful of this and try to work with comfortable positions for them.
- Prepare the wound site appropriately, ensuring that the wound is not contaminated, it is clean and that the surrounding skin is dry.
- Collect all bandaging materials and necessary equipment before you start and place in a clean receptacle (such as a clean litter tray or trug).
- Wash hands or, if hands are already clean, use alcoholic hand gel.
- Open dressing pack aseptically and apply in aseptic manner.
- Do not use the dressing if contaminated in any way.
- Check each layer of bandaging *before* applying the next layer. Monitor the tension throughout.

Introduction

Bandages and dressings are frequently applied for a range of injuries and conditions. The most important consideration is that the patient benefits from the application and that they are comfortable.

© CAB International 2018. *Veterinary Clinical Skills Manual* (eds N. Coombes and A. Silva-Fletcher)

A bandage that is incorrectly applied can often lead to patient interference, as it may be too tight. The first remedial action when patients are interfering with their bandages should always be to investigate the bandage. It should *not* be the placement of an Elizabethan collar, punishment, bitter spray or chemical restraint.

It is important to remember that bandages and dressings are two different things. There are also many different uses for the different dressings; one size does not fit all.

13.1 What is a Wound Care Dressing?

A dressing is used to help a wound to heal and help to prevent further complications such as infection or dehiscence. Dressings should be handled aseptically, as they are designed to be in direct contact with the wound. This distinguishes them from bandages, which are layers that hold the dressing in place and do not have to be aseptically handled, though hands should be clean.

The two terms are often used interchangeably by veterinary staff and although dressings are used as the first layer of a bandage, it is important that the differences are made clear to students.

13.1.1 Dressings

Dressings serve a variety of purposes, depending on the type, severity and position of the wound (Table 13.1). Aside from the major function of reducing the risk of infection, dressings play a vital role in:

- Arresting haemorrhage whilst minimizing the introduction of further infection.
- Absorbing any exudate such as blood, serous fluid or pus.
- Wound debridement.
- The commencement of the healing process.

13.1.2 Bandages

Bandages consist of four layers and it is important that the student understands the action of each layer in order to prevent an iatrogenic injury.

 Never tear bandage material, as this will cause unwanted tension to the bandage. Always use scissors to cut.

 Key points about how to avoid iatrogenic injuries

Iatrogenic injuries are not uncommon and are most often created by one or more (and often all) of the following factors:

- Poor wound handling prior to dressing.
- Inappropriate selection of dressings.
- Inappropriate handling of dressings prior to application.
- Inadequate padding.
- Inadequate protection of vulnerable areas such as joints.
- Poor application of bandage layers, most commonly by using too much pressure, uneven pressure and/or by leaving gaps between the layers.
- Ill-judgement or laziness regarding how often the dressings should be changed and the bandage checked.
- Poor home-care advice for clients.

It may be helpful to provide students with instructions in the practice area, to remind them of the components of good wound management and bandaging technique (Table 13.2).

13.2 Protecting Bony Prominences

Homemade 'doughnuts' (Fig. 13.1) are simple to make from cotton wool and padding materials, and are hugely effective at protecting vulnerable areas from pressure sores. They are applied directly over the area to be protected, most commonly a bony prominence such as an elbow or hock, and are incorporated into the bandage with the primary layer.

13.3 Advanced bandages

There are advanced bandage techniques such as the Robert Jones bandage or haemostatic pressure bandages. These methods are not considered as Day One skills and are not described here. However, if students wish to practise these skills, it should be under the supervision of a member of staff who can critique the bandage throughout the process and give relevant advice.

It is most important that students understand the principles of bandage application, how to recognize a poor application and how to avoid iatrogenic injury.

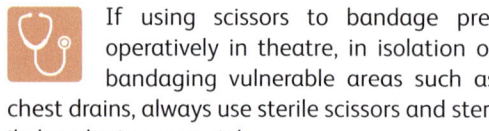

If using scissors to bandage pre-operatively in theatre, in isolation or bandaging vulnerable areas such as chest drains, always use sterile scissors and sterile bandaging material.

13.4 Applying a bandage to a small animal

Effective wound management in small animals depends on accurate assessment of the site, size and nature of the wound. The most important to consider here is the patient and the wound: it is important to

Table 13.1. Types of common impregnated dressings used in veterinary wound management.

Type	Description
Hydrocolloid	Hydrocolloid dressings are used on burns, light to moderately draining wounds, necrotic wounds, under compression wraps, pressure ulcers and venous ulcers
Hydrogel	This type of dressing is for wounds with little to no excess fluid, painful wounds, necrotic wounds, pressure ulcers, donor sites, second-degree or higher burns and infected wounds
Alginate	Alginate dressings are used for moderate to high amounts of wound drainage, decubitus ulcers and to pack wounds
Collagen	A collagen dressing can be used for chronic wounds, ulcers, surgical wounds, burns and wounds with large surface areas
Manuka honey	A light net dressing coated with Manuka honey. Has excellent antibacterial properties. Most useful in the granulation/epithelialization stage of wound healing and can be used on any wound type
Silver antimicrobial	There are many dressings that contain antimicrobial silver preparation. The type of dressing that is used should be tailored to the wound and needs to be in direct contact with the wound bed. Flamazine is a commonly used and highly effective silver sulphadiazine preparation that can be used in burn cases or for wounds that may be in areas of the body that are difficult or impossible to apply a dressing to

Table 13.2. Details of the different layers in bandaging a wound.

Layer	Action	Appearance
Contact layer (often referred to as the 'dressing' layer)	Sterile dressing, which is in immediate contact with the wound	Varies but should be in sterile packs that are in-date
Primary layer (sometimes referred to as the intermediate padding layer)	Holds the dressing in place Provides padding and support	Cotton wool or a soft padded roll
Secondary layer (often referred to as the conforming layer)	Provides support and some light pressure in order to keep the primary and contact layers *in situ*	A mesh appearance, often with elasticity
Tertiary layer (often referred to as the top or protective layer)	Provides protection	A springy, rough surface texture in a variety of colours

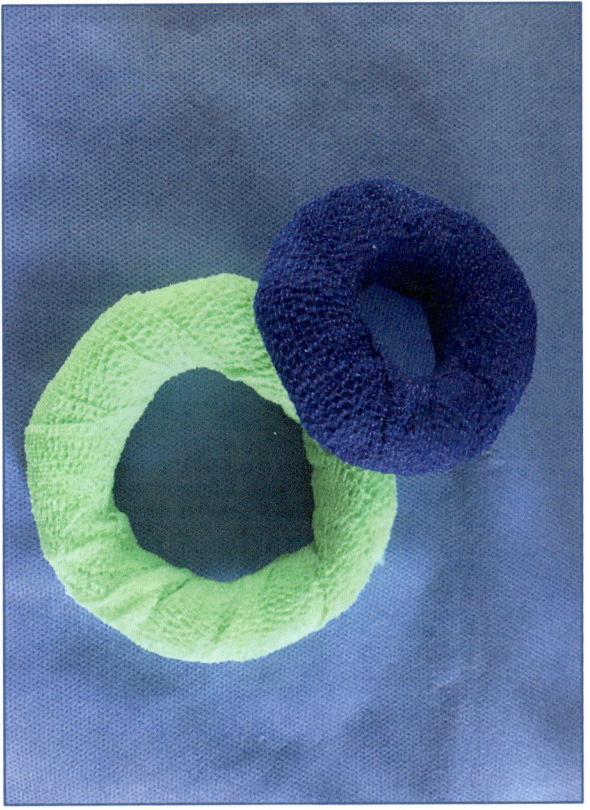

Fig. 13.1. Homemade 'doughnuts'.

think about the individual patient whilst bandaging, rather than seeing the bandaging as being a 'blanket' technique that is easy and requires little thought. Limbs are relatively easy places to apply a bandage, as there is a natural contour.

 SS 13.33 Go through the clinical skills sheet on canine forelimb bandage that describes the indications for use and the method in detail

SS 13.34 To apply a bandage to the main body of an animal compared to a limb, different points must be taken to account. The clinical skills sheet on chest drain bandage offers guidance on how to bandage a chest drain

SS 13.35 Another common site of injury where a bandage is required in a small animal is the ear. Further details are given on the clinical skills sheet

SS 15.40 Applying a lower-limb protective bandage to an equid. This technique is slightly different so students need to be aware of the difference

 V 13.1 The video on ear bandage demonstrates the procedure; for detailed guidance please watch this video

V 13.1 video.cabi.org/bkmvv

Further Reading: Calder, C. (2014) Gold-standard bandaging. *Veterinary Nursing Journal* 29(6), 198–202.

Lima, A., Mesquita, J., Mega, A.J. and Nobrega, C. (2011) How to apply a foot bandage. *The Veterinary Nurse* 2(8), 476–479.

Pritchard, P. (2015) The nurse's role in the management of equine limb wounds. *The Veterinary Nurse* 6(2), 90–93.

Clinical Skills Sheet

13.33. Applying a canine forelimb bandage

Task:

Apply an appropriate bandage to the patient's left forelimb following surgical repair of a minor wound on the dorsal aspect of the limb.

Indications for use:

- First-aid treatment for the control of limb/foot haemorrhage (e.g. cut pad).
- Postoperative limb/foot support following a surgical procedure.
- Light dressing for anchoring intravenous fluids.
- Protection of a limb/foot wound from patient interference.

Method
Select and prepare (unwrap) all the equipment and materials required: • Scissors. • Dressing material (e.g. Melolin, Zorbopad, Rondopad). • Padding layer (e.g. Orthoband). • Conforming layer (e.g. Knitfix). • Protective outer layer (e.g. Vetrap). 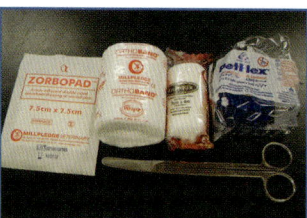
Position the patient into lateral recumbency with the affected limb uppermost and ask an assistant to support the limb to facilitate bandaging.
Wash your hands or use alcoholic hand rub.
If a wound is present, cover this with a sterile, absorbent, non-adhesive dressing (e.g. Melolin). If applicable, ensure that the shiny side is placed down over the wound.
Apply interdigital padding between the toes using strips of cotton wool. If this is not available, alternative padding material (such as Soffban) will suffice. 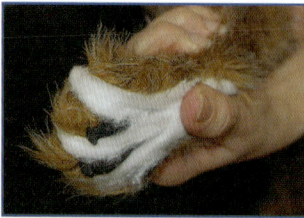

Method
Select the padding layer (e.g. Soffban). Apply the padding layer over the paw covering the dorsal and palmar area.   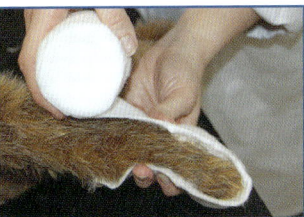
Once these two aspects of the paw are covered, twist the bandage to cover both the medial and lateral surfaces of the paw.   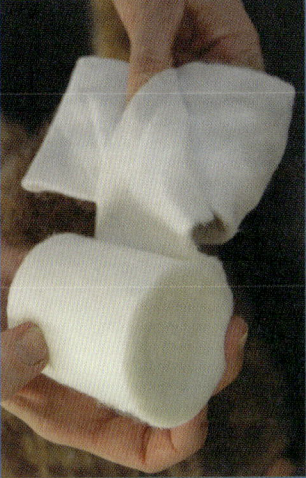
Once the paw is fully enclosed, continue up the limb, working from distal to proximal, spiralling up the leg in a neat and even manner.
For ease of application, ensure that the bandage material is kept uppermost during application.   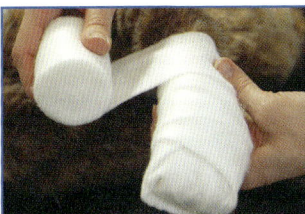
Continue up to and include the next joint (carpus or elbow).
Repeat this for the conforming and cohesive layers.
Check suitable tension of the bandage (i.e. not too loose or too tight).

Method
Check the bandage is neat (e.g. no pieces of padding showing). 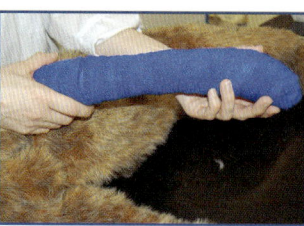

Question:

What pieces of advice should you give to the owner of this patient regarding care of the bandage?

Answer:

Protect from wet and dirt by covering when out; prevent patient interfering with bandage (Elizabethan collar if necessary); return as advised for removal/change; observe for evidence of: movement, bad odour, sores, discharge.

© RVC

Clinical Skills Sheet

13.34. Applying a canine chest drain bandage

Task:

Apply a thoracic bandage around an indwelling chest drain.

Indications for use:

- To provide stability for the drain.
- To maintain asepsis of the surgical site.
- To prevent injury and infection from self trauma.

Method

Select and prepare all the materials required :
- Sterile dressing scissors.
- Non-sterile gloves.
- Primary dressing (e.g. Melolin, Rondopad, Alleveyn).
- Padding layer (e.g. Orthoband).
- Conforming layer (e.g. Knitfix).
- Outer layer (e.g. Easifix, Vetrap).

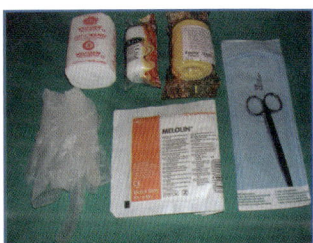

- Wash your hands thoroughly or put on non-sterile gloves.
- Open the sterile scissor pack aseptically.
- Remove the dressing pad in an aseptic manner.
- Fold the dressing in half with contact sides together, cut a small arc along the fold then open the dressing and cut a straight line up from one edge to the hole. This will allow you to place the dressing around the drain.

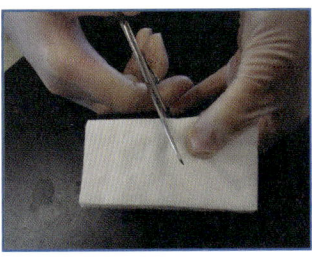
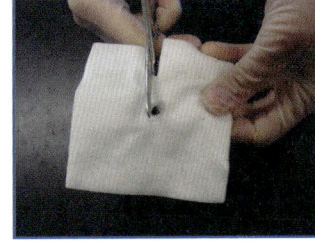
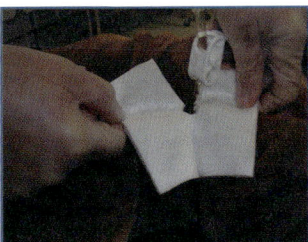
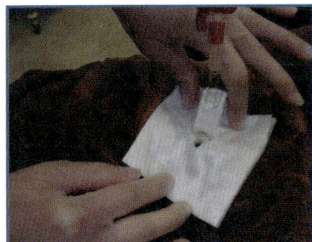

Method

- Secure the opening with a small strip of Elastoplast or Micropore.
- Select an appropriate size of padding material and apply to the thorax in a figure-of-eight around the forelimbs. The important points are that:
    - the correct size of padding is used;
    - there are at least two layers of padding on all aspects of the bandage;
    - there is a criss-cross pattern on the back of the neck and across the cranial chest to distribute the tension and avoid putting any pressure on the throat (the bandage should never encircle the neck);
    - there is adequate padding coverage in the axillae; and
    - there should be no gaps in the padding layer.

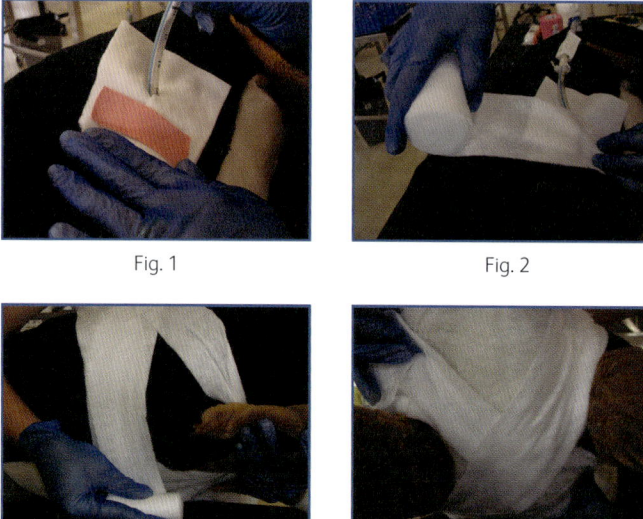

Fig. 1   Fig. 2

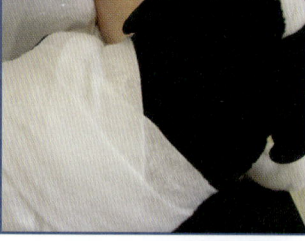
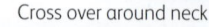

Fig.3

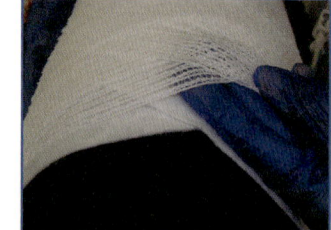
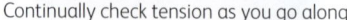

Fig. 4 Crisscross over sternum

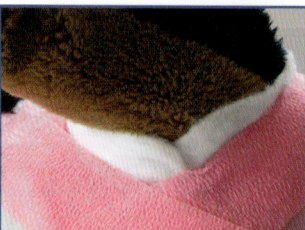
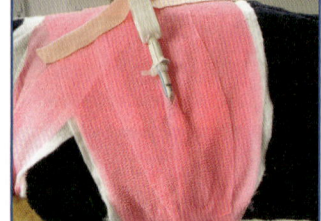

Cross over around neck   Continually check tension as you go along

Check Vetrap is not on fur or skin, especially in axillae

- Repeat this pattern with a layer of conforming bandage (Knitfix) and a layer of cohesive bandage (Vetrap). Remember to release the tension in the Vetrap before placing.
- Check all around the bandage to ensure it is not too tight and not restricting breathing or movement.
- Tape the drain against the chest using Elastoplast. Ensure there are no kinks and no potential to become kinked.

Method

Important considerations:

- The incorrect size of dressing materials will give a poor bandage.
- The bandage should not be ruched – it will be uncomfortable for the patient.
- Conforming or cohesive dressings should never be resting directly on the fur or skin.
- Check the tension of the bandage continually as you go along and consider the vital structures in your bandage area.
- Wet and soiled dressings should always be changed promptly.
- RELEASE THE TENSION in the Vetrap before placing it on the patient. It should mould on to the animal – if it bunches up there is still tension in it.

© RVC

Clinical Skills Sheet

13.35. Applying an ear bandage

Task :

Apply a bandage to the patient's left ear pinna following surgery to repair an aural haematoma.

Indications for use :

- As a first-aid measure to control haemorrhage from the ear pinnae following injury.
- To control haemorrhage post-operatively following aural surgery.

Method
Select and prepare (unwrap) all the equipment and materials required: • Scissors. • Dressing (e.g. Melolin). • Cotton wool. • Padding layer (e.g. Orthoband). • Conforming layer (e.g. Knitfix). • Protective outer layer (e.g. Vetrap). • Permanent marker pen. 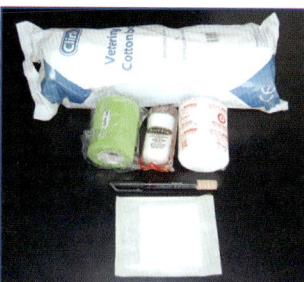
Position the patient into sternal recumbency (conscious patient) or lateral recumbency (anaesthetized or sedated patient).
Ask an assistant to support the head.
If a wound is present, cover this with a sterile, absorbent, non-adhesive dressing (e.g. Melolin). If applicable, ensure that the shiny side is placed downwards over the wound. 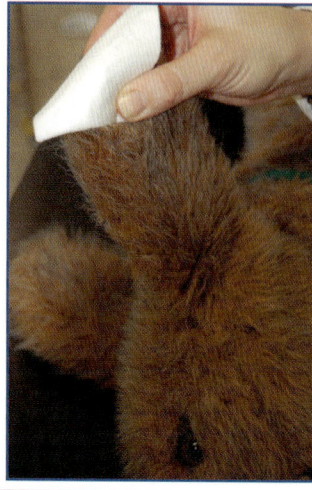

Method
Apply the dressing in a sterile manner, i.e. touching it only at the edges.
Place a wedge of padding on top of the head.
Fold the affected ear pinna up on to the padding.
Cover the ear with further padding. 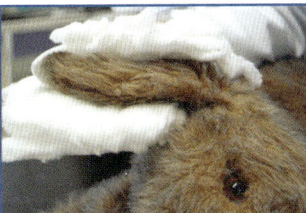
Apply a layer of synthetic padding material (e.g. Soffban) in a figure-of-eight pattern around the head with the unaffected ear left exposed. 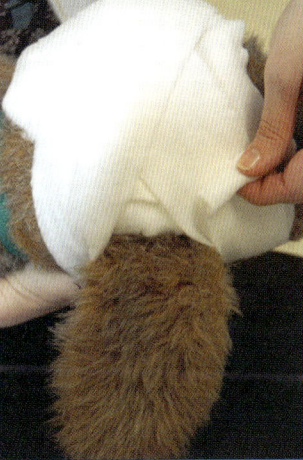
For ease of application, ensure that the bandage material is kept uppermost during application. 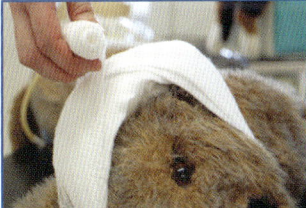
Apply conforming bandage in a figure-of-eight fashion, taking care to check the tension.
Apply protective layer in a figure-of-eight fashion. 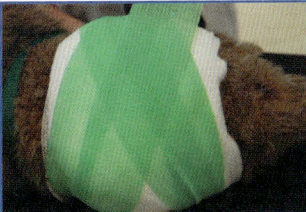

Method
Use a marker pen to indicate on the outer layer the position of the pinna. 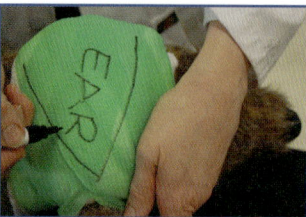
Check that the eyes are not covered by the bandage. 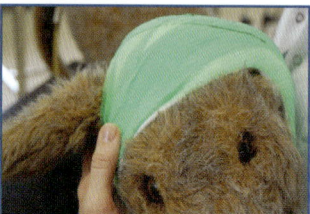
Check that the patient can still open its mouth fully.
Check suitable tension of the bandage (i.e. not too loose or too tight) and ensure that the airway is not restricted. 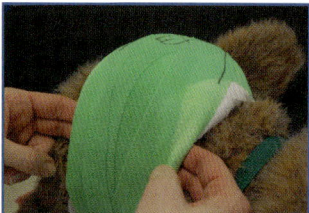 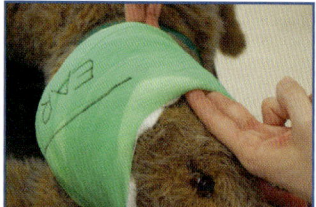
Check that the bandage is neat (i.e. no pieces of padding showing).
Question: Why is it important to mark the position of the ear pinna on the outer layer of the bandage?
Answer: To avoid cutting through the ear pinna when the bandage is removed.

© RVC

14 Pharmacy

Hilary Orpet

The Royal Veterinary College, London

Learning objectives

By the end of this chapter, students should be able to:

- Identify the relevant legislation and guidelines associated with storage and dispensing of veterinary medication.
- Utilize relevant legislation and prepare a written prescription for veterinary drugs.
- Interpret written prescriptions or drug orders and calculate the required dose.
- Handle medications safely to reduce risk of accidental injection, absorption or ingestion.
- Dispose of medication according to relevant legislation and guidelines.
- Dispose of equipment used in the administration of medication according to relevant legislation and guidelines.

Introduction

Most veterinary practices dispense medication from their own pharmacy, despite the increase of online veterinary pharmacies. It is essential that all veterinary professionals are aware of the relevant legislation with regard to storing and dispensing veterinary medications. In addition, accurately calculating doses can ensure good welfare of the animals in our care. There are potential health and safety risks in handling medications licensed for animal use, and care must be taken to avoid accidental injection, absorption or ingestion.

There are various online sources of information regarding veterinary pharmaceuticals and some of these are suggested at the end of this chapter; they are cross-referenced in the main text as, for example: '*(online: Government guidance)*'.

14.1 Relevant Legislation

The Veterinary Medicines Directorate (VMD) is a government body under the Department for Environment, Food and Rural Affairs (DEFRA). It sets out to protect public health, animal health and the environment and to promote animal welfare by assuring the safety, quality and efficacy of veterinary medicines in the UK.

Since new legislation in 2005, veterinary medicines have been considered separately from the Medicines Act 1968 and there are revisions from a European directive. The Veterinary Medicines Regulations (VMR) (SI No 2745) first came into force on 30 October 2005 and are updated annually.

Thus the main legislation that now covers the storage, handling, use and supply of veterinary medicinal products (VMPs) in veterinary practice is:

- The Veterinary Medicines Regulations *(online: Government guidance)*.

Controlled drugs (CD) (see Section 14.7 below) are still covered by:

- The Misuse of Drugs Act 1971
  - The Misuse of Drugs Regulations 2001.
  - Misuse of Drugs (safe custody) Regulations 1973.

14.2 Registration of Premises

All premises from which VMPs are dispensed are required to be registered. As the Royal College of Veterinary Surgeons (RCVS) maintains a register of all veterinary practices as 'Registered Veterinary Practice Premises', this serves as a way of complying with the VMD requirements and ensuring there is traceability of controlled drugs, and that veterinary surgeons are compliant with the Veterinary Medicines Regulations *(online: RCVS advice)*.

© CAB International 2018. *Veterinary Clinical Skills Manual* (eds N. Coombes and A. Silva-Fletcher)

14.3 Health and Safety

Further legislation regarding the handling of medicines mainly concerns health and safety aspects:

- The Health & Safety at Work Act 1974.
- The Control of Substances Hazardous to Health Regulations 2002 (COSHH).
- Management of Health & Safety at Work Regulations 1999 (risk identification).

Drugs may enter the body in different ways:

- Absorption across the skin.
- Absorption across mucous membranes.
- Accidental ingestion.
- Inhalation.
- Accidental injection.

Data sheets should contain information regarding any hazards that may present to the operator *(online: NOAH)*. A COSHH assessment should be produced, especially for hazardous drugs (anaesthetic agents, chemotherapy drugs, controlled drugs). If common-sense rules are followed, there should be little danger of hazard to the health and safety of employees.

14.3.1 Safe handling

- Wear gloves when handling medication, to avoid self-absorption or any moisture affecting the tablet or capsule.
- When counting tablets, use the 'no-touch' method and a 'tablet counter' (if tablets are round). Counting the number of rows will give the total number of tablets.
- To avoid needle-stick injuries, keep the needle cap on at all times until injection.
- Never remove needle caps with teeth: drugs may be present on or in the cap.
- Avoid recapping needles – dispose of needles and syringes directly into the 'sharps' box.

14.3.2 Cytotoxic drugs

Take care when preparing cytotoxic drugs.

- Prepare and administer toxic drugs in well-ventilated and low-traffic areas.
- Wear correct protective clothing and equipment (face mask with eye protection or face mask and goggles, double gloves, apron).

- Administer through intravenous catheter to ensure that the drug enters the vein.
- Use incontinence sheets to prepare the drug on and administer; potential spills may be absorbed immediately.
- The incontinence sheets and equipment may then be disposed of in clinical waste bags. Double bag all waste.

14.4 Record Keeping, Stock Control and Storage

The practice may be visited by the VMD to check that accurate records are being kept and that the optimum conditions for storage are available. Always follow manufacturers' instructions on storing medications. Information may be found on the drug datasheet or the National Office of Animal Health (NOAH) website *(online: NOAH)* and a Summary of Product Characteristics (SPC) is available from the VMD database *(online: VMD)*.

Regular stock control ensures that there are no surplus stocks and that out-of-date drugs are disposed of promptly.

14.5 Disposal

Out-of-date drugs may be disposed of into DOOP (destruction of old pharmaceuticals) bins or, as they are now called, 'pharmaceutical waste' bins as a category of 'healthcare waste' (new term for 'clinical waste'), which are collected by licensed carriers of special waste. Further details of disposal of sharps, pharmaceuticals and cytotoxic drugs are given in Chapter 9. Full descriptions of colour coding for veterinary waste disposal facilities are available in the BSAVA Medicines Guide *(online: BSAVA)*.

14.5.1 Cytotoxic and carcinogenic drugs

If these need to be disposed of, they must be put in blue or purple rigid lockable plastic containers.

14.5.2 Controlled drugs

There are strict guidelines on the storage and disposal of controlled drugs *(online: RCVS Publications)*.

Additional sources of information that will help to shape the management of medicinal waste include:

- British Veterinary Association (BVA) Waste Guidelines.
- Department of Health guidance booklet *Safe Management of Healthcare Waste*.
- Special Waste Regulations 1996 and Collection and Disposal of Waste Regulations 1998.
- The practice's waste contractor's systems and processes.

14.6 Prescribing and Dispensing Categories

There are four main classes of veterinary medications (Table 14.1).

Further guidance is given by the RCVS *(online: RCVS advice)* and from the VMD *(online: Government guidance)*.

14.7 Controlled (Dangerous) Drugs

The Home Office has overall responsibility for controlled drugs and legislation that relates to both veterinary and human medicines *(online: Government guidance)*. Under the Misuse of Drugs Regulations 2001, controlled drugs are divided into five schedules (Table 14.2). Veterinary surgeons are permitted to prescribe from Schedules 2–5.

14.8 Prescribing Cascade

If there is no veterinary medicine authorized to be used for a specific condition, veterinary surgeons may use an off-label medication in order to treat the animal and avoid suffering. Detailed online guidance is available *(online: RCVS advice; BSAVA)*.

14.9 Dispensing and Labelling of Medicines

The Royal Pharmaceutical Society *(online: RPharmS)* suggests that medications repackaged from bulk containers should be in appropriate containers both for the product and for the user (Rock, 2007). Generally, loose tablets should be dispensed in child-proof tablet pots. Exceptions may be made in the case of elderly clients who find child-proof pots difficult to open. Drugs

Table 14.1. Details of prescribing categories.

Prescribing category	Prescribed by
POM-V (Prescription Only Medicines –Veterinary) Controlled Drugs (CD) are a sub-category of POM-Vs	May be prescribed and dispensed only by a **veterinary surgeon (VS)** and only for animals under their care *OR* by a pharmacist under the instruction of a veterinary prescription CDs may only be prescribed by a **VS**
POM-VPS (Veterinarian, Pharmacist and SQP)	Products supplied only by • **Veterinary Surgeons** • **Pharmacists** • **Suitably Qualified Persons (SQPs)** to animals under their care
NFA-VPS (Non-Food Animal – Veterinarian, Pharmacist or SQP)	Products supplied only by • **Veterinary Surgeons** • **Pharmacists** • **Suitably Qualified Persons (SQPs)** For use in non-food animals only Drugs used routinely to prevent or limit endemic disease in non-food animals
AVM-GSL (Authorized Veterinary Medicine – General Sales List)	Products may be supplied by any supermarket or pet shop

Table 14.2. The five schedules of controlled drugs and legislation.

Schedule	Examples	Controls
Schedule 1	Addictive drugs (e.g. cannabis, LSD, mescaline)	Possession requires Home Office licence Not routinely used in veterinary medicine
Schedule 2	Opiate analgesics (e.g. methadone, morphine, etorphine, pethidine, fentanyl and now also ketamine)	Drugs must be kept locked up and records kept of supply and use Must follow CD prescription writing requirements
Schedule 3	Barbiturates (e.g. pentobarbitone, phenobarbitone, opiate analgesics, e.g. buprenorphine, pentazocine, midazolam, tramadol)	Drugs must be kept locked up Records do not need to be kept Must follow CD prescription writing requirements
Schedule 4	Benzodiazepines (e.g. diazepam)	Do not need to be kept locked up or records kept Must still follow CD prescription writing requirements
Schedule 5	Certain preparations of cocaine, codeine and morphine that only contain small quantities of the drug (e.g. codeine cough linctus, kaolin and morphine suspension)	Do not need to be kept locked up or any records except invoices kept

should be kept in their original containers until they are dispensed. Package-insert leaflets should also be handed out with the drugs.

14.9.1 Labelling

The Medicines (Labelling) Regulations 1976 state that the label must be printed or written in indelible ink. All medicines that are dispensed should be clearly labelled and the label should not obscure any expiry date or other important information on the packaging (*online: BSAVA; Government publications*).

Legal requirements for a drug label (Fig. 14.1) include:

- owner's name and address of where the animal is kept.
- pet identification.
- date.
- name and address of veterinary surgeon/practice.
- 'For Animal Treatment Only'.
- 'Keep Out Of Reach Of Children'.
  As well As:

- quantity and strength and name of drug.
- dosing instructions.
  Additional information may include:

- 'For External Use Only'.
- 'WEAR GLOVES when handling drugs'.
- 'Give with food'.
- 'Give before food'.

> 12.7.17 Mr J Jones BVetMed MRCVS
> 20 High Street, Upnorth, Yorks
>
> Spotty Brown
> 2 Main Road, Upnorth, Yorks.
> 21 x Ceporex 250mg tablets
> Give one tablet twice daily for five days

Fig. 14.1. Example drug label.

14.10 Prescriptions

The veterinary surgeon may write out a prescription for an animal under their care. The client can then obtain the drug from any pharmacy.

The following must be on a legal prescription (Fig. 14.2):

- Name of veterinary surgeon (printed and signature) and qualification.
- Name and address of the practice (and tel. no.).
- Name and address of the owner.
- Name (and breed) of animal.
- Date (when prescription is written).
- Drug name and form (tablet, capsules, liquid).
- Strength of drug.
- Amount needed (in words and figures).
- Dosage instructions.
- 'For animal treatment only'.
- 'This animal is under my treatment'.
- 'Keep out of reach of children'.

Fig. 14.2. Example of a prescription.

> **Mr J Jones BVetMed MRCVS**
> **20 High Street**
> **Upnorth**
> **Yorks**
> **YO23 2NL Tel: 0123 456789**
>
> **Date**: *12th July 2017*
>
> **Owner**: *Mr Brown's dog 'Spotty'*
> **Address**: *2 Main Road, Upnorth, Yorks*
> **Patient**: *'Spotty'*
> **Species:** *Canine*
>
> R_x *Tablets - Amoxicillin 200mg Send 10 (ten)*
> Label: *Give one tablet twice daily for 5 days*
>
> This animal is under my care   Signed *J Jones* MRCVS

Key points:

- A prescription is needed for a POM-V or POM-VPS drug.
- It must be written in ink.
- It must be used within 6 months.

Prescriptions are legal documents. It is an offence to alter a prescription unless instructed by the prescriber. Misuse of a veterinary prescription may be reported to the VMD *(online: Government publications).*

14.10.1   Repeat prescriptions

The animal must be seen by the veterinary surgeon at least every 6 months for a health check-up before more medicines are issued. *All* repeat prescriptions must be checked with a veterinary surgeon.

14.10.2   Terms used in prescription writing

Many shorthand terms are used when writing up a patient's medication needs and these are often used on hospital charts and prescriptions (Table 14.3). It is important to understand the different terms that are used and interpret them correctly.

14.11   Drug Administration

When administering any drug, the '5 Rights' must be followed to avoid medication errors (Box 14.1).

Table 14.3. Different terms used in prescription.

Abbreviations used	Latin / Greek	Meaning
b.i.d., bid	*bis in die*	twice daily
t.i.d., tid	*ter in die*	three times daily
q.i.d., tid	*quater in die*	four times daily
s.i.d., sid	*semel in die*	once a day
q4h	*quaque 4 hora*	every 4 hours
q8h	*quaque 8 hora*	every 8 hours
e.o.d., eod		every other day
'ad lib'	*ad libitum*	as much as one desires
o.m., om	*omne mane*	every morning
o.n., on	*omne nocte*	every night
a.c., ac	*ante cibum*	before meals
p.c., pc	*post cibum*	after meals
prn	*pro re nata*	as needed
po	*per os*	oral, by mouth
od	*oculus dexter*	right eye
os	*oculus sinister*	left eye
ou	*oculus uterque*	both eyes

> **Box 14.1. The '5 Rights' in drug administration**
>
> 1.   RIGHT ANIMAL – which black cat?
> 2.   RIGHT DRUG – what strength is the drug?
> 3.   RIGHT DOSE – correct calculation?
> 4.   RIGHT TIME – bid, q6h?
> 5.   RIGHT ROUTE – oral or topical?

This means you should have knowledge of the drug and how it may be given as well as ensuring that the dosage is calculated correctly.

14.12 Drug Calculations

Most drug doses in the UK are expressed in terms of metric weights and volumes (Table 14.4).

Injectable drugs are usually solutions where the amount of drug is expressed as weight per volume (w/v). For example, buprenorphine is available as a 0.3 mg/ml solution. Some injectable drugs are presented as powders that need to be reconstituted; for example, cefuroxime is available as 250 mg, 750 mg or 1.5 g to which sterile water is added to reconstitute the drug as a solution. This means cefuroxime can be made up to different-strength solutions, depending on the amount of water added.

A drug formulary will indicate the dosage required by a particular species. This is usually expressed as the number of milligrams per kilogram bodyweight (mg/kg).

14.12.1 Calculating the required amount to give

A simple formula can be used to work out how much the animal needs:

$$\text{Dose} = \frac{\text{dosage}\left(\text{mg/kg}\right) \times \text{bodyweight}\left(\text{kg}\right)}{\text{concentration of the drug}}$$

Let's use an example and work this out in stages.

 Example:

A 20 kg dog requires an injection of methadone using a dosage of 0.2 mg/kg.

Step 1: Calculating the amount of drug required

$$\text{weight of the animal} \times \text{dosage}$$

$$20 \, \text{kg} \times 0.2 \, \text{mg / kg} = 4 \, \text{mg methadone}$$

Step 2: Calculating how much in volume needs to be injected

We know our patient needs 4 mg of methadone. We have a vial that contains 10 mg/ml of methadone in solution.

If you know that an animal needs a certain amount (**mg**) of a drug, but you do not know how many **ml** that is, then use the following formula to work it out:

$$\text{amount in ml} = \frac{\text{dose prescribed or required (mg)}}{\text{dose per ml (mg / ml)}}$$

So, for this patient: 4 mg/10 mg/ml = **0.4 ml** is the volume that needs to be drawn up to be injected.

 Sometimes the solution is presented as a percentage solution.

Example:

A 10 kg dog requires an injection of enrofloxacin and you have a bottle of 2.5 % Baytril

The dosage for a dog is 5 mg/kg, so the patient needs 10 kg × 5 mg/kg = **50 mg** of enrofloxacin. But how many millilitres is this?

Firstly, 'per cent' means 1 in 100. When referring to drug percentage solutions we mean 'weight per volume' or 'g/ml' or 'mg/ml'. So a 1 % solution = 1g in 100 ml. Our formula requires that the strength is described as 'mg/ml' so we need to describe our percentage solution as how many mg/ml it is.

We know that	1 %	= 1 g in 100 ml
This equates to	1 %	= 1000 mg in 100 ml
Which is equivalent to	1 %	= 10 mg in 1 ml or 10 mg/ml

For the example above:

$$\begin{aligned} a \, 2.5 \, \% \, \text{solution} &= 2.5 \, \text{g in} \, 100 \, \text{ml} \\ \text{Or} &= 2500 \, \text{mg in} \, 100 \, \text{ml} \\ \text{Or} &= \mathbf{25 \, mg/ml} \end{aligned}$$

So now we can use the formula:

$$\text{amount in ml} = \frac{\text{dose prescribed or required (mg)}}{\text{dose per ml (mg / ml)}}$$

The dog requires 50 mg / 25 mg / ml = **2ml**

The same formula can be used for calculating the number of pills to give.

Example:

A 5 kg Yorkshire terrier requires ampicillin at a dose of 20 mg/kg, divided into two equal doses daily for 5 days. The tablet sizes available are 50 mg, 100 mg, or 250 mg.

Which tablet size is most suitable and how many tablets would you dispense?

$$Dose = \frac{dosage\,(mg\,/\,kg) \times bodyweight\,(kg)}{concentration\,of\,the\,drug}$$

The dog weighs 5 kg and needs 20 mg/kg, so 5 kg × 20 mg/kg = 100 mg of the drug. This amount is to be divided into two equal doses per day, so it makes sense to use the 50 mg strength of the drug in order to give whole tablets and avoid the need to split the tablet. So:

$$Dose = \frac{20\,mg\,/\,kg \times 5\,kg}{50\,mg}$$
$$= 100\,mg\,/\,50\,mg$$
$$= 2\,tablets\,per\,day$$

The dog requires a 5-day course, so 2 × 5 days = ten 50 mg tablets to be dispensed.

 If you like working with formulae, you might find the following easy to remember.

Depending on what you need to work out, use the appropriate formula. Note the weight measurements are in 'g', not 'mg'.

$$\%SOLUTION = \frac{weight\,(g) \times 100}{vol.\,of\,solution\,(ml)}$$

$$VOL.OF\,SOLUTION\,(ml) = \frac{weight\,(g) \times 100}{\%solution}$$

$$WEIGHT\,(g) = \frac{volume\,of\,solution \times \%}{100}$$

14.13 Route of Administration

The route of administration depends on the formulation of the drug, how quickly it needs to have an effect and how often the drug needs to be given.

14.13.1 Enteral administration

This means that drugs are administered via the gastrointestinal tract. Some guidance is given in Table 14.5.

14.13.2 Parenteral administration

Some drugs have to be administered using one of several routes, the most common being subcutaneous, intramuscular and intravenous. Some guidance is given in Table 14.6.

14.13.3 Topical administration

These are compounds for external administration only; some details are given in Table 14.7.

Online Resources

AHWLA:

http://www.ahwla.org.uk/site/tutorials/BVA/BVA02-Introduction.html

BSAVA:

https://www.bsava.com/Resources/BSAVA MedicinesGuide

BVA:

https://www.bva.co.uk/member-documents/handling-veterinary-waste-england/

Government guidance:

https://www.gov.uk/guidance/legal-controls-on-veterinary-medicines

https://www.gov.uk/guidance/the-cascade-prescribing-unauthorised-medicines

Government publications:

https://www.gov.uk/government/publications/best-practice-in-the-labelling-and-packaging-of-medicines

Table 14.4. Details of how drugs can be supplied in metric weights and volumes.

Most drugs are expressed in measurements of weight	Some are supplied in volumes
1 kilogram (kg) = 1000 grams (g) 1 gram = 1000 milligrams (mg) 1 milligram = 1000 microgram (mcg or μg)	1 litre = 1000 millilitres (ml) 1 centilitre (cl) = 10ml 1 decilitre (dl) = 100ml 1 ml = 1 cubic centimetre (cc)

Table 14.5. Details of oral drugs and guidance on administration.

Oral preparations	Method of administration
• Convenient • Slower absorption • May be absorbed by stomach/small intestine • Some drugs act locally in the intestine • Not recommended for vomiting patients • Drug may be destroyed by gastric acid	• Open mouth and place at back of tongue, close mouth and wait for animal to swallow • Add to *small* amount of food • Use 'sticky' food (squeezy cheese?) • Insert into 'pill poppa' treat; or cold sausage works well

Table 14.6. The three routes of parenteral administration and guidance on administration.

Route	Site	Method of administration
Subcutaneous route		
• Least painful • Absorption is slower (30 – 40 min) as poor blood supply • Large volumes maybe injected	Any area of loose skin (scruff)	• Swab area with surgical spirit • Insert needle at 45 degrees into loose skin • Withdraw plunger slightly to check not in vessel • Inject and massage area to disperse drug
Intramuscular route		
• Inject small amounts otherwise painful • Depending on drug effect takes place 20–30 min • Always withdraw plunger to check not in vessel	• Quadriceps • Triceps • Dorsal lumbar (epaxial muscles)	• Swab area with surgical spirit • Insert needle 90 degrees into muscle body • Withdraw plunger slightly to check not in vessel • Inject and massage area to disperse drug
Intravenous route		
• Drug absorbed quickly as directly into blood stream • Highest peak plasma concentration But: • Drug concentration decreases more rapidly – so given more often	Veins commonly used: • Cephalic • Saphenous • Jugular Could also use marginal ear vein on rabbits	• Clip appropriate area over selected vein • Clean with chlorhexidine and surgical spirit • Assistant to raise vein • Stabilize vein with thumb • Insert needle with bevel upwards into vein • Withdraw plunger slightly – should see blood in hub of needle • Inject slowly • Withdraw needle putting pressure on injection site with a swab

Table 14.7. Some examples of drugs for topical use and guidance on administration.

Drug formulations	Precautions
• Creams/ointments • Powders • Lotions • Medicated shampoos • Aerosol sprays • Eye medications • Ear medications • 'Spot-ons'	• Wear gloves • Apply as directed • Avoid overdosing • Eye drops: leave 5 min between administrations • Ear drops: clean ear first

https://www.gov.uk/government/publications/report-prescription-misuse-animal-medicine

NOAH:

http://www.noahcompendium.co.uk

RCVS advice:

https://www.rcvs.org.uk/advice-and-guidance/code-of-professional-conduct-for-veterinary-surgeons/supporting-guidance/veterinary-medicines

RCVS publications:

https://www.rcvs.org.uk/publications/controlled-drugs-guidance

RPharmS:

http:/www.rpharms.com/home/home.asp

VMD:

http://www.vmd.defra.gov.uk/ProductInformation Database

https://www.gov.uk/government/organisations/veterinary-medicines-directorate

Further Reading: Rock, A. (2007) *Veterinary Pharmacology: A Practical Guide for the Veterinary Nurse.* Butterworth-Heinemann, Oxford, UK.

Rock, A. and Ackerman, N. (2010) Practical notes on pharmacy management: Part 1. *Veterinary Nursing Journal* 25(6), 30–33.

Rock, A. and Ackerman, N. (2010) Practical notes on pharmacy management: Part 2. Pharmaceutical waste disposal. *Veterinary Nursing Journal* 25(7), 27–29.

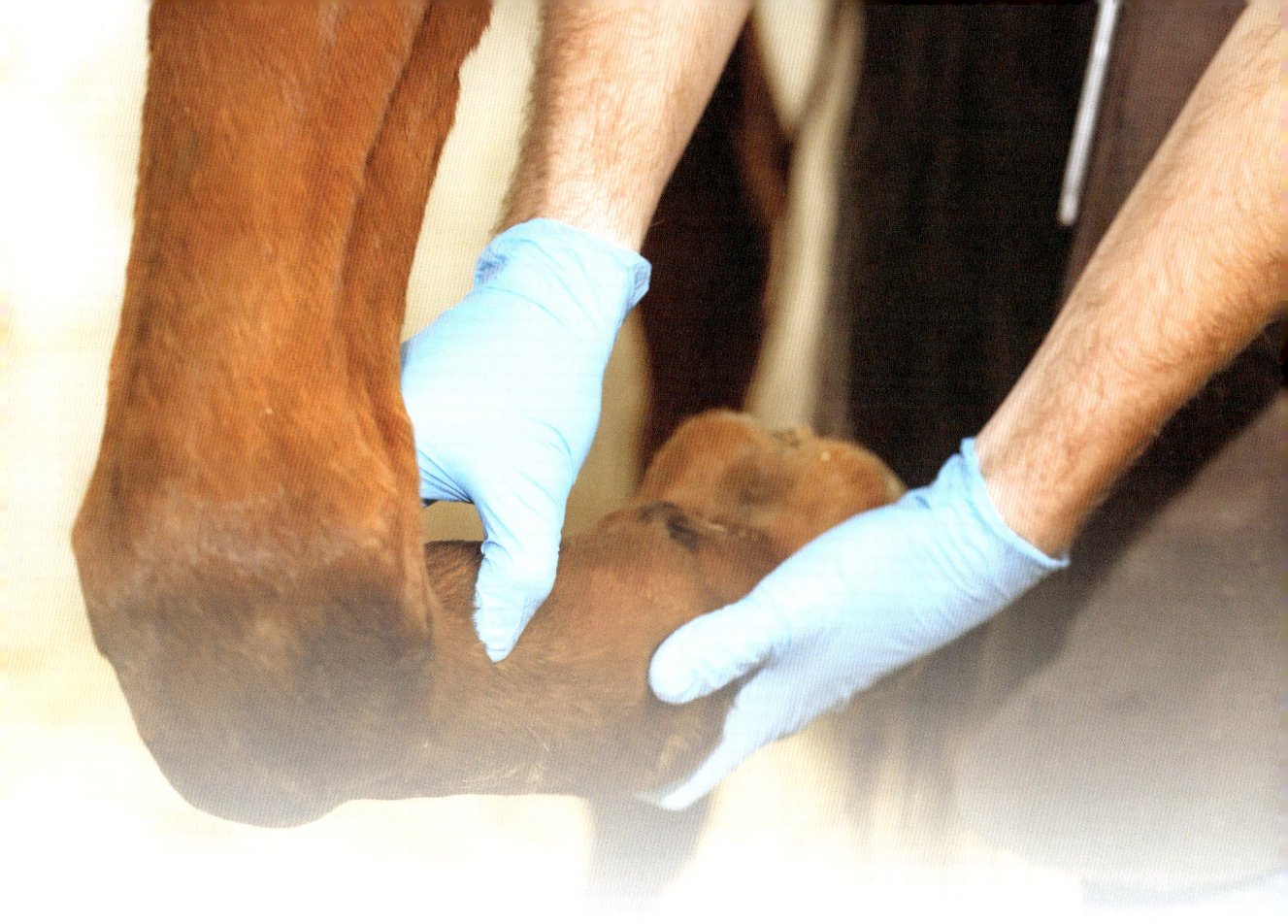

Patient Handling and Diagnostics

Section Editor: Isobel Vincent

Introduction

Diagnostic imaging is a rapid, safe procedure to 'look inside' an animal. Today, radiography and ultrasound are conducted as common procedures in most veterinary practices. Therefore a thorough understanding of the basics, how to image accurately and what not to do is essential. Imaging an animal requires safe handling and restraint. Without adequate knowledge and skills in approaching, handling and controlling an animal it is not possible to position an animal correctly for imaging. The student also needs to understand the welfare issues in animal handling and how to handle a variety of species.

The aim of this section is to provide that basic knowledge required to start handling and restraining the animal for diagnostic imaging. Within this section there are three chapters:

Chapter 15: General Principles of Animal Handling

Chapter 16: Diagnostic Imaging

Chapter 17: Equine Radiography-Example Tarsus

Within each chapter you will find pictures and tips about how to conduct relevant basic Day One skills. Each chapter will also detail key points for each set of skills and point out the health and safety considerations, which are critical to good practice.

An overview of all the learning outcomes is presented below and the more detailed learning outcomes are presented under each chapter.

Learning objectives

After studying this section, students should be able to:

- Demonstrate principles of safe and responsible handling and physical restraint of small and large animals.
- Address welfare issues associated with learning skills.
- Position an animal for diagnostic imaging.
- Explain and discuss film faults and digital radiology artefacts.
- Obtain an ultrasound and interpret an ultrasound image.
- Position and acquire images in a safe manner for all radiographic views of the tarsus.

What You Will Need

Clinical skills sheets (SS)

Twenty-one clinical skills sheets will be used in this section. Reference will be made to each skills sheet at the relevant point within the chapter. Clinical skills sheets for the following 12 accompany this section:

SS 15.36 Rugging up a horse

SS 15.37 Tying up a horse using a quick-release knot

SS 15.38 Putting a tail bandage on a horse

SS 15.39 Putting a stable bandage on a horse

SS.15.40 Applying a lower-limb protective bandage on a horse

SS 15.41 How to halter a cow

SS 16.42 Imaging BVA/KC hips

SS 16.43 Imaging caudo-cranial stifle

SS 16.44 Ultrasound (U/S) set-up

SS 17.45 Radiographic help sheet: understanding radiographic projections

SS 17.46 Radiographic projections of the foot

SS 17.47 Radiographic projections of the tarsus

A further nine skills sheets are used that have also been used in other chapters and cross-references are made in this section:

SS 9.18 Venepuncture techniques: blood collection by Vacutainer

SS 9.19 Venepuncture techniques: blood collection by syringe + needle

SS 12.29 Ophthalmalogy practical: eye examination

SS 12.31 Catheterizing a limb

SS 13.33 Applying a canine forelimb bandage

SS 13.34 Applying a canine chest drain bandage

SS 13.35 Applying an ear bandage

SS 18.48 Bovine sterile milk sampling method

SS 18.49 California Milk Test (CMT) sampling method

Videos (V)

Seventeen videos will be used in this section and reference will be made to each video at the relevant point within the chapter. Videos will be hyperlinked and the following accompany this section:

V 15.1 Restraint of a cat (out of a basket, jugular/cephalic blood sampling & wrapping cat in a towel)

V 15.2 Crush cage

V 15.3 Handling a cat

V 15.4 Check chain – dog

V 15.5 Restraint of a large dog for injection

V 15.6 Restraint techniques for a small to medium dog

V 15.7 Restraint of a large dog for jugular and cephalic sampling

V 15.8 Hamster handling

V 15.9 Rat handling

V 15.10 Rabbit lifting and carrying

V 15.11 Chicken handling

V 15.12 Rugging up a horse

V 15.13 Quick-release knot

V 15.14 Lead rope over neck & put on head collar

V 15.15 Tying up a cow

V 15.16 Sheep handling including 1 & 2 person method

V 15.17 Lambing

General Principles of Animal Handling

15

Isobel Vincent
The Royal Veterinary College, London

Learning objectives

By the end of this chapter, students should be aware of:

- Principles of safe and responsible handling.
- Sensory perception in animals.
- Handling and physical restraint of small animals.
- Handling and physical restraint of large animals.
- Addressing welfare issues associated with learning skills.

Clinical skills sheets (SS)

Six clinical skills sheets will be used in this chapter, along with nine skills sheets from other chapters. They can be found at pages 135–139, 179–180, 183–185, 194–202, 229–248 and 296–297. Reference will be made to each skills sheet at the relevant point within the chapter. The details of the clinical skills sheets used are as follows (in numerical order):

SS 9.18 Venepuncture techniques: blood collection by Vacutainer
SS 9.19 Venepuncture techniques: blood collection by syringe + needle
SS 12.29 Ophthalmology practical: eye examination
SS 12.31 Catheterizing a limb
SS 13.33 Applying a canine forelimb bandage
SS 13.34 Applying a canine chest drain bandage
SS 13.35 Applying an ear bandage
SS 15.36 Rugging up a horse
SS 15.37 Tying up a horse using a quick-release knot
SS 15.38 Putting a tail bandage on a horse

SS 15.39 Putting a stable bandage on a horse
SS 15.40 Applying a lower-limb protective bandage on a horse
SS 15.41 How to halter a cow
SS 18.48 Bovine sterile milk sampling method
SS 18.49 California Milk Test (CMT) sampling method

Videos (V)

Seventeen videos will be used in this chapter to demonstrate how to perform the clinical skills. They are:

V 15.1 Restraint of a cat (out of a basket, jugular/cephalic blood sampling & wrapping cat in a towel)
V 15.2 Crush cage
V 15.3 Handling a cat
V 15.4 Check chain – dog
V 15.5 Restraint of a large dog for injection
V 15.6 Restraint techniques for a small to medium dog
V 15.7 Restraint of a large dog for jugular and cephalic sampling
V 15.8 Hamster handling
V 15.9 Rat handling
V 15.10 Rabbit lifting and carrying
V 15.11 Chicken handling
V 15.12 Rugging up a horse
V 15.13 Quick-release knot
V 15.14 Lead rope over neck & put on head collar
V 15.15 Tying up a cow
V 15.16 Sheep handling including 1 & 2 person method
V 15.17 Lambing

© CAB International 2018. *Veterinary Clinical Skills Manual* (eds N. Coombes and A. Silva-Fletcher)

NB: Throughout this chapter the term 'handler' will be used to signify veterinary surgeon, student, veterinary nurse, owner, farmer if the information is of generic nature.

15.1 Objective 1: Principles of Safe and Responsible Handling

15.1.1 Introduction

Competence in a broad range of animal handling skills is important for achieving best care and welfare appropriate for the individual species. It is essential to be able to restrain or control a patient effectively in order to carry out veterinary or husbandry procedures, some potentially painful. You need to be able to recognize signs of agitation and aggression. Failure to address such a fundamental issue can result in serious injury or even fatality for handler or animal. There is a wealth of published information on normal and abnormal animal behaviour and body language from aggressive, to territorial, to maternal and so on (Grandin, 2006; Atkinson *et al.*, 2012; Broom and Fraser, 2015). These behavioural signs will not be covered in detail here other than as a reminder for approach, capture and restraint.

15.1.2 CSC laboratories

Whilst a clinical skills centre laboratory is not primarily an environment for handling the live animal, adapted manikins can provide important visual and tactile cues for learning. They do not necessarily need to be 'high fidelity' as long as there are key focal points for the student to concentrate on; for example, catheter placement. Using a standing manikin dog can facilitate consolidation of a skill by repetition, without the concern of welfare issues that would arise from over-handling individual animals; an example is learning how to use an ophthalmoscope and correctly holding a dioptic lens. Another well tested example is the use of a simulator ewe to aid teaching and learning of lambing skills (Vincent and Thompson, 2011). Indeed, building confidence in one's dexterity in a clinical skills environment is more likely to produce success when carrying out the skill with a real-live non-compliant patient.

SS 12.29 for eye examination, including use of an ophthalmoscope
SS 12.31 for details of catheter placement

15.1.3 Environment

The environment the animal finds itself in will have a huge impact on how it behaves. The 'white coat' surroundings of a consultation room or a strange loosebox will more likely elicit measurable levels of stress (elevated heart rate, blood pressure) when compared with a familiar home or enclosure. Additionally, in a clinical setting, if the patient is not used to a cage or the confines of a stable it may exhibit a heightened 'fight or flight' response, which is potentially dangerous for the inexperienced handler.

15.1.4 Species-specific and individual behaviour

In order to be able to handle an animal, large or small, farm or exotic, you need knowledge of that animal's species-specific behaviour. For example, a dog might welcome a pat on the head, but for a ram that would be threatening. Humans interact best with animals under their care when they recognize that those animals have individual as well as species characteristics. This comes with experience; in fact, research has shown that canine temperament, assessed by an experienced handler, can be linked to cardiovascular response (Vincent and Michell, 1996).

Exposing animals, preferably early on in their life, to a wide variety of experiences, sensations and other species in a non-threatening way allows habituation to occur. Animals well handled from an early age are easier to treat and are less stressed by husbandry and veterinary procedures. For example, training very young foals to load on to a trailer by encouragement and reward is of great benefit as they mature. In reality, however, the veterinary surgeon or handler may often have to deal with results of uninformed training, which means that patients are more likely to be unpredictable.

All animals can be unpredictable, of course, and this is magnified when they are under situations of stress. For example, no animal likes being turned on its back (dogs and cats may tolerate it in play, or where they trust the handler); for some species it can have an effect on heart function (e.g. birds and rabbits), or result in increased cortisol levels (e.g. sheep).

15.1.5 Behaviour assessment

You should always assess overall behaviour before approaching and handling an animal. The Queen Mother Hospital for Animals (QMHA) of the Royal Veterinary College (RVC) is introducing a 'PAWS' (Pause; Assess; Welfare; Seek assistance) recording system in order to reduce incidence of bites and scratches when students are not aware that the animal is indicating warning signs of fear or aggression.

Risk of accident to the handler is increased when a creature is frightened or injured, or receiving potentially painful veterinary intervention. The RVC 'TREAT' policy aims to raise awareness by reminding the veterinary surgeon that they should have sufficient **T**ime, **R**estraint (physical or chemical), **E**quipment (for personal protection), **A**ssistance and **T**raining appropriate to the level of risk in the task they are to perform.

No animal (or human) likes their 'personal space' invaded without invitation. This 'critical' or 'flight' distance varies from species to species and individual to individual. A well handled (or unthreatened) animal will have a greatly reduced flight distance when compared with a poorly handled (or nervous) one. Remember, any animal approached within its perceived territory may guard it ferociously (e.g. hamsters in a nest).

Animals can feel threatened by body language and react in fight or flight mode. Some species are threatened by a direct stare (dogs, sheep) and this needs to be taken into account on approaching different species. Recent research (Smith *et al.*, 2016) has gone some way to proving that horses, along with dogs and chimpanzees, recognize and respond to human facial expressions such as anger or pleasure.

Many animals prefer to be in a group, particularly large animal domesticants, and they can become stressed if separated from other conspecifics (sheep, cattle).

15.1.6   Handler behaviour

Some creatures can be controlled by our voices (dog, horse), others by food reward measures (sheep) and others by the 'less is more' type of contact (cats).

You should let the animal know of your presence by voice first, unless they are elderly and possibly hard of hearing, in which case make sure that they can see you before touching them. If the patient is to be palpated, move your hand along from a less sensitive body area to the possibly more sensitive area to be touched, e.g. running a hand along a cow's flank towards a teat. Sudden movements can produce a startle reaction, which could result in injury.

So, talk to the animal (keeping your voice low pitched); maybe stroke a dog, cat, or equid; walk around them calmly if bovine or ovine species. Never turn your back on large animals. Large animals weigh considerably more than we do – use their weight to help you to move them and others as a group.

There are overarching generic points to bear in mind, though: a high-pitched human voice will alert or excite many animals (cf inter- and intra-species alarm calls, common between bird and small mammal species) while a low calm voice promotes a more peaceful aura. Unexpected movements or touch by the handler are more likely to result in a protective kick, bite or scratch from the patient. However, when catching a sheep in a pen, you need to act with alacrity if the opportunity presents itself to restrain an individual while it wedges itself between its flockmates.

Animals respond much better to firm (not too firm, and do not 'overhandle') confident handling rather than a feeling of being 'tickled by an insect', or non-committed catching/holding/restraint (Grandin, 2006). It is better and less stressful to carry out a procedure *once* than to make repeated half-hearted attempts. On the other hand, over-tight restraint can stress/overheat the animal (and handler). Some individuals can be very sensitive to touch on certain parts of the body (horse: ears, behind girth, belly; dog: hindquarters, tail; cat: feet, tail, etc.). Never pull tails, ears or hair/fleece to catch or restrain an animal – it hurts them.

15.2   Objective 2: Sensory Perception in Animals

Our five senses can be very differently calibrated compared with other species. In fact, animals may have a whole battery of extrasensory and physical abilities to perceive and interact with their environment.

15.2.1   Touch

Animals have tactile sensations detected mainly by mechanoreceptors, thermoreceptors and nociceptors in their skin (much as we do) and muzzle and extended through vibrissae. Those whose muzzle is permanently moist (dog, cat, cow) are particularly sensitive to touch in that area.

15.2.2   Sight

We can see colour across the visual spectrum (750–400 nm) via a trichromatic battery of photoreceptors (cones) in the retina. In contrast, many other mammals have dichromatic facilities and cannot perceive red as we can, rather similar to red–green colour blindness in humans. Unlike us, many of our mammalian domesticants have a higher concentration of light-sensitive photoreceptors (rods) and also a reflective layer behind the retina (tapetum lucidum) as they evolved from twilight-living forebears. This layer harnesses any available light and allows them to see at very low light intensities. Rods are most sensitive to light and dark changes, shape and movement. Rods are more numerous than cones in the periphery of the retina.

This means in reality that domestic mammals are more sensitive than we are to peripheral activity, sudden movement and sharp contrast between light and dark environments. Horses, cattle and sheep are less able to adjust to sudden changes of light than are humans, such as when moving from a bright day into a dark barn. This is a consideration during training, as certain tasks, such as loading into a trailer, may frighten a horse simply because it cannot see adequately. They are predominantly monocular with a visual field of over 300 degrees (good for spotting predators in their peripheral vision) and a restricted degree of binocular vision, which is important for depth perception (about 60 degrees, compared with 140 degrees in humans). These species have a 'blind spot' just in front of the face and so it is important to approach these creatures at an angle when in close proximity to avoid a 'startle' reflex.

Many of our domesticated species are very sensitive to motion, as motion is usually the first alert that a predator is approaching. Such motion is usually first detected in their periphery, where they have poorer visual acuity, and so they will usually act defensively and run/fly off if something suddenly moves into their peripheral field of vision. One animal in a group spooking will often cause a chain reaction in others as a safety mechanism.

It is worth remembering that birds have a highly developed ability to see colour (and this extends into the ultraviolet spectrum) and sometimes tend to peck at brightly coloured objects (e.g. nail varnish, jewellery, hair clips).

15.2.3 Hearing

Humans can hear in the range 20–20,000 Hz (about 10 octaves). Outside our auditory range we term 'infrasound' at the long wavelength end (which elephants, for example, use to communicate over great distances) and 'ultrasound' at the short wavelength end. Bats hear between 14,000–100,000 Hz and utilize the top end to echolocate in their habitat at close distances.

Dogs can hear in the range 67–45,000 Hz (9 octaves) and cattle in the range 23–35,000 Hz.

In practice it is important to bear in mind that sounds may be distracting or upsetting to an animal; for example, a water tap will emit ultrasonic noise if not turned off properly and this can be irritating if the animal cannot escape it (e.g. in a kennel environment). Sudden sounds, like sudden movements, can also spook animals and cause them to flee or fly, regardless of whether they are prey or predator species.

Vocalizations are an important mode of communication amongst many species and can provide information on the age, sex, dominance status and reproductive status of the caller.

15.2.4 Olfaction

Animals have a range of odiferous glands over their body, including interdigital, infraorbital, inguinal and sebaceous glands, indicating that olfaction plays a large role in their social life. Both the primary olfactory system using the olfactory bulbs and the secondary olfactory system using the vomeronasal organ are used. This latter olfactory system is used in the *flehmen* response (seen in rams, cats).

Many animals communicate by smell and taste: they release pheromones (hormone-like compounds) into the environment that affect the behaviour or physiology of others of its species. Pheromones play an important part in reproduction and other social behaviour. They are used by many animals, including insects, wolves, deer, and even humans. They are a vital part of dam–offspring bonding and the principle can be utilized to encourage fostering practices in the sheep industry. We also know that pheromones can affect behaviour of non-conspecifics. Prey species show specific adaptations that allow recognition, avoidance and defence against predators. For many mammalian species this includes sensitivity towards predator-derived odours. The typical sources of such odours include predator skin and fur, urine, faeces and anal gland secretions. Avoidance of predator odours has been observed in many mammalian prey species, including rats, rabbits and sheep (Apfelbach *et al.*, 2005). The presence of these volatile substances can affect animal behaviour, including in the clinical environment where animals are in close proximity in waiting room areas. It is worth remembering the potential stress for a mouse being handled in the consulting room straight after a cat has been treated in the same room.

Human beings have in the region of 10 cm² olfactory epithelium; in comparison, dogs have 170 cm². The dog's olfactory capabilities are awesome. They can be trained to pick up a chemical trace sometimes down to single molecules. Thus it is not surprising to consider that strong perfumes in, for example, cosmetics or cleaning fluids can be really disorientating to a dog and in fact to many animals that rely on olfactory signals to communicate and to find food, etc. in their environment. We have found in rat-handling classes that use of hand-cleansing gels results in an increased risk of bites to the handler.

15.3 Objective 3: Handling and Physical Restraint of Small Animals

15.3.1 Introduction

Animals much smaller than us can be physically overpowered by us – theoretically. Their first instinct, in an unfamiliar scenario, will be to escape capture. Therefore, if catch and restraint are carried out incorrectly, the handler will be bitten and scratched and the resulting wounds may be very serious. Although it is important to be in control of the 'biting end' of the patient, some animals will become more fractious if they are restrained too fiercely by a new handler in the first instance. On the other hand, restraint that is too feeble for the temperament of the patient (particularly in a stressful environment) can result in a sudden bite or attempt to escape. That balance of handling comes only with experience, so be guided by the owner, or by experienced professionals in the consulting room, hospital or kennels.

15.3.2 Personal protective equipment (PPE)

Gauntlets may be necessary for handling small animal biters and scratchers.

15.3.3 In the consultation clinic

Some species can feel uncomfortable or over-excited by other species – for example, the dog versus cat scenario. To have separate waiting areas or barriers separating these animals works well and addresses the potential stressfulness of the environment. Proper restraint techniques and equipment will help the handler to feel more in control, and so more relaxed and confident, thus the patient may also relax as a consequence.

Restraint methods and equipment need to be used efficiently, but always keeping the animal's welfare in mind. Remember that a determined dog could pull off a correctly-fitted muzzle in less than 15 seconds (personal observation). In the laboratory environment, rats and mice may be restrained by holding the base of their tails (Atkinson *et al.*, 2012), but this is not what the pet owner wants to observe during a consultation.

In order to give oral medication or check teeth or ventral body, for example, it may be necessary to 'scruff' a small patient such as a rodent (Atkinson *et al.*, 2012). It is preferable wherever possible to incorporate medication into feed, or sedate (chemically restrain) patients who are unwilling to have their mouth (armed with dental weapons) interfered with.

Cages and vivaria come in all shapes and sizes and these environments quickly become the territory and personal space of the animal contained within. This can be the case even if the cage is 'hospital accommodation'. Bear this in mind as you remove the occupant.

15.3.4 Risk points to consider when handling different small animal species

- **Cats** are lithe but you should not 'over-hold' them. Wounds they inflict are punctures and so there is a high risk of infection. You may need a towel or other wrapping restraint, or a crush cage to contain those who will not settle (e.g. for vaccination). Correct restraint for venepuncture ensures success with minimal injury risk.

- **Dogs** and their ancestors are the species with the longest known interaction with humans. They watch our body movements and our facial expression for cues to our intentions. There are numerous breeds and a wide variety of behaviours, some innate, some owner- or environment-taught. Some behave well with the owner present, some quite the reverse. Correctly applied slip leads or check chains and, if necessary, muzzles (Atkinson *et al.*, 2012), are appropriate restraints. Dogs up to 15 kg can be lifted on to an examination table; if heavier, they are probably safer on a floor for assessment. They can also be placed in lateral recumbency for palpation. Correct restraint for venepuncture ensures success with minimal injury risk.

- **Small rodents** are protective of cages, so do not poke fingers through bars or into their nests. Wait for them to come to the cage door and let them come out on to your hand, or reach into the main cage area and lift them out firmly and support them under their body.

- **Rabbits** have powerful defensive hind legs to kick and scratch; they can bite too. You need to maintain a firm nestled hold, restraining those hind legs if necessary. Never pick up a rabbit, or indeed any animal, by its ears and no animal should be picked up by its legs (with the exception of neonate lambs; see sheep handling section).

- **Guinea pigs** are ideal pets for children but if poorly handled they can exhibit defensive biting and hind leg scratching. When being picked up they should be supported under their body.

- **Birds** peck and scratch. Ducks can be caught by the neck but then the body should be supported. Catch small turkeys and hens with your hands either side of the wings. Do not turn birds upside down to handle – it is a big strain on the lungs and heart and they may become comatose. In fact, it is stressful for any animal to be turned on its back, as they feel vulnerable.

- **Exotics** handling is not covered in this chapter. They are specialist pets, so be guided by the owner as to their response to handling. There can be deep-seated misconceptions regarding animal intelligence; for example, fish do not just have a 15-second memory (Balcombe, 2016) as some believe.

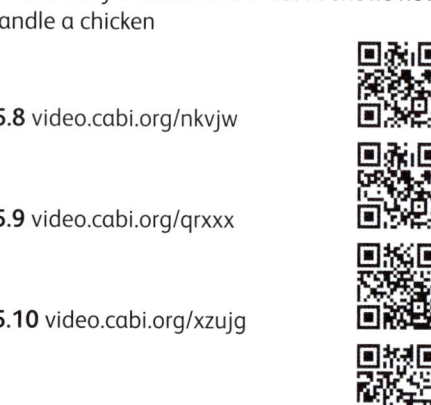

V 15.5 video.cabi.org/mwpob

V 15.6 video.cabi.org/ifxro

V 15.7 video.cabi.org/bdjmr

V 15.8 shows how to handle a hamster, **V 15.9** shows how to handle a rat, **V 15.10** shows how to lift and carry a rabbit and **V 15.11** shows how to handle a chicken

V 15.8 video.cabi.org/nkvjw

V 15.9 video.cabi.org/qrxxx

V 15.10 video.cabi.org/xzujg

V 15.11 video.cabi.org/judqh

 V 15.1, **V 15.2** and **V 15.3** show how to handle and restrain a cat

V 15.1 video.cabi.org/luojw

V 15.2 video.cabi.org/uhdxk

V 15.3 video.cabi.org/fvmuc

V 15.4, **V 15.5**, **V 15.6** and **V 15.7** show how to restrain a dog

V 15.4 video.cabi.org/dnbrf

15.4 Objective 4: Handling and Physical Restraint of Large Animals

15.4.1 Introduction

Domesticated livestock species are prey animals and instinctively want to flee at the first sign of danger or if you come closer than their natural 'flight distance'. They are also social with clear-cut hierarchies within their groups; such hierarchies can affect handling and movement. When needing to separate a single animal for treatment, it is usually easier to corral a small group in a pen (and maybe a race) before attempting to capture them. Guide them with arms held wide and continuous encouraging voices (preferably not shouting).

It is important to remember that there are great behavioural differences between species; for example, ewes and their lambs stay close for the first few weeks, but a cow will leave her calf hidden while she rejoins the herd, coming back to suckle maybe only four to six times during the day. Heifers left in close confinement (a stall) with their calf may show aggression towards it. Bottle-fed livestock species have a much-reduced fear of humans and thus can be more challenging or dangerous as adults.

15.4.2 Personal protective equipment

Sturdy footwear is essential for all large animal work. Helmets (and gloves) for working with horses is also advised; it is a subject under hot debate at the moment (Butterworth, 2016).

Key safety advice

- Beware of single entire males – large weight, aggression (particularly in reproductive season); bulls need a nose ring.
- Always have an escape route from a pen/ stable.
- When not in a field, move livestock groups in small cohorts, in single file, through races or chutes – no sharp edges, no sudden change of light/dark/light.
- Avoid slippery floors, change of floor surface, slippery ramps, swinging chains or light fittings.
- When handling the individual animal, you must have control of its head.

15.4.3 Risk points to consider when handling different large animal species

Horses

Horses are social and prefer to be within sight and sound of others. Donkeys, however, are known to break away from feral groups and function independently if resources are scarce.

Horses are very flighty animals, trained to accept 'tack' and other clothing but can still be ear-shy, head-shy, etc. They may be very sensitive to being touched behind the 'saddle' area, i.e. rump, dock, groin. They

can rear, buck, bite and kick – all with potentially serious or lethal consequences. They should be tied up securely before any procedures are carried out. If the horse will not tolerate a procedure such as blood sampling, further restraint using a nose twitch may be employed.

SS 15.36 for rugging up a horse
SS 15.37 for making a quick-release knot
SS 15.38 for applying a tail bandage
SS 15.39 for applying a stable bandage
SS 15.40 for applying a lower-limb bandage to cover a wound or surgical incision

V 15.12 for rugging up a horse and **V 15.13** for making a quick-release knot

V 15.12 video.cabi.org/wdxdw

V 15.13 video.cabi.org/xfrzl

Their long and close association with humankind has meant that, like dogs, horses are responsive to modulations in the human voice and nuances in our body language. They can also very quickly sense a handler's nervousness and will exploit a lack of competence and 'play up'. It is important that they are treated with the correct mix of sensitivity and firmness.

In the hands of an experienced trainer, of course, they are capable of the most amazing feats of speed, endurance and agility. 'Horse whisperers' utilize their profound knowledge of the subtleties of equine behaviour in order to encourage tractability. Sadly, a lack of ability to control a horse is often compensated for by use of more fierce or restrictive tack, especially bits. Nevertheless, with a difficult or young animal an anti-rearing or Chifney bit is advised for the handler's safety (Atkinson *et al.*, 2012).

Horses can be 'captured' when out at grass and a head collar and lead rope applied, by judicious use of a food reward, or familiarity with the owner. However, remember that the horse has *chosen* to let itself be caught and controlled because of its trust in the handler. Therefore sensitive handling of this species is essential to obtain the best human–animal bond. Training should start at an early age; a horse-breeder friend of the author's trains foals a few days old to load successfully on to a trailer by following their dams.

 **V 15.14** for placing a lead rope and head collar

V 15.14 video.cabi.org/niybt

Cattle

Cattle may chase and trample a dog (or goose) straying into their field. Never pick up your dog in such a scenario. Also it is best not to run from cows in a field (and do not enter a field with a bull in it); instead, face them and shout or flap your arms – they are usually just being curious and will back off if you stand your ground. They can mostly defend themselves from a rogue dog, unlike sheep or alpacas.

Cattle are not just 'bigger sheep' but can be territorial and aggressive, their sheer size and unpredictability making them a potential danger. They might not be used to much handling but can certainly be trained to accept a halter. Horns are an added risk and are often disbudded early on. Cattle can kick in any direction, and head butt, and can crush in small spaces. They should be tied securely before procedures are performed. Alternatively,

they should be restrained in a cattle crush (Fig. 15.1), or samples can be collected in the milking parlour.

 SS 15.41 for haltering a cow
SS 18.48 and **SS 18.49** for carrying out milk test sampling

 V 15.15 for tying up a cow

V 15.15 video.cabi.org/brhoi

Sheep

Sheep are primarily flight animals. Move sheep as a group in the field; singling out an animal makes it much harder, if not impossible, to capture. It is easier to catch them once they are in a small penned group. Never grab them by the fleece, but by a hand under the lower jaw, mid-mandible. You can restrain them against a wall or fence using your legs against their torso and a hand under the mandible. In this position they can be aged by teeth, scored for body condition (by palpation of the lumbar vertebrae) or venepuncture samples can be taken. Sheep can also be 'cast' (turned over to sit on their haunches) to check udders, trim feet or for shearing.

Sheepdogs have a co-evolutionary link with sheep dating back hundreds of years. Sheep learn to recognize

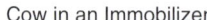
Cow in an Immobilizer

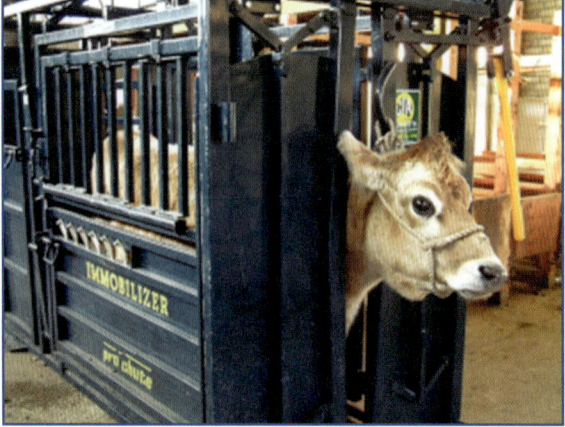

Fig. 15.1. Restraint of cattle using a crush.

'their' dogs and even very large flocks can be herded safely and effectively by just one shepherd and a dog. In contrast, lambs, and more primitive breeds such as the Hebridean, may scatter on sighting a dog of any description.

 SS 9.18 and **SS 9.19** for venepuncture techniques

 V 15.16 for sheep handling

 V 15.16 video.cabi.org/ropgq

Outside the mating season, rams can be kept peaceably in groups, but at tupping time these same animals may fight by charging and butting, with sometimes fatal consequences (a broken neck). Around lambing, even ewes can become aggressive, particularly towards dogs – a dam with her young will stand and fight if necessary. Neonate lambs may be picked up by two front legs to move them to a mothering-up pen; this allows the dam to follow the lambs' scent. By a few days old, they should be picked up with hand/s under the ribs/belly and supported against the handler's body.

 V 15.17 for lambing

 V 15.17 video.cabi.org/lixts

Goats

Goats are full of curiosity and are profligate chewers and adept at escape. They are friendly (unless suspicious) and would rather be led by collar and lead than driven like cattle or sheep. They will not usually respect a well trained dog and will face up to them and can butt. They are also able to reach all parts of their body, so bandages, etc. will not stay on long. Foot trimming is carried out with the goat upright and tethered – unlike sheep, which are cast.

Camelids

Old world camels and New World llamas and alpacas need handling from an early age to become tractable.

They can be trained to wear a halter/head collar to move them. As with a horse, you can assess camelid docility by ear set, vocalization and head and neck position. If feeling threatened, llamas and alpacas can kick with hind limbs or forelimbs in any direction (including forwards and outwards, like a cow).

Camelids may vocalize during restraint and llamas may scream if restrained even though no pain has been inflicted. They can bite and may also spit foul-smelling stomach contents if stressed or threatened. Chutes and corrals should be fenced to a height 1.8 m or more.

Deer

Deer are very flighty and nervous. They are not domesticated as such but can be tamed. They are most dangerous at rutting and when calves are present. They can jump traditional-height fences and so penning needs to be at least 14 ft (4.3 m) high. Antlers and kicking and jumping are injury risks. Reindeer can be trained to accept a head collar and harness to facilitate moving them.

Pigs

The usual husbandry of grouping pigs of similar sex, age and size does not make for harmony. Newly mixed piglets may fight for hours until they achieve some semblance of hierarchy. The introduction of a boar penned nearby, or even boar pheromone, can make a marked difference. Their natural grouping would be the extended family – several sows and their young. Pigs may be moved by droving boards, paddles, or flags, but quietly.

Neonate and very young piglets may be picked up and bodily supported, as with lambs or indeed most other small mammals.

15.5 Objective 5: Addressing Welfare Issues Associated with Learning Skills

15.5.1 Pain

One of the reasons for catching/restraining an animal might be to assess and dress a wound, or maybe to collect a blood sample by venepuncture. There will inevitably be a pain element to be factored into such procedures. Pain can cause an otherwise tractable animal to behave fearfully and/or aggressively, especially in an alien environment. The patient may also have a memory of past fearful events and will in consequence be more stressed next time the procedure is repeated.

SS **13.33** for bandaging a forelimb
SS **13.34** for chest drain bandaging
SS **13.35** for bandaging an ear
SS **15.38**, **15.39** and **15.40** for applying bandages to a horse
SS **9.18** and SS **9.19** for venepuncture techniques

The potential Health & Safety consequences of intractable patient behaviour correlate with increasing body mass, species (and thus its 'weapons'), aggressive characteristics, sex, breeding stage and whether or not it is in pain or feeling threatened.

Of course restraint may be to assess a source of pain or discomfort and thus it is important to be able to recognize pain behaviour in different species (D'Andrea and Sjogren, 2014). However, as livestock are prey species it is not to their evolutionary advantage to advertise that they are vulnerable. In consequence their pain markers may be very subtle, such as the 'grimace' response (NC3RS, accessed online November 2016) or abnormal standing posture. Recent research findings by Dyson et al. (2017) suggest that horses have a raft of facial expressions that may be under-interpreted by horse owners. Ear positions ranging from flattened back (fear or anger) to upright or forward-pointing (relaxed, curious) are more recognizable, but a horse exposing its teeth in a 'grin', or 'yawning', can be signs of pain.

15.5.2 Development of a lamb manikin for elastration practice

Certain husbandry practices need good dexterity to be carried out effectively. One such practice is tailing and castrating of lambs using a tight rubber ring to cut off blood supply (Fig. 15.2). The ring is applied (to the scrotal neck and one-third of the way down the tail) using a hand-held metal 'elastrator'. The procedure must be carried out before the animal is 7 days old (DEFRA, accessed online December 2016). It is recognized as painful (Pizzey et al., 2016) and thus should be performed by someone who has received training in this skill. The author has made simple manikins for use in first-year student lamb-handling

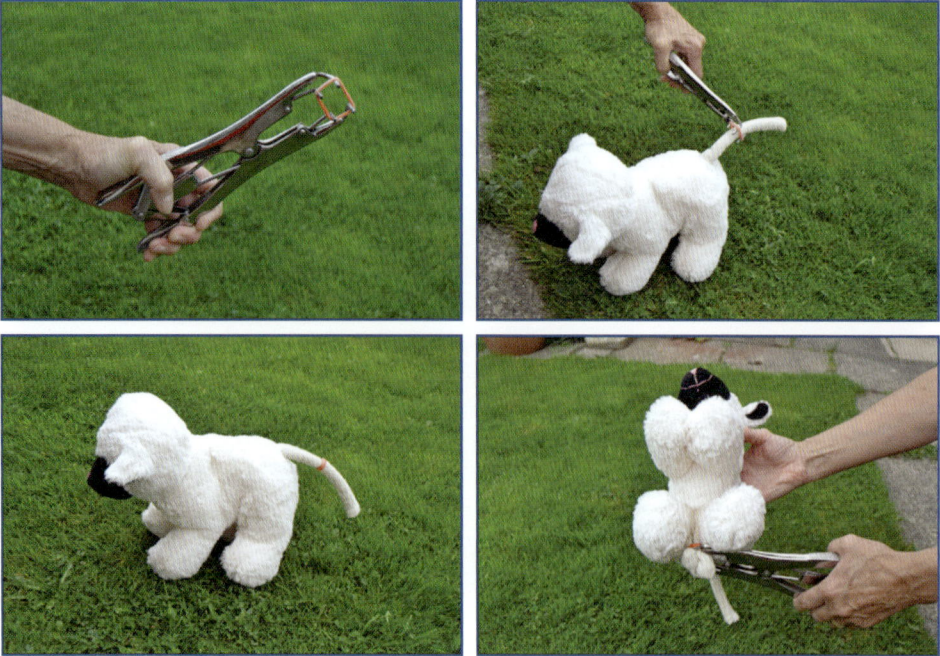

Fig. 15.2. Use of a manikin lamb to demonstrate the application of a rubber ring to tail dock and castrate.

sessions to complement real-life elastration of lambs in the RVC commercial flock. Crepe bandage around rubber tubing simulates a tail; two marbles in a crepe bandage pouch simulate the testicles. These artefacts are sewn sturdily on to a toy lamb and have proved robust enough for multiple use by students (Fig. 15.2).

15.5.3 Development of a cow tail-vein manikin

An RVC student has developed a model to facilitate learning how to take blood from the coccygeal vein of a cow (Fig. 15.3). The results from this research project indicated strongly that students felt more confident when sampling from a live animal after practising on this model.

15.5.4 Future ideas and widening participation

The idea of a CSC does not have to remain within a dedicated laboratory. Many skills can be portable or field based, such as bandaging manikins and hand ties. Currently the RVC CSC provides learning opportunities by verbal, visual and touch methods. It may be worth considering the use of olfactory stations to identify 'healthy' versus 'unhealthy' odours (e.g. in urine). Also auditory stations could be set up where, for

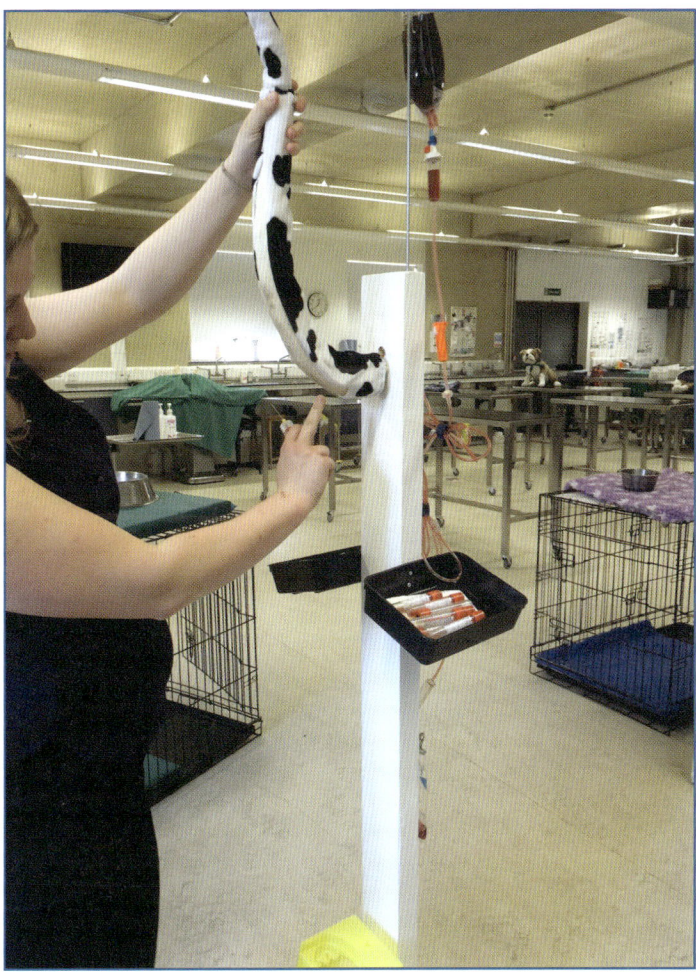

Fig. 15.3. Cow tail vein model.

example, a student could learn the signature bleat of a hungry lamb, or the warning whinnies of a horse. Maybe manikins could be created that are more mobile and lifelike and could be placed in postures to denote fear or pain, aggression or pleasure.

References and Further Reading: Apfelbach, R., Blanchard, C.D., Blanchard, R.J., Hayes, R.A. and McGregor, I.S. (2005) The effects of predator odors in mammalian prey species: a review of field and laboratory studies. *Neuroscience and Biobehavioral Reviews* 29(8), 1123–1144.

Atkinson, T., Devaney, J. and Girling, S. (2012) Animal handling, restraint and transport. In: Cooper, B., Mullineaux, E. and Turner, L. (eds) *BSAVA Textbook of Veterinary Nursing 5th edition*. BSAVA, Gloucester, UK.

Balcombe, J. (2016) *What a Fish Knows. The Inner Lives of our Underwater Cousins*. Scientific American/Farrar, Strauss and Giroux, New York.

Broom, D.M. and Fraser, A.F. (2015) *Domestic Animal Behaviour and Welfare*, 5th edn. CAB International, Wallingford, UK.

Butterworth, J. (2016) Think ahead: safety first for equine vets. *Veterinary Record* 178(12), 295–296.

D'Andrea, A. and Sjogren, J. (2014) *Veterinary Technician's Large Animal Daily Reference Guide*. Wiley Blackwell, Chichester, UK.

DEFRA (2016) Codes of Recommendations for the Welfare of Livestock. Sheep. Available at: https://www.gov.uk/government/uploads/system/uploads/attachment_data/file/69365/pb5162-sheep-041028.pdf (accessed December 2016).

Dyson, S., Berger, J.M., Ellis, A.D. and Mullard, J. (2017) Can the presence of musculoskeletal pain be determined from the facial expressions of ridden horses (FEReq)? *Journal of Veterinary Behavior: Clinical Applications and Research* 19, 78–89.

Grandin, T. (2006) *Animals in Translation*. Bloomsbury, London.

National Centre for the Replacement Refinement & Reduction of Animals in Research (NC3RS) Grimace scales. Available at: https://www.nc3rs.org.uk/grimacescales (accessed November 2016).

Pizzey, R., Prior, S., Logan, Z., Thompson, J. and Vincent, I. (2016) *The use of subcutaneous meloxicam injections in reduction of pain related behaviours and improvement of growth rates in neonatal lambs*. Paper presented at Recent Advances in Animal Welfare Science V: UFAW Animal Welfare Conference, York, UK, 23 June 2016, p. 85.

Smith, A.V., Proops, L., Grounds, K., Wathan, J. and McComb, K. (2016). Functionally relevant responses to human facial expressions of emotion in the domestic horse (*Equus caballus*). Available at: http://rsbl.royalsocietypublishing.org/content/12/2/20150907?ref=curiositydotcom (accessed May 2017).

Vincent, I.C. and Michell, A.R. (1996) Relationship between blood pressure and stress-prone temperament in dogs. *Physiology and Behaviour* 60(1), 135–138.

Vincent, I. and Thompson, J. (2011) Use of an articulating manikin lamb and ewe simulator to enhance and supplement teaching of ovine obstetrics. In: *Proceedings of the 2nd Veterinary Education (VetEd) Symposium, Nottingham University*, 13–14 July 2011, pp. 19–20.

Webster, J. (2011) *Management and Welfare of Farm Animals*. UFAW, Wheathampstead.

Clinical Skills Sheet

15.36. Rugging up a horse

The method described is a recommended safe way of rugging for all circumstances, particularly if you do not know how the horse is going to react.

It is important to maintain awareness of health and safety issues at all times when working around horses.

Method
View of left side of folded rug: 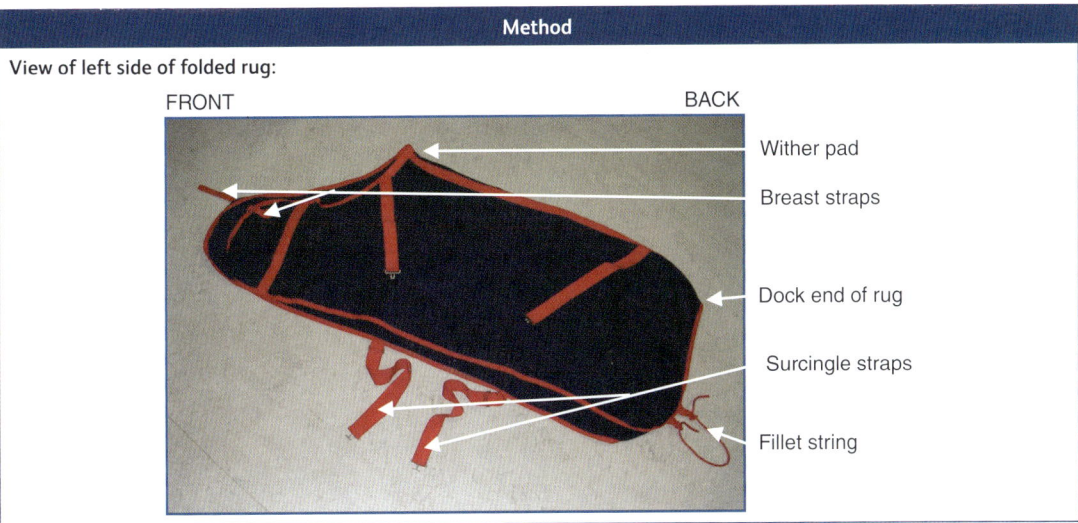
First check that the surcingle (belly) straps are tied together and leg straps (where present) are clipped to their D-rings. 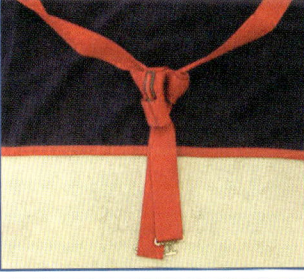
Fold the rug in half widthways, **inside out**, withers (base of neck) to dock (tail end).
Hold the rug so the wither pad (if present) and dock end are held, withers uppermost, in your left hand, and the mid-fold is in your right hand (creating a second fold). 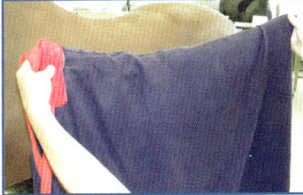

Method

Gently approach the horse's left shoulder, verbally reassuring it.

Please remember that many horse-handling activities are traditionally performed on the horse's left (near) side.

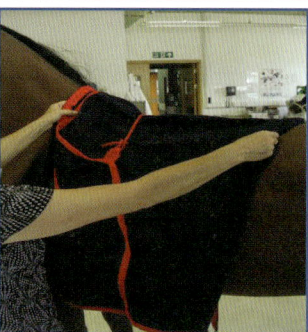

Place the folded rug gently across the withers, in front of the desired position. The open folds should be facing the neck, and the wither pad should be in contact with the horse.

Now do up the front fasteners, over the breast.

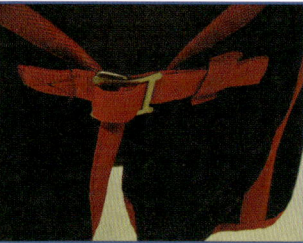

Unfold the rug over the horse's back, sliding the rug caudally into position if necessary. **Do not** pull the rug forwards against the lie of the coat.

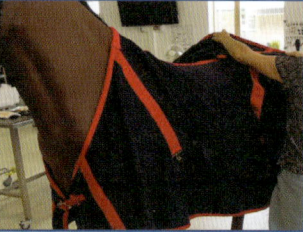

Go round the front of the horse to the right side; untie the surcingles and let them hang gently. Come back to the near side and secure them (rear strap to front clip, front strap to rear clip) so they cross under the belly.

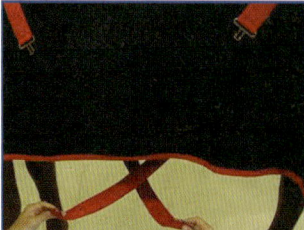 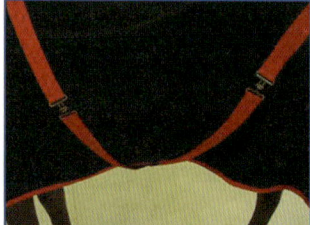

Method
Standing by the left hindquarters, lift the tail over the fillet string (if present) at the dock end of the rug. *Remember to avoid standing directly behind the horse.* 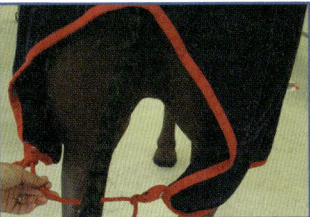
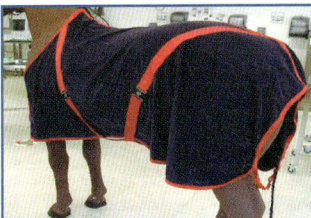
If the rug has hind leg straps, secure them now: pass the left strap around the medial aspect of the left leg and clip to the left-hand-side D-ring. Then pass the right strap around the medial aspect of the right leg, **looping it through the left leg strap, and clip it to the right-hand-side D-ring.**
Removing the rug: First undo any leg straps and clip them to the D-rings to prevent them dangling. You can lift the fillet string back over the tail at this stage.
Then undo the surcingles, letting them hang gently. Go round the front of the horse to the offside to tie these together for safety.
Finally, undo the front fasteners, then fold the rug backwards and remove gently by pulling the rug towards the tail and off at the nearside hip/buttock area.

© RVC

Clinical Skills Sheet

15.37. Tying up a horse using a quick-release knot

It is important to maintain awareness of health and safety issues at all times when working around horses.

Method
Remember never to tie a horse directly to a fixed object (e.g. fence, metal ring). For safety, tie up to string attached to the fixed object. This is so the string would break rather than injury being caused, in the event of the animal pulling back and panicking.
Feed the end of the lead rope through the string loop, leaving about 0.5 m between it and the horse's head. 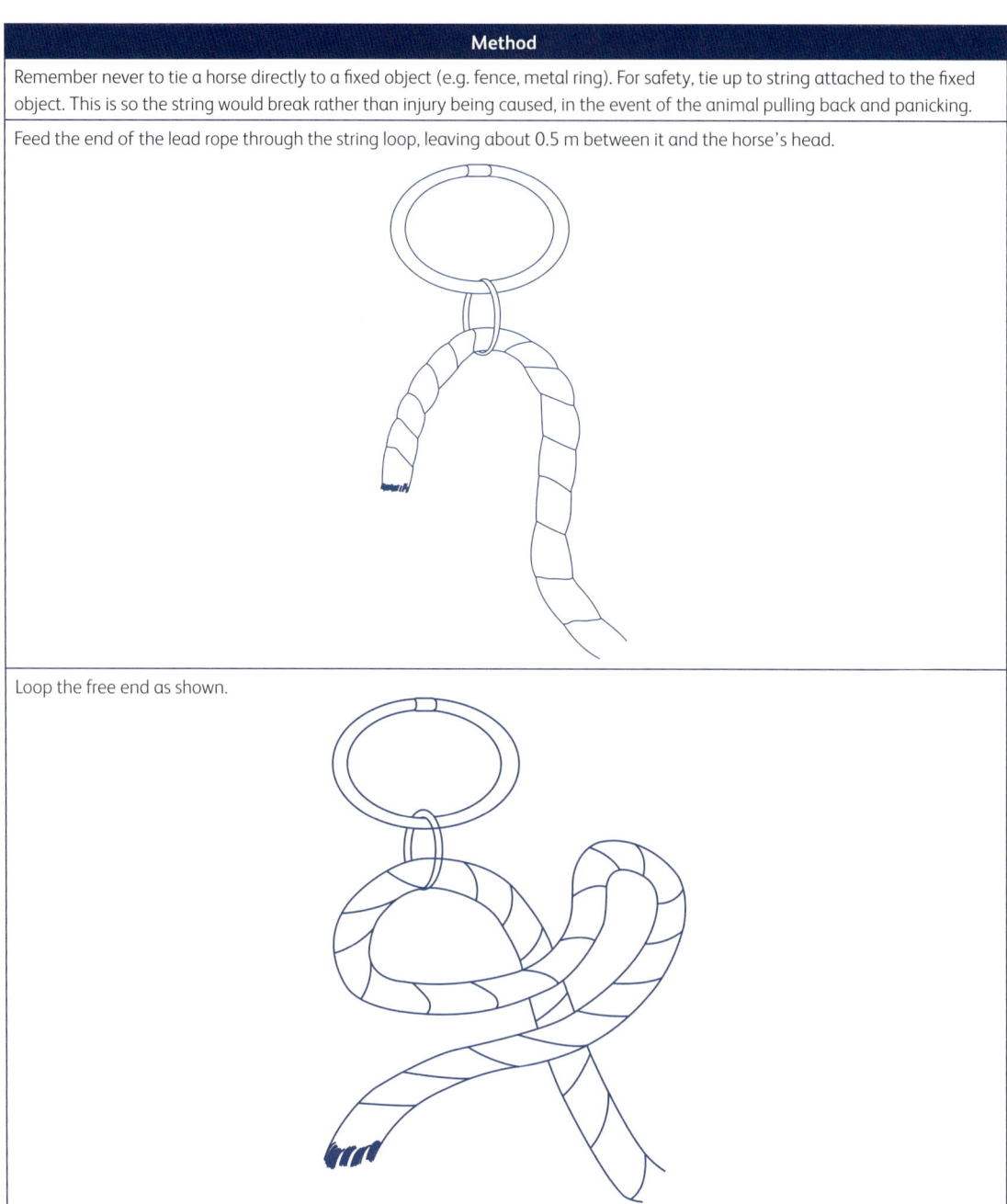
Loop the free end as shown.

Method

Feed the loop around the rope and through the circular gap. Secure the knot by holding the loop while pulling tight the lead rope on the 'horse' end.

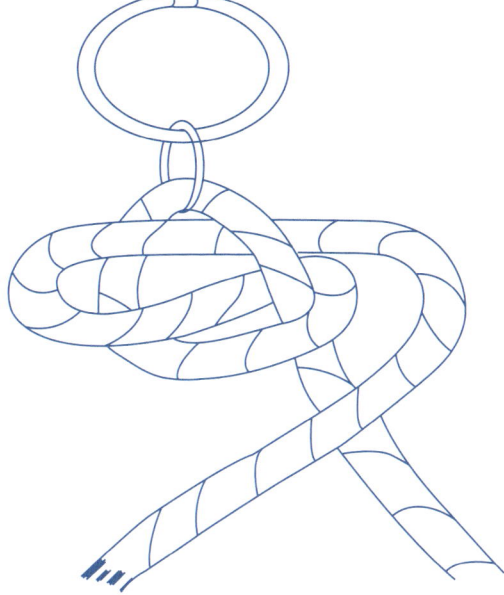

Some horses learn to pull the end of the rope to undo it! In that situation you can feed the end of the rope through the loop. This must be taken back through the loop before release.

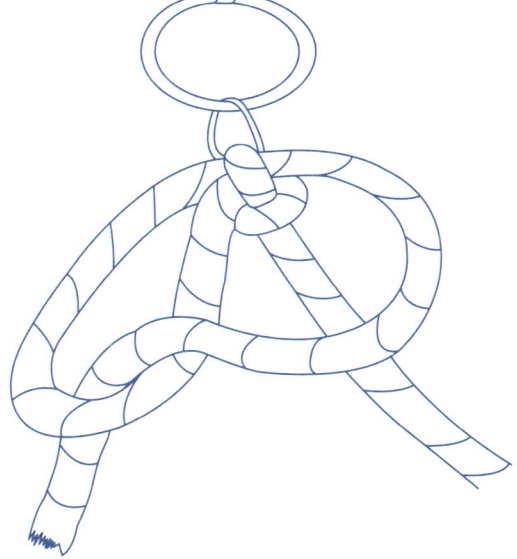

To release the knot, just pull on the end of the rope!

© RVC

Clinical Skills Sheet

15.38. Putting a tail bandage on a horse

It is important to maintain awareness of health and safety issues at all times when working around horses.

Method
Tail bandages can be used: • for protection during travel. • to neaten the tail after washing. • if a mare is to be covered (mated). A tail bandage should not be left on for longer than 4 h.
You will need one stable bandage (correctly rolled, with fastenings in the middle of the roll).
Please practise on the model tail only, as the manikin horses' tails are just for show.
With a real horse you will need to reassure it by voice and touch and monitor its behaviour, because this skill is necessarily performed directly behind the horse.
Take the bandage, with the roll on the outside, and place 10–15 cm of the bandage above the tail on the hindquarters. 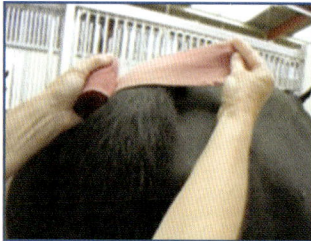
Wrap the bandage under the dock (base of tail) as far up as possible and firmly around itself a couple of times to secure it. 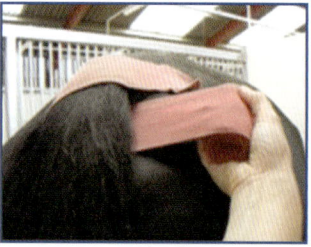 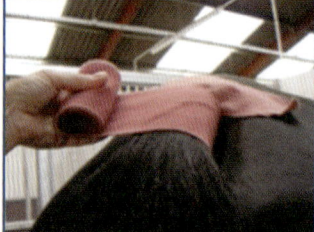
The flap can then be folded down and concealed behind the next turn. 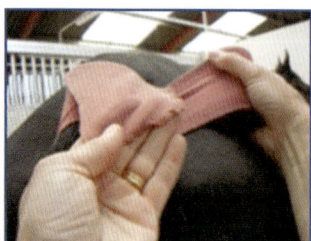 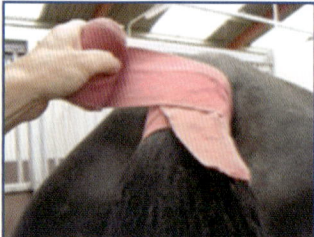

Method

Continue rolling the bandage down the tail, using an even pressure, overlapping the previous turn by a half. Wrap to just *above* the end of the caudal bones.

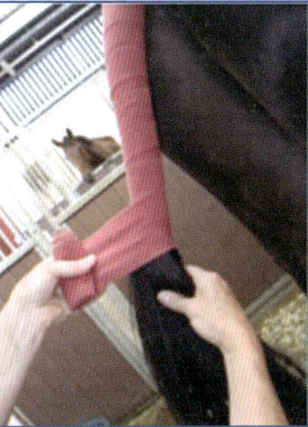

The bandage is now wrapped back up the tail, continuing an even pressure and half overlap, until the tape fastenings are reached. These are wrapped around the tail and tied in a firm bow on the outside, tucking the ends neatly into the bandage layer. If desired, fold down the previous bandage turn over the ties for neatness.

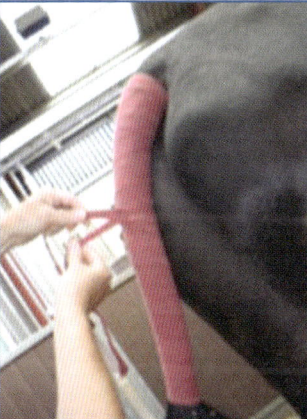

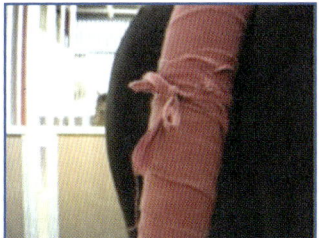 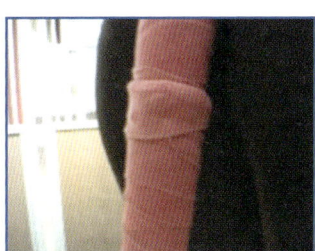

Method
(During travel, the fastening should ideally be on the lateral side of the tail in case of rubbing against the back of the trailer, causing pressure injury or loosening of the ties.)
Finish by getting hold of the bandaged tail and bending it slightly into the shape of the horse's rump (don't do this with the model tail!). 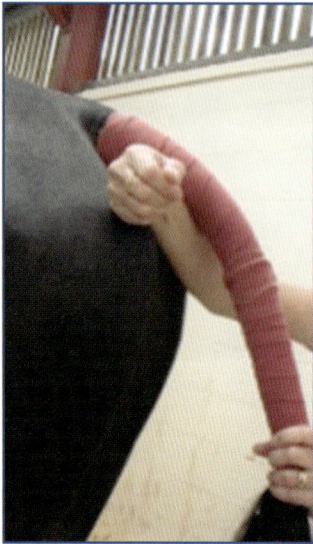
Removing the bandage: Undo the tapes, hook your fingers over the top of the bandage by the dock and pull the whole bandage downwards and off the tail in a smooth movement. Step away from the horse. 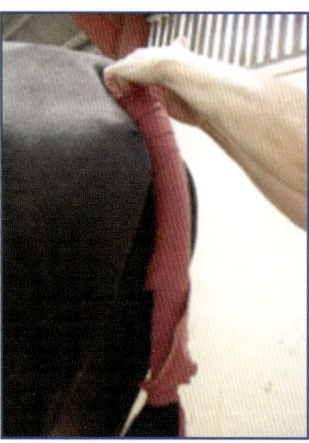 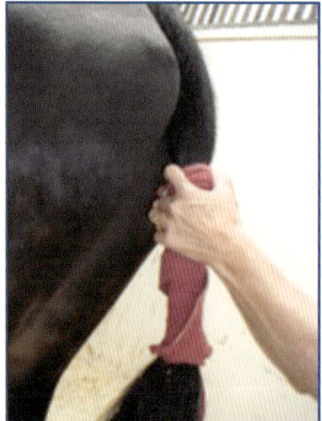
(Removing the bandage from the model tail: Undo the tapes and completely unwrap the bandage, as the model is not smooth enough to slide the bandage off.)
Unroll the bandage fully, fold the tapes neatly and then reroll the bandage around them, ready for next use.

© RVC

Clinical Skills Sheet

15.39. Putting a stable bandage on a horse

It is important to maintain awareness of health and safety issues at all times when working around horses.

Method
Stable bandages are used: • For warmth and aiding circulation. • To prevent the legs from 'filling' (becoming oedematous). • To assist in drying off wet legs. • As support for a sound leg when the opposite one is being treated for injury. • To protect the legs while travelling. • For keeping poultices in position.
Collect the equipment you need: • Padding layer (Fibregee or Gamgee) long enough to cover the leg from knee/hock to just below the coronet (around the top of the hoof) and wide enough to wrap around the leg with a comfortable overlap. • Stable bandage (correctly rolled, with fastenings in the middle of the roll).
Squatting down (***never kneeling or sitting***), wrap the padding layer around the leg, ideally with the outside edge facing to the rear. The subsequent bandage must be applied in the same direction as this padding layer. 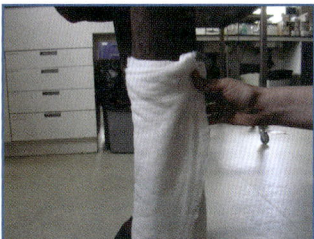
Take the stable bandage, with the roll on the outside, and begin the bandaging just below the knee, leaving an exposed margin of padding.
There are two effective ways of securing the end of the bandage – choose your preference, A or B! **A: The 'flap' method** Wrap the bandage around the leg once, leaving a small flap. 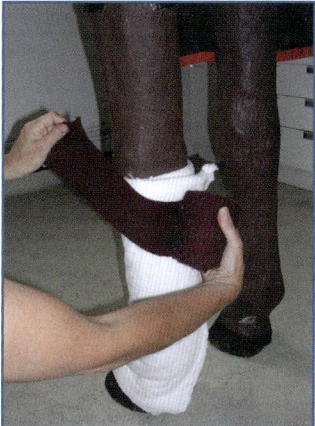

Method

The flap can then be folded down and concealed behind the next turn.

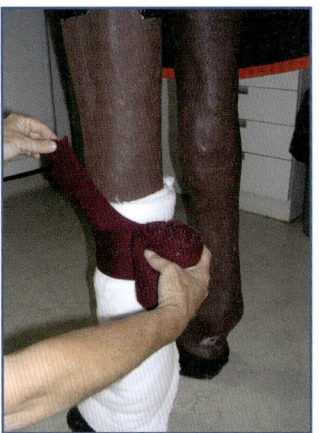 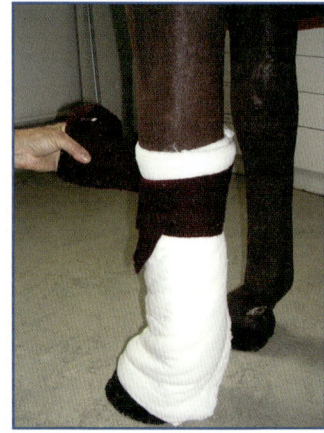

B: The 'tuck' method

Take the bandage and place the end inside the padding layer, securing it with the thumb of your other hand.

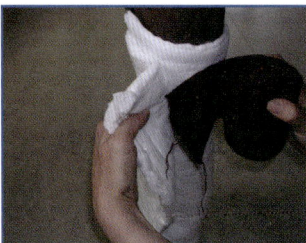 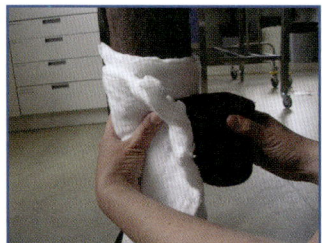

Wrap the bandage around itself once to secure the end hidden behind the padding layer.

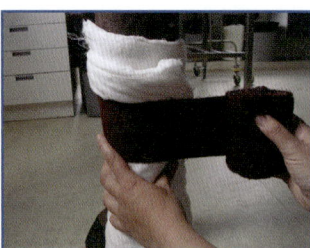

Method

Once you have secured the bandage by either method, continue rolling the bandage down the leg, using an even pressure, overlapping the previous turn by a half to two-thirds. Wrap over the fetlock and pastern until you reach the top of the hoof.

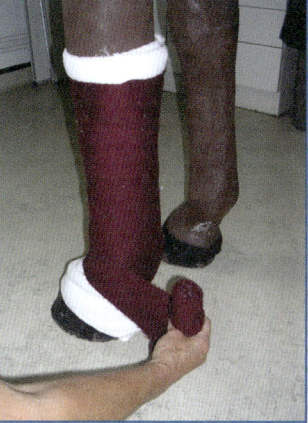

Leaving a margin of padding exposed over the hoof, start to wind the bandage back up the leg, continuing an even pressure and half to two-thirds overlap, until the fastenings (Velcro or tapes) are reached.

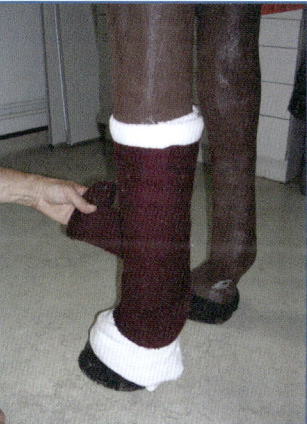

Ideally, the fastening should be on the lateral side of the leg, half to two-thirds of the way up the leg. Secure the Velcro, or tie tapes into a firm bow, tucking the ends neatly into the bandage layer.

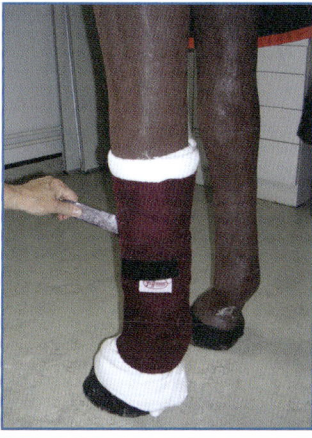 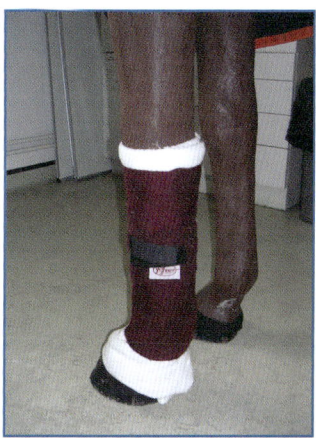

Method
Test the firmness of the bandage by placing a finger down between the padding layer and the horse's leg. There should be room for one finger's width only.
Removing the bandage: Undo the fastenings, then unwrap the bandage by passing it quickly from hand to hand around the leg (*don't waste time carefully reversing the rolling process!*). Collect the wad of bandage in one hand, remove the padding layer with the other hand and step away from the horse. 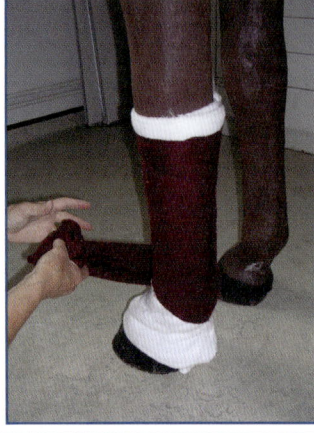
Unroll the bandage fully, and rewind it with all fastenings on the inside ready for next use. 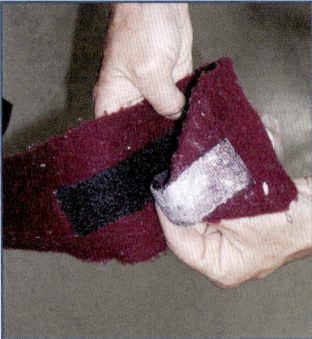

© RVC

Clinical Skills Sheet

15.40. Applying a lower-limb protective bandage on a horse to cover a wound or surgical incision

Method
Select and collect all the items you require for the bandage before commencing:

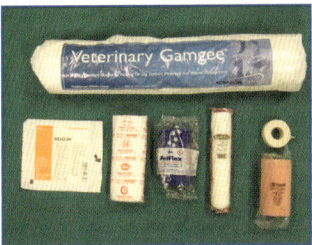

or

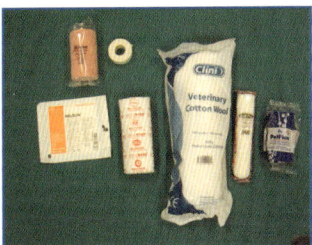

Primary dressing:
- Non-adherent wound dressing, 1–2 pads (e.g. Melolin).

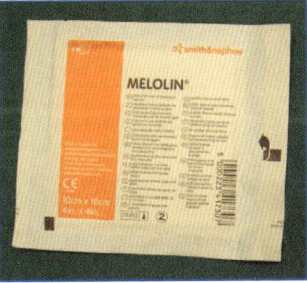

Method

Padding layer:
- Orthopaedic padding, 1 roll (e.g. 15 cm Orthoband).
- Cotton wool (1 roll) *or* Gamgee bandage (1 pad).

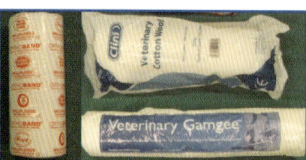

Conforming layer:
Conforming bandage, 1–2 rolls (e.g. Knit-Fix).

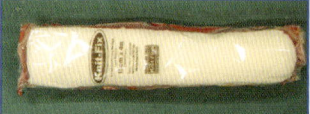

Shell layer:
Cohesive bandage tape, 1–2 rolls (e.g. 10 cm Vetrap).

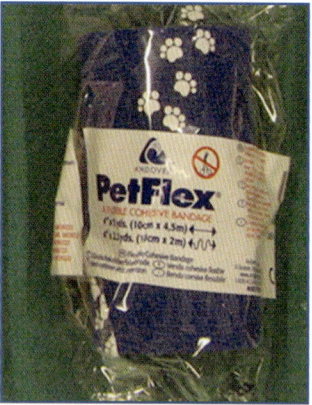

Top and/or bottom seal:
Adhesive bandage tape (e.g. 10 cm Elastoplast).

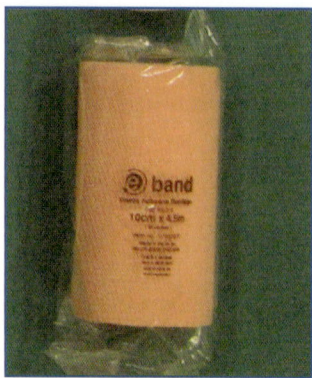

Method
Scissors.
White tape.
Procedure
Place the primary dressing (non-adherent = 'shiny' surface towards the wound or incision) and hold in place.

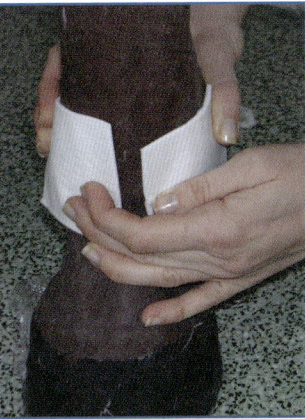

Secure the primary dressing in place by applying a layer of orthopaedic padding.

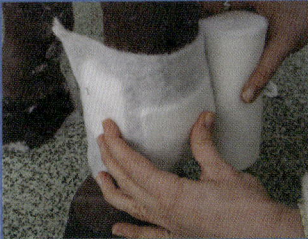

Continue to wrap the orthopaedic padding around the limb, working distally to the hoof and then proximally, ideally finishing just below the carpus.
Note: use the entire roll.

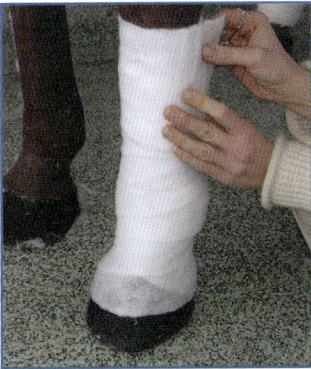

Method

Wrap the cotton wool or Gamgee bandage around the limb from just below the carpus to halfway down the hoof. Ensure that the heel is covered.

Note: wrap in the same direction as the orthopaedic padding.

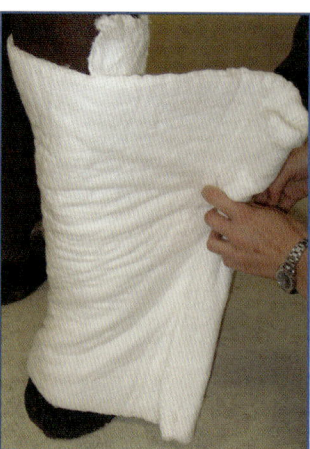
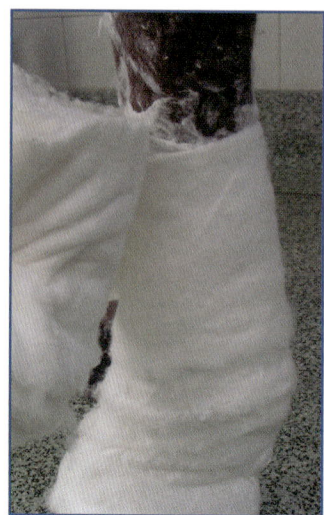

Starting just below the carpus, apply a layer of conforming bandage over the cotton wool or the Gamgee bandage.

Note: wrap in the same direction as the cotton wool or the Gamgee bandage.

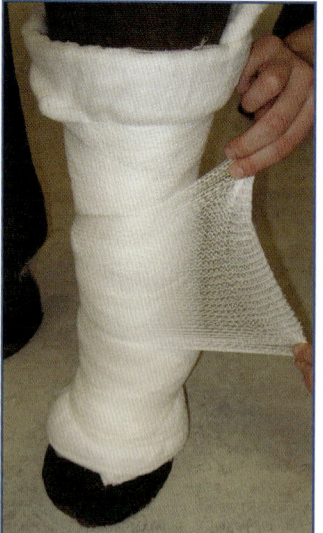
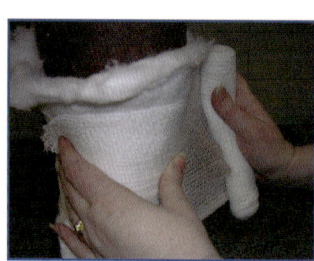

As you apply this layer, overlap two-thirds of the width of the conforming bandage. Compress the underlying padding with even pressure by applying tension to the conforming bandage.

Leave a margin of the underlying padding exposed at the top and distal end of the bandage.

Note: This acts as protection to prevent the bandage cutting into the horse's leg.

Method

Apply the shell layer = cohesive bandage tape (e.g. 10 cm Vetrap) over the conforming bandage.

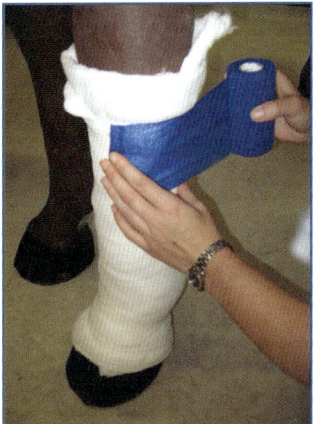 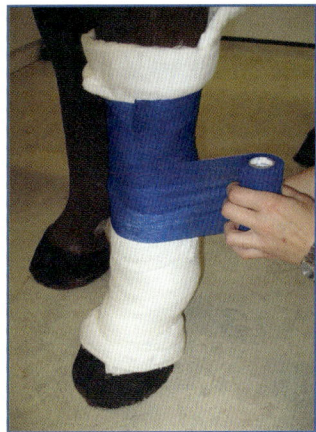

As you apply this layer, overlap half of the width of the cohesive bandage tape.

Leave a margin of the underlying padding exposed at the top and distal end of the bandage.

Note: wrap in the same direction as the conforming bandage.

Seal the top and/or bottom of the bandage by applying a layer of adhesive bandage tape (e.g. Elastoplast) so that it overlaps the edges of the bandage and sticks to the hair and/or hoof, respectively.

This prevents dirt or debris from entering the bandage.

Note: do not put any tension on the adhesive bandage tape, as it will constrict circulation.

Secure the ends of the adhesive bandage tape with strips of white tape.

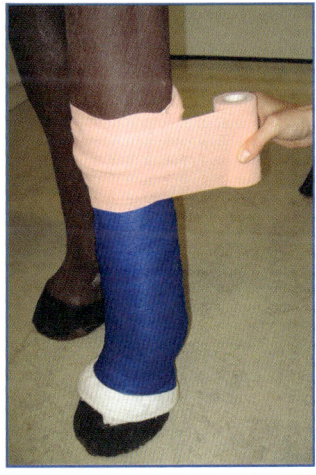 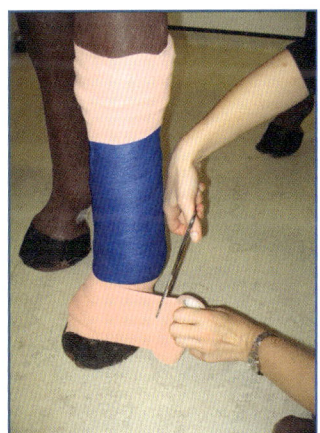 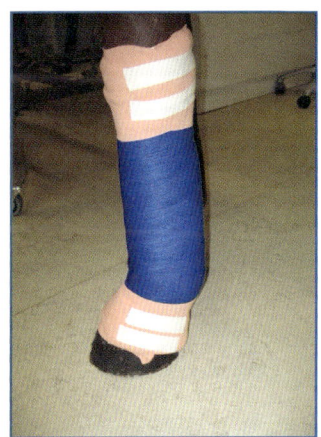

Your completed bandage should be even in thickness and pressure with no pieces sticking out.

The key to a good protective bandage is to apply the conforming layer firmly and to ensure that the bandage is even throughout.

© RVC

245

Clinical Skills Sheet

15.41. How to halter a cow

It is important to maintain awareness of health and safety issues at all times when working around large animals.

Method
A halter put on correctly has the short fixed part of the rope placed over the nose. The halter tightens under the chin with the metal ring (or loop) usually on the left side. The cow is then led from her left-hand side. 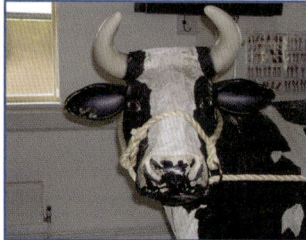
To begin, stand on the left side of the animal, with the halter opened up sufficiently to go over the cow's head. 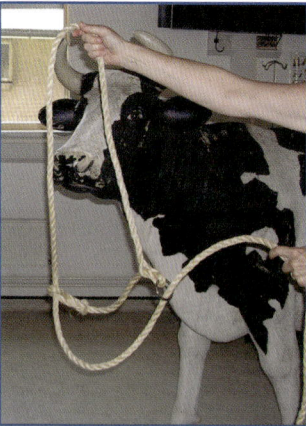
Place the halter over the far ear and horn first, then over the near ear and horn. 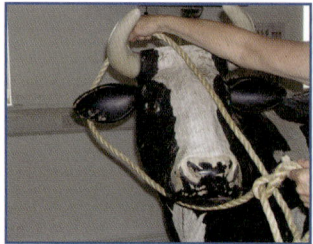 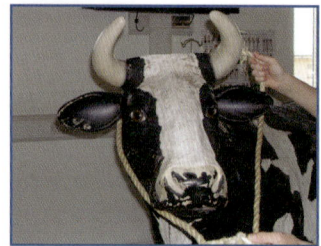

Method

Holding the short fixed noseband piece in your right hand, place it over the cow's nose …

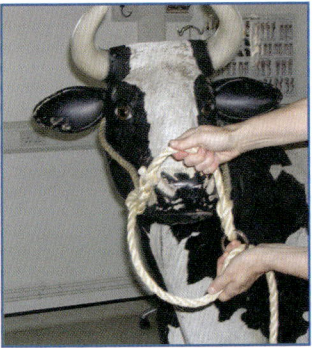 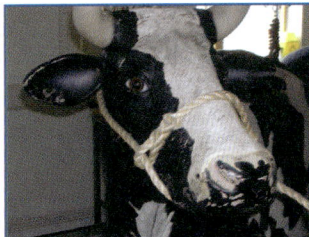

… and tighten/adjust as necessary through the metal ring or loop.

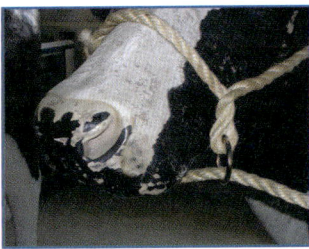

Putting on a halter – supplementary information

Arrange rope to look like this:

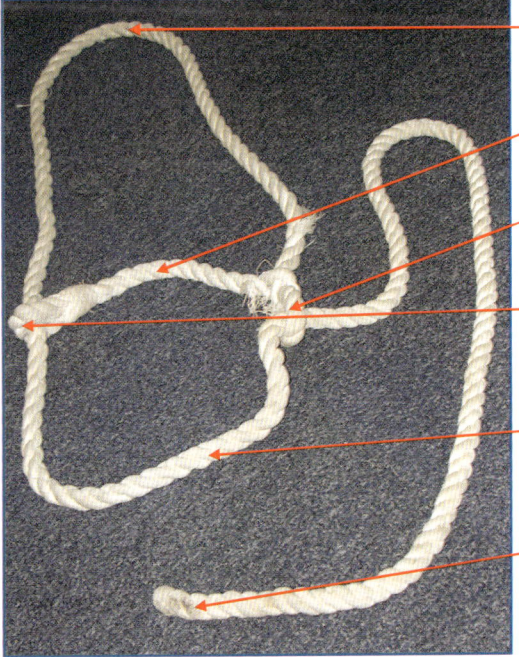

This goes behind the horns and ears.

Fixed noseband goes **over** nose.

Fixed attachment of noseband.

Slip attachment of noseband, placed on right side of cheek.

This goes *under* the lower jaw, and tightens on left-hand side cheek.

End of rope held on left-hand side of animal

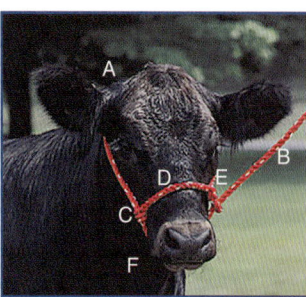

A	Poll part of halter placed behind horns (where present) and ears
B	Rope end
C	Slip attachment of noseband
D	Noseband = short, fixed-length piece of rope
E	Fixed attachment of noseband
F	Halter tightens under lower jaw

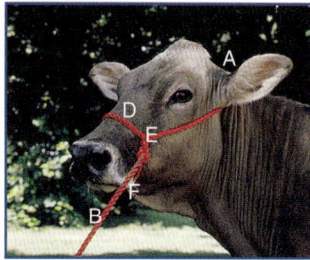

© RVC

Diagnostic Imaging

Panagiotis Mantis[a] and Victoria Watts[b]

[a]Dick White Referrals, Newmarket; [b]The Royal Veterinary College, London

Learning objectives

By the end of this chapter, students should be able to:

- Demonstrate how to position an animal for diagnostic imaging.
- Explain how common film faults occur.
- Identify common digital radiology artefacts.
- Understand the basic physics of ultrasound and the functional parts of an ultrasound machine.
- Recognize the normal appearance of the heart and major abdominal organs.

Clinical skills sheets (SS)

Three clinical skills sheets will be used in this chapter and these can be found at pages 263–271. Reference will be made to each skills sheet at the relevant section within the chapter. The details of the clinical skills sheets used are as follows:

SS 16.42 Imaging BVA/KC hips
SS 16.43 Imaging caudo-cranial stifle
SS 16.44 Ultrasound (U/S) set-up

16.1 Radiographs

16.1.1 Positioning: rules and terminology

- Radiographic projections are named based on the direction in which the X-ray beam enters the body, followed by the exit point.
- For lateral recumbency projections of the thorax and abdomen, the projection can also be named by the side that the patient lies on (recumbent side).
- For limb projections, the projections are named as mediolateral or lateromedial.
- While in the body the terms cranial, caudal, medial and lateral are used, for the head the term cranial is replaced by rostral.
- In the limbs, the terms cranial and caudal are used until proximal to carpus and tarsus. From the carpus and tarsus, the terms dorsal and palmar (front limbs) or plantar (hind limbs) are used.
- The term oblique is added in views where the X-ray beam passes obliquely through the body; for example, dorsolateral–plantaromedial oblique view.

16.1.2 General guidelines

- Two views of each anatomical area, taken at right angles to each other, are considered the minimum recommended views.
- Each view should be labelled with a left/right marker and, if required, an appropriate scaling device for accurate measurements (e.g. radiopaque ruler).
- The part of the image closer to the cassette will be the less distorted.
- When the area under examination is thicker than 10 cm, a grid is used.
- For **thoracic views**, centre at the caudal edge of the scapula and expand the collimation to include just caudal to the last rib. For ventrodorsal (VD) or dorsoventral (DV) projections, expand to the lateral edges of the thorax. For the lateral views, expand ventrally to the sternum and dorsally to the thoracic spine. Two points to note: (i) the DV or VD should be acquired first to prevent atelectasis forming when recumbent; and (ii) if possible the exposure should take place at peak inspiration (general anaesthesia is ideal for providing the means to achieve this).

© CAB International 2018. *Veterinary Clinical Skills Manual* (eds N. Coombes and A. Silva-Fletcher)

- For **abdominal views**, centre on the last rib and expand caudally to include the coxofemoral joints. For VD or DV views, expand to the lateral edges of the abdomen. For the lateral views, expand ventrally to include the most ventral aspect of the abdomen and dorsally to include the lumbar spine. Two points to note: (i) the diaphragm can extend quite high into the thorax (e.g. during expiration) and the distal third of the sternum should be included within the collimation to avoid missing part of the cranioventral abdomen; and (ii) if the animal is particularly long, two views, one for the cranial abdomen and one for the caudal abdomen, should be acquired, ensuring that there is overlap of structures to avoid missing any anatomy

- For **limb views**, when radiographing long bones, make sure that the leg is parallel to the cassette and to include the joints on both sides.

- For **limb views**, when radiographing joints, align the long side of the cassette with the distal long bone and centre through the joint.

- For the **lateral view of the cervical spine**, keep head in true lateral projection and use foam under the neck to keep it parallel to the cassette where needed.

- For **skull** radiographs, keep nose parallel to the cassette and centre at the lateral canthus of the eye extending to include the skull.

> **SS 16.42** describes the positioning for a ventrodorsal radiograph of the hip
>
> **SS 16.43** describes the positioning for a caudo-cranial radiograph of the stifle

16.1.3 Common film faults

Positioning

- Avoid or minimize superimposition and rotation (Fig. 16.1).

- Area of interest should be centred on the radiograph to avoid geometric distortion.

Movement

- Reducing the animal's stress and the use of sedation or general anaesthesia will reduce movement of the patient that results in motion blur (Fig. 16.2).

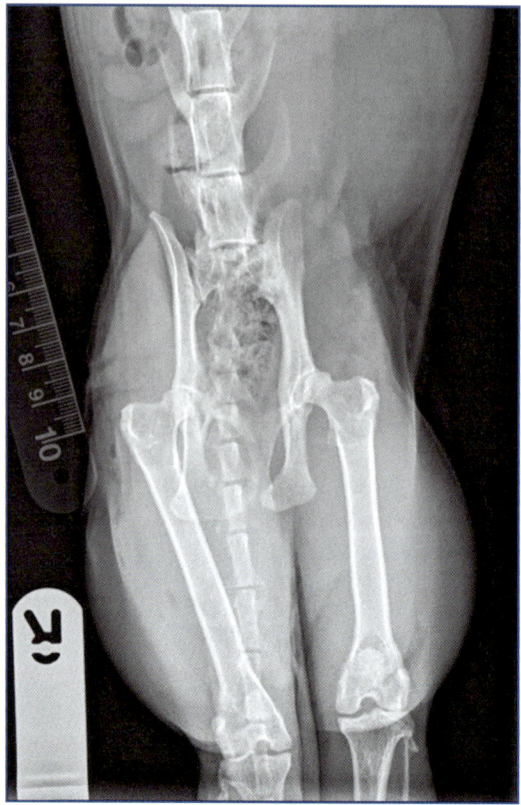

Fig. 16.1. Rotated pelvic radiograph from a skeletally mature cat. The left side is closer to the cassette, resulting in the left wing of the ileum appearing wider, the left obturator foramen smaller and the left coxofemoral joint space wider than it is.

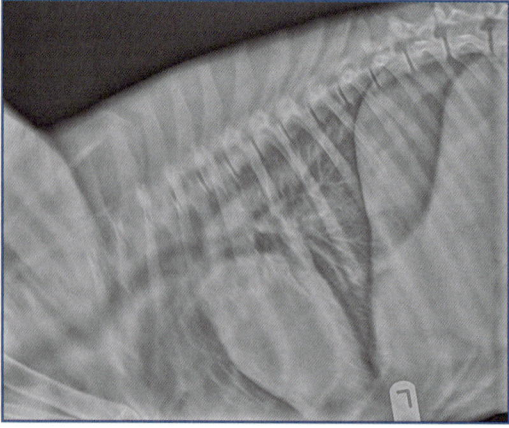

Fig. 16.2. Radiograph with marked motion blur. The structures are unclear due to the blur.

- Generally, the shortest time possible for a given milli-ampere-seconds (mAs) should be chosen to reduce or avoid motion blur, especially on thoracic radiographs.

- In larger patients, the use of fast screen/film combinations may also aid in the reduction of motion blur.

16.1.4 Radiographic contrast

- Poor contrast results in images with little difference between opaque and lucent structures.

- Factors affecting the radiographic contrast include:

  - Development, and especially underdevelopment. In underdevelopment, holding the film on light you should not be able to see your fingers behind the film when they are in the background area of the film. This is caused commonly by exhausted developer and/or low developer temperature (Fig. 16.3).

  - Fogging is the darkening of the film when it is exposed to light or X-rays (Fig. 16.4) and usually it is seen when there is light leakage in the darkroom.

  - A high peak kilovoltage (kVp) and low mAs results in a radiograph with low contrast and is preferred for thoracic radiographs. A low kVp and high mAs results in a radiograph with high contrast and is preferred for abdominal radiographs and musculoskeletal radiographs (Fig. 16.5).

16.1.5 Exposure

- Overexposure will result in too dark radiographs (Fig. 16.6). To correct, reduce the exposure. (*Tip*: reducing the exposure by 10 kVp or halving the mAs will halve the exposure.)

- Underexposure will result in too light radiographs (Fig. 16.7). To correct, increase the exposure. (*Tip*: increasing the exposure by 10 kVp or doubling the mAs will double the exposure.)

- Incorrect exposures are compensated more easily in computed radiography (CR) and digital radiography (DR) systems. Significant over- or underexposure can lead to artefacts in DR and CR systems and these may not be able to be corrected.

- Double exposure (Fig. 16.8) happens when two exposures are made in the same cassette.

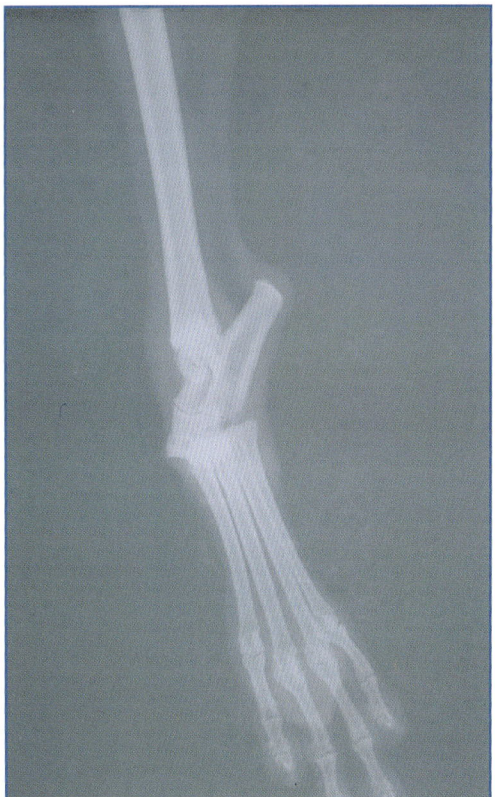

Fig. 16.3. Underdeveloped radiograph. Watch the more opaque background around the exposed part of the radiograph. If you place a finger behind that part you can see it clearly, something that is not possible in a properly exposed and developed radiograph.

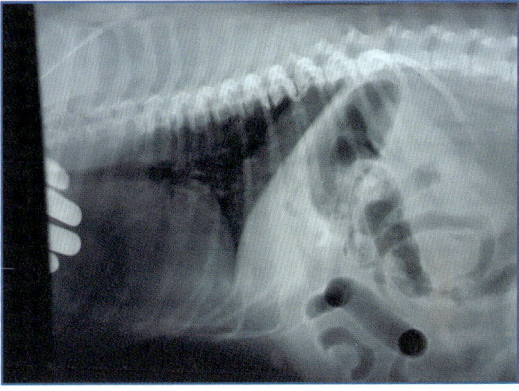

Fig. 16.4. Fogging evident, especially in the left side of the radiograph, where we can also see the outline of the processing hand.

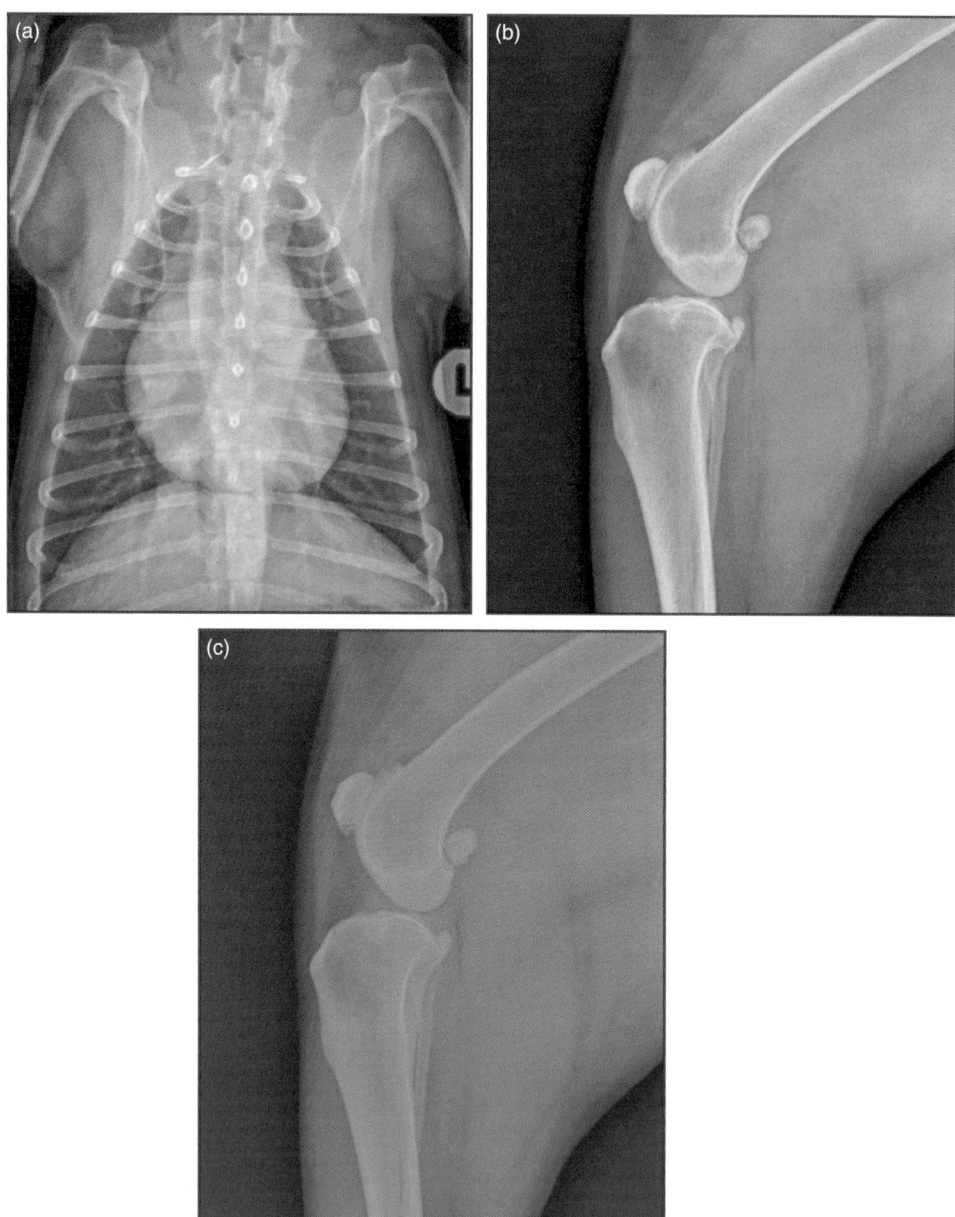

Fig. 16.5. (a) A DV thoracic radiograph with high kVp and low mAs, resulting in low contrast. (b) A lateral radiograph of a canine stifle with low kVp and high mAs, resulting in more contrast. (c) The same radiograph as (b) with low contrast.

16.1.6 Film marks

- Crescent-shaped artefacts: dark lines are created by rough handling of X-ray film (fingernail pressure or excessive bending) (Fig. 16.8) and white lines are created by cracked intensifying screen.

- Electrostatic artefacts are created when films are rubbed or unwrapped forcibly or secondary to excessive bending. They appear as black lightning strikes (Fig. 16.9).

- The presence of hair, dust and other particles in the cassette will stop exposure of the film/plate in

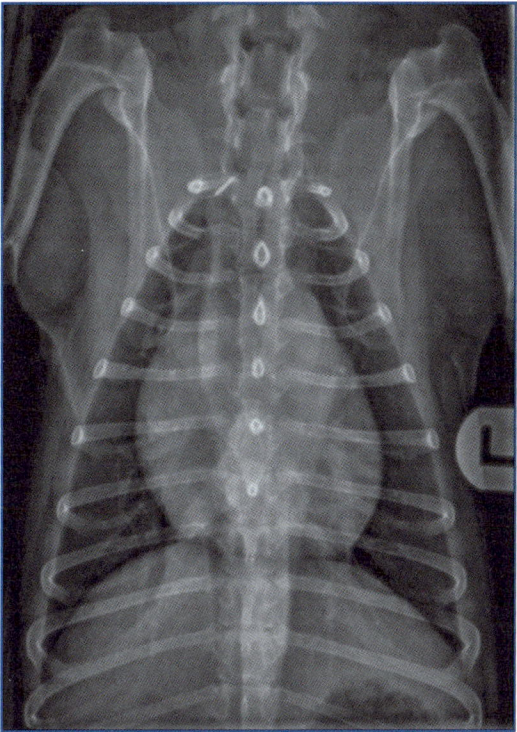

Fig. 16.6. Overexposed DV thoracic radiograph. The whole radiograph appears darker. Reducing the exposure by 10 kV will result in an optimally exposed radiograph (see Fig. 16.5a).

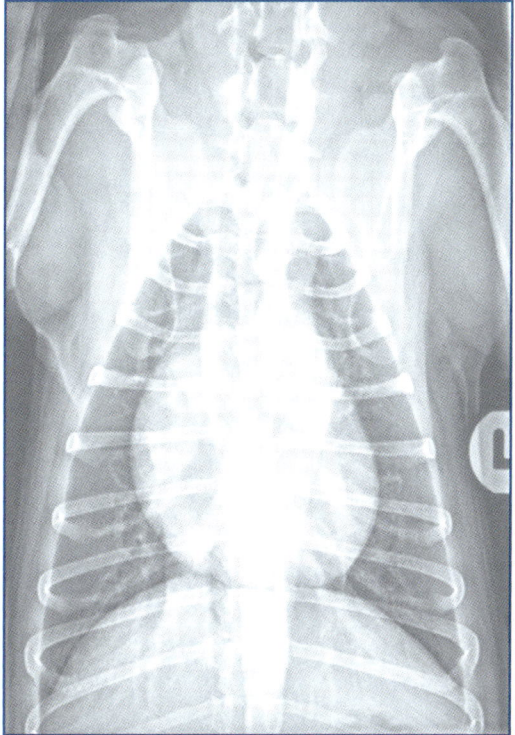

Fig. 16.7. Underexposed thoracic radiograph. Compare with Fig. 16.5a (properly exposed) and Fig. 16.6 (overexposed).

that area, resulting in unexposed flecks on the radiograph (Fig. 16.10). (*Tip*: screens should be regularly examined and cleaned.)

- Streaking artefacts from the automatic processor. The automatic processor should be cleaned regularly.
- Chemical splashes from developer or fixer are usually seen with manual processing (Fig. 16.10). (*Tip*: white splashes are fixer and black splashes are developer artefacts.)

16.1.7 Common digital radiology artefacts

- *Uberschwinger* artefact appears as a radiolucent halo around metal or where there is a large density difference between adjacent structures. It can be mistaken as implant loosening or pneumothorax (Fig. 16.11).

- The graininess/pixelation (Fig. 16.12) observed in underexposed digital radiographs comes from statistical uncertainty in adjacent pixels (there is not enough data for a complete image).
- Calibration marks errors:
  - Inhomogeneous tabletops may produce stipple that is not visible using film/screen. The calibration should be performed with the detector on top of the table, or the table should be moved away between each calibration exposure.
  - DR systems are susceptible to radio frequency interference. These artefacts have a periodic pattern characteristic of the cause.
- Ghost images can be produced by DR systems. Stimulated photodiodes trap charge and release that charge even after the readout. These look like a double exposure.
- CR ghost images happen when effective saturation of the image receptor is present.

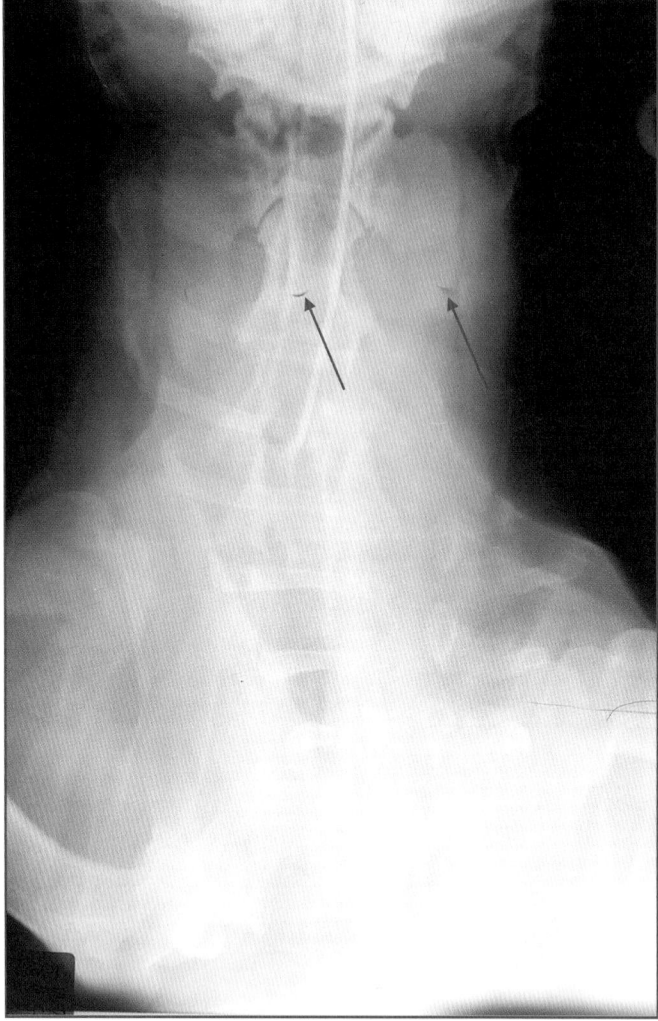

Fig. 16.8. Double exposure with ribs visible over the neck. There are also crimps (arrows).

- Saturation occurs when digital radiographs are overexposed (Fig. 16.13).

- A light-bulb artefact is present when the outer portions of the film are darker than the remainder of the image.

- Grid lines can show when used incorrectly, for example when not removed for an extremity radiograph (Fig. 16.14).

- Improper look-up table assignment can lead to alteration of the image contrast and density. If that is the case, change to appropriate post-processing values.

- Reader artefacts can occur when one or more light guides is dirty – the light is blocked and a white line across the image results (Fig. 16.15).

- CR imaging plates are more susceptible to fogging than X-ray films, because they have an opening/closing system.

- Foreign bodies in cassettes occur only with CR systems because the cassette is opened during processing/reading (Fig. 16.16).

- If foreign bodies show on the image and a cause is not found on/in the cassette or on the detector, check the table, mattress, animal and X-ray tube.

Fig. 16.9. Electrostatic artefact appears as black lightning strikes.

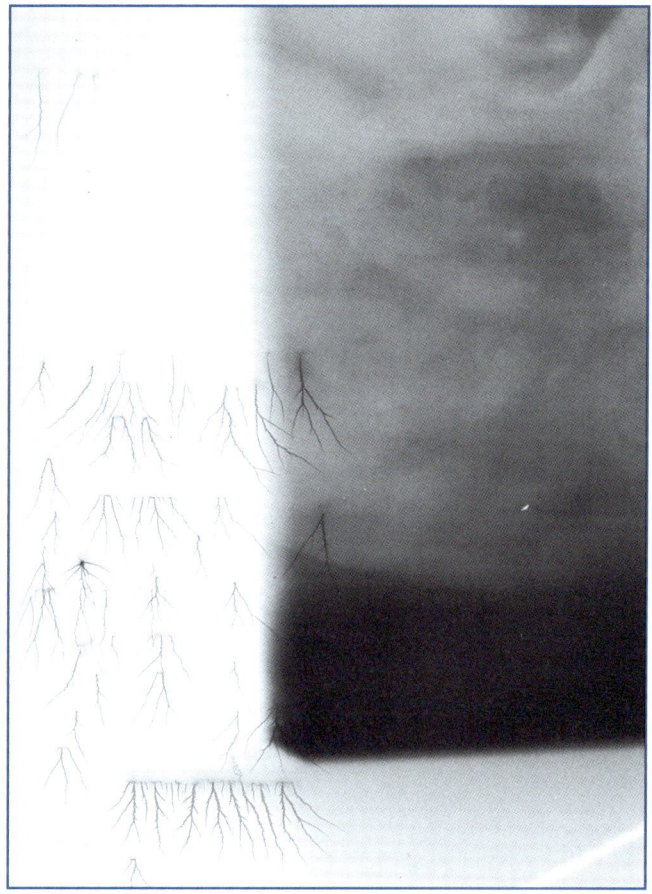

Fig. 16.10. Dirty screen artefacts (arrows) and chemical spill artefact from fixer (*).

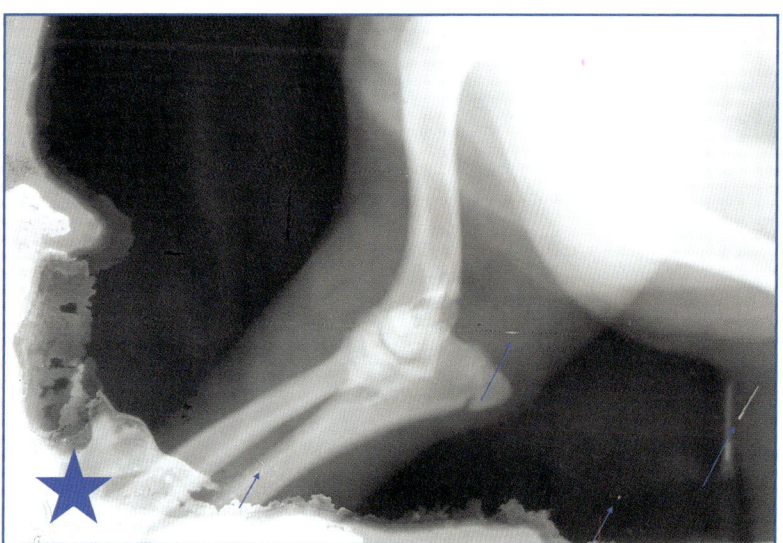

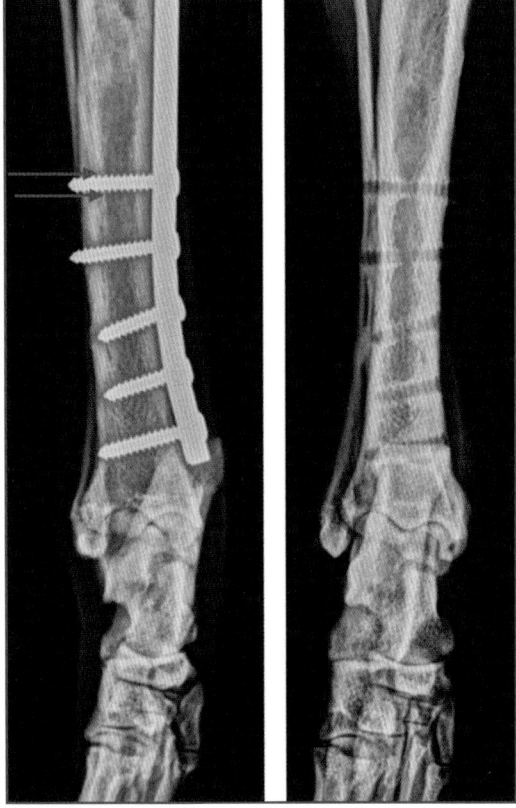

Fig. 16.11. *Uberschwinger* artefact appears as a radiolucent halo around metal (arrows around first screw but the artefact is visible around all screws). Left image with implants and right image after implant removal.

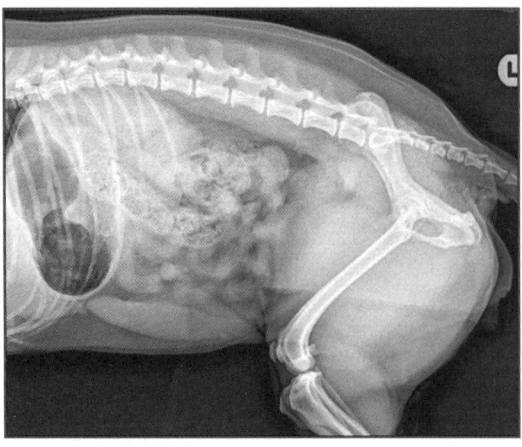

Fig. 16.12. Observe the graininess in this canine lateral abdominal radiograph.

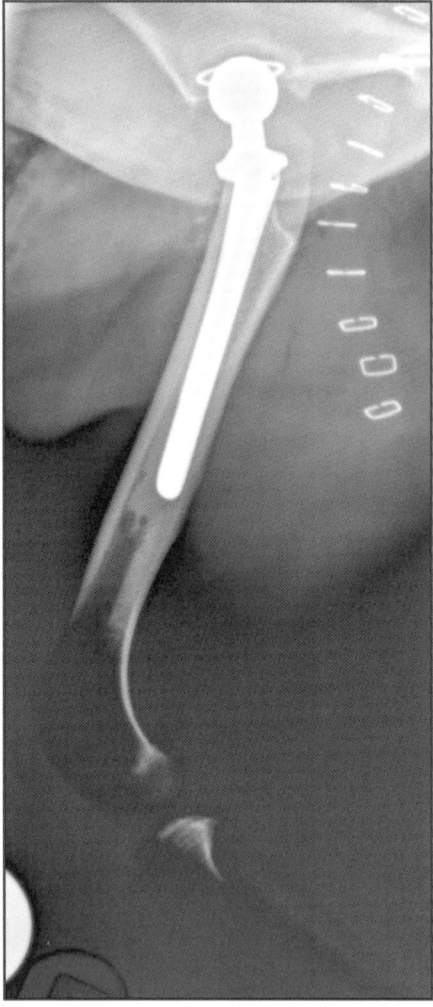

Fig. 16.13. Overexposed lateral radiograph of a canine femur with evident saturation.

16.2 Ultrasound

16.2.1 Basic physics

- Ultrasound employs high-frequency sound waves that are travelling through the body, reflected on interfaces and the reflected sound is analysed and recorded by a computer to provide cross-sectional images of organs.

- Diagnostic ultrasound uses the pulse-echo principle: short pulses of sound are transmitted into the body.

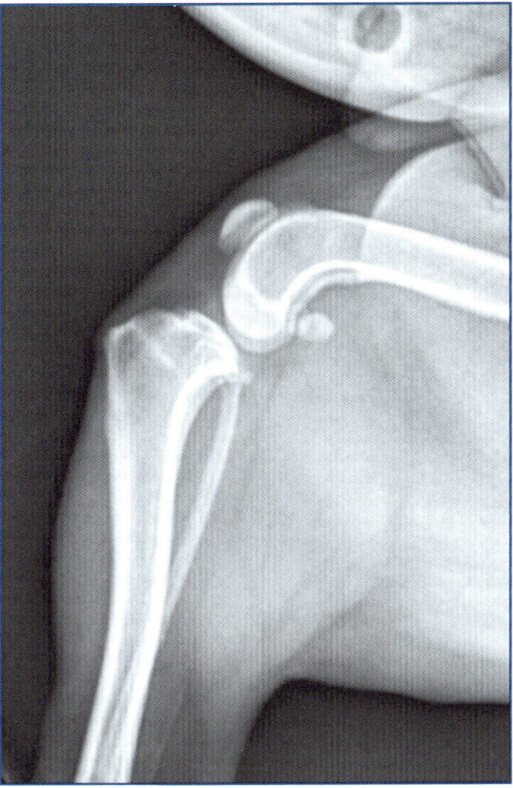

- The speed of the sound is different in different tissues and is affected by the density and elasticity of the tissues. The sound propagation velocity increases with higher stiffness and decreases with higher density. The propagation velocity in the soft tissues of the body is similar and the ultrasound machine assumes a constant velocity of 1540 m/s.

- The depth to which the sound reaches is inversely proportional to the frequency of the sound. Lower frequencies reach deeper; however, the resolution is reduced with lower frequencies. That is why you should always employ the highest possible frequency for the depth you need to examine.

- The product of sound velocity and tissue density is called acoustic impedance (Z). The difference in acoustic impedance between tissues is what determines the amount of the sound that is reflected.

- When the sound encounters gas or bone, most of the sound is reflected and very little is available to image deeper.

- Ultrasound is not specific. A normal ultrasound does not exclude the presence of disease.

Fig 16.14. Lateral radiograph from a canine stifle. The grid lines are evident.

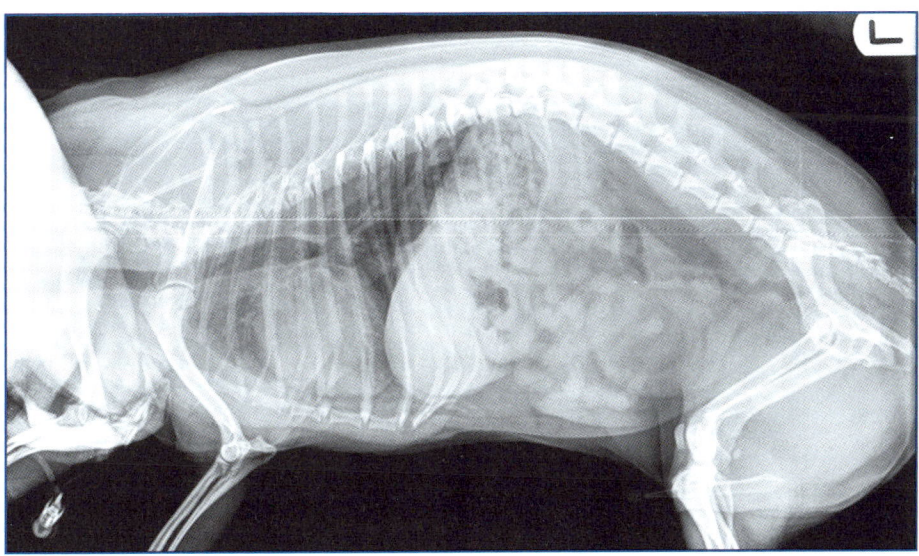

Fig. 16.15. Reader artefact. Two white lines are seen across the screen.

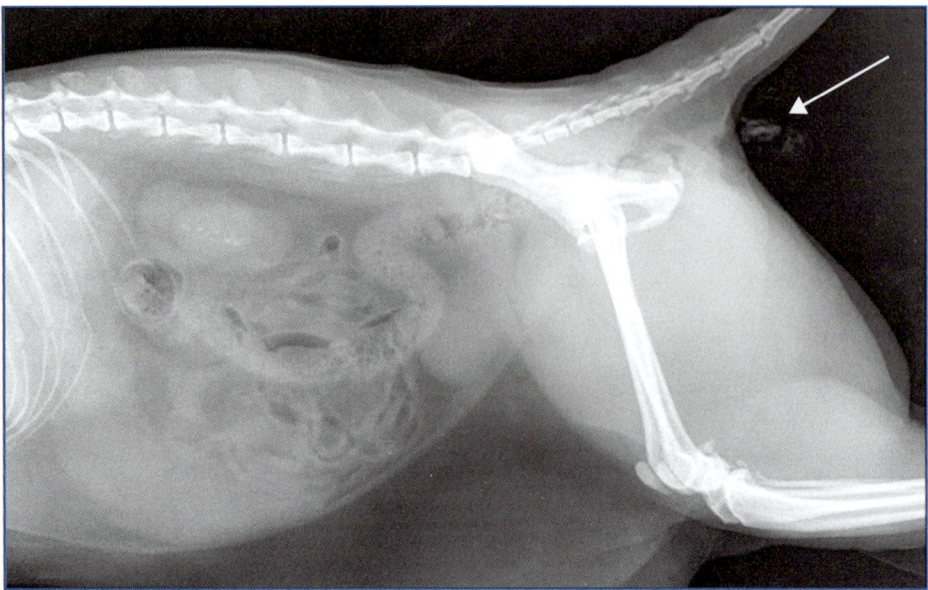

Fig. 16.16. Lateral feline abdominal radiograph. The dirt in the cassette is visible (arrow).

16.2.2 Machine knobs and buttons

The most commons controls used on ultrasound are the following (Fig. 16.17).

- Patient details button (1): to input the patient details – these are recorded in every saved image and clips.

- Exam preset button: to choose the type of examination (e.g. cardiac, abdomen, eye). Sometimes you choose the preset when you select probe (3).

- Freeze button (2): to freeze the image. In most recent machines, it allows you to move through several frames.

- Probe selection button (3): to select the transducer you are going to use. You can also change the frequency of the probe (3A).

- Depth button (4): to change the depth of the image during the examination. The rule is that the organ under examination should occupy three-quarters of the screen.

- Save buttons (5, 6): usually one for the images and one for the clips.

- Measure button (7): to perform linear measurements.

- Time gain compensation (series of buttons or knobs) (8): to adjust returning echo amplification differently in different depths.

- Overall gain knob (9): amplifies or de-amplifies all returning echoes regardless of depth.

- Focal zone button/knob (10): the focal zone is the area in your image with the higher resolution and in new machines can be moved to different depths or have more than one.

16.2.3 Transducer

- The transducer has a marker/indicator that is displayed on the screen.

- Ideally hold the transducer with the thumb or index finger in the marker so you know your orientation without the need to look at the transducer.

Movements of the transducer:

- Sliding (Fig. 16.18a).

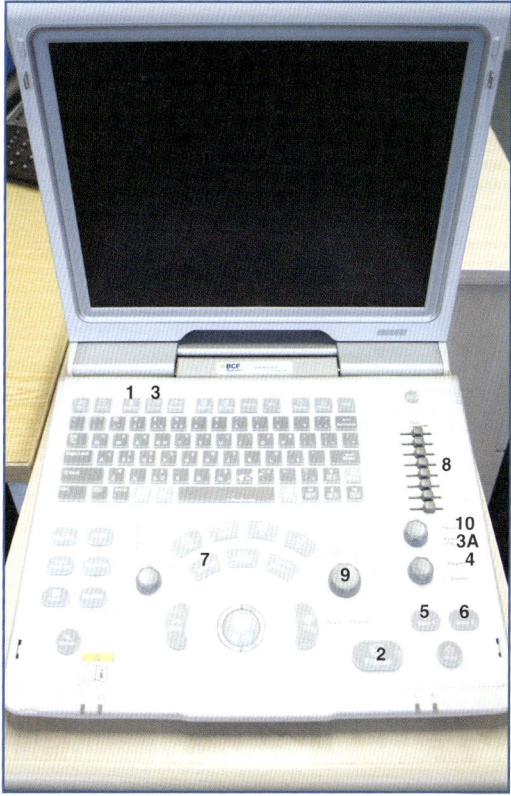

- Echogenicity on ultrasound is described, usually in comparison with other organs in the same animal, as: hyperechoic (whiter), hypoechoic (greyer), isoechoic (equal echogenicity), anechoic (black) or mixed echogenicity (mixed areas of increased, decreased echogenicity possibly with anechoic areas).

- Many organs are examined by ultrasound, including: skin, thyroid and parathyroid glands, salivary glands, lymph nodes, eyes, muscles, tendons, joints, thoracic and abdominal organs.

- Most commonly ultrasound in small animals is used to evaluate the heart and the abdominal organs.

 SS 16.44 for detailed procedure on how to set up an ultrasound machine

Further Reading: Brown, M. and Brown, L. (2013) *Lavin's Radiography for Veterinary Technicians*, 5th edn. Elsevier Health Sciences, London.

Kremkau, F.W. (2014) *Sonography Principles and Instruments*, 8th edn. Elsevier Saunders, St Louis, Missouri, USA.

Mantis, P. (2016) *Practical Small Animal Ultrasonography*. Editorial Servet, Zaragoza, Spain.

Mattoon, J.S. and Nyland, T.G. (2015) *Small Animal Diagnostic Ultrasound*, 3rd edn. Elsevier Saunders, St Louis, Missouri, USA.

Owens, J. and Biery, D. (1998) *Radiographic Interpretation for the Small Animal Clinician*, 2nd edn. Williams & Wilkins, Hagerstown, Maryland, USA.

Penninck, D. and d'Anjou, M.A. (2015) *Small Animal Ultrasonography*, 2nd edn. Wiley-Blackwell, Ames, Iowa, USA.

Sirois, M. (2011) *Principles and Practice of Veterinary Technology*, 3rd edn. Elsevier Mosby, St Louis, Missouri, USA.

Sirois, M., Anthony, E. and Maugaris, D. (2009) *Handbook of Radiographic Positioning for Veterinary Technicians*. Delmar Engage Learning Inc., New York.

Smallwood, J.E., Shively, M.J., Rendano, V.T. and Habel, R.E. (1985) A standardized nomenclature for radiographic projections used in veterinary medicine. *Veterinary Radiology* 26(1), 2–9.

Thrall, D.E. (2012) *Textbook of Veterinary Diagnostic Radiology*, 6th edn. Elsevier Saunders, St Louis, Missouri, USA.

Thrall, D.E. and Robertson, I.D. (2016) *Atlas of Normal Radiographic Anatomy and Anatomic Variants in the Dog and Cat*, 2nd edn. Elsevier, St Louis, Missouri, USA.

Fig. 16.17. Image of a portable ultrasound machine. Basic keys are indicated: patient details button (1), freeze button (2), exam preset button and probe selection button (3), change the frequency of the probe (3A), depth button (4), save buttons (5, 6), measure button (7), time gain compensation (series of buttons or knobs) (8), overall gain knob (9), focal zone button/ knob (10).

- Rotation (Fig. 16.18b).
- Pressure (Fig. 16.18c).
- Rocking (Fig. 16.18d).
- Fanning (Fig. 16.18e).

16.2.4 Normal ultrasonographic appearance

- On ultrasound, an organ's echogenicity (Table 16.1) is evaluated in comparison with other organ(s) in the same animal. The echotexture (how grainy an organ looks on ultrasound) is a more subjective evaluation.

Table 16.1. Echogenicity of different organs

Organ	Echogenicity
Heart (Fig. 16.19)	The ventricles and atria of the heart along with the atrioventricular valves and the aorta and pulmonic artery along with their valves are visible
Liver (Fig. 16.20a)	The liver is normally hypoechoic to the falciform fat and the spleen. With the renal context, it is commonly hyperechoic or isoechoic to the renal cortex; however, it can also normally be mildly hypoechoic
Gallbladder (Fig. 16.20b)	Anechoic with thin wall. In older animals, it normally appears thicker and slightly irregular due to mucinous gland hyperplasia
Spleen (Fig. 16.20c)	Hyperechoic to the other organs
Stomach (Fig. 16.20d)	The wall layers are seen with a hypoechoic mucosa, hyperechoic submucosa, hypoechoic muscularis and hyperechoic serosa
Duodenum (Fig. 16.20e)	The thicker loop of small intestine that can be up to 5 mm thick. The wall layers are visible: hypoechoic mucosa, hyperechoic submucosa, hypoechoic muscularis and hyperechoic serosa
Jejunum and ileum	The wall layers are visible and are the same echogenicity as in the duodenum. The ileum is distinguished by its location and its wagon-wheel appearance when viewed transversely
Colon	Very thin wall. Can be followed from dorsal to the bladder. The wall layers have the same echogenicity as the small intestine but it measures much thinner
Kidneys (Fig. 16.20f)	Typical appearance with hyperechoic cortex and hypoechoic medulla. The normal renal pelvis is not visible
Adrenals (Fig. 16.20g)	Visible in their location craniomedial to the kidney. The left adrenal has a 'monkey-nut' appearance while the right kidney is more arrow-shaped. A hypoechoic cortex and hyperechoic medulla can be occasionally seen
Pancreas (Fig. 16.20h)	Difficult to see and slightly hypoechoic to the surrounding tissues
Urinary bladder (Fig. 16.20i)	Thin wall with the layers (hypoechoic mucosa, hyperechoic submucosa, hypoechoic muscularis and hyperechoic serosa) occasionally seen. The urine is normally anechoic
Lymph nodes (Fig. 16.20j)	Varied in location and size. A hypoechoic cortex and hyperechoic medulla can be occasionally seen
Prostate (Fig. 16.20k)	The normal prostate is oval and uniformly hypoechoic seen caudal to the bladder neck in dogs
Uterus (Fig. 16.20l)	Seen between the urinary bladder and colon; very small in anoestrus and may not be possible to follow it throughout
Ovaries (Fig. 16.20m)	Difficult to see in anoestrus. Easier if they contain follicular cysts. They are normally seen up to 2 cm caudal to the respective kidney

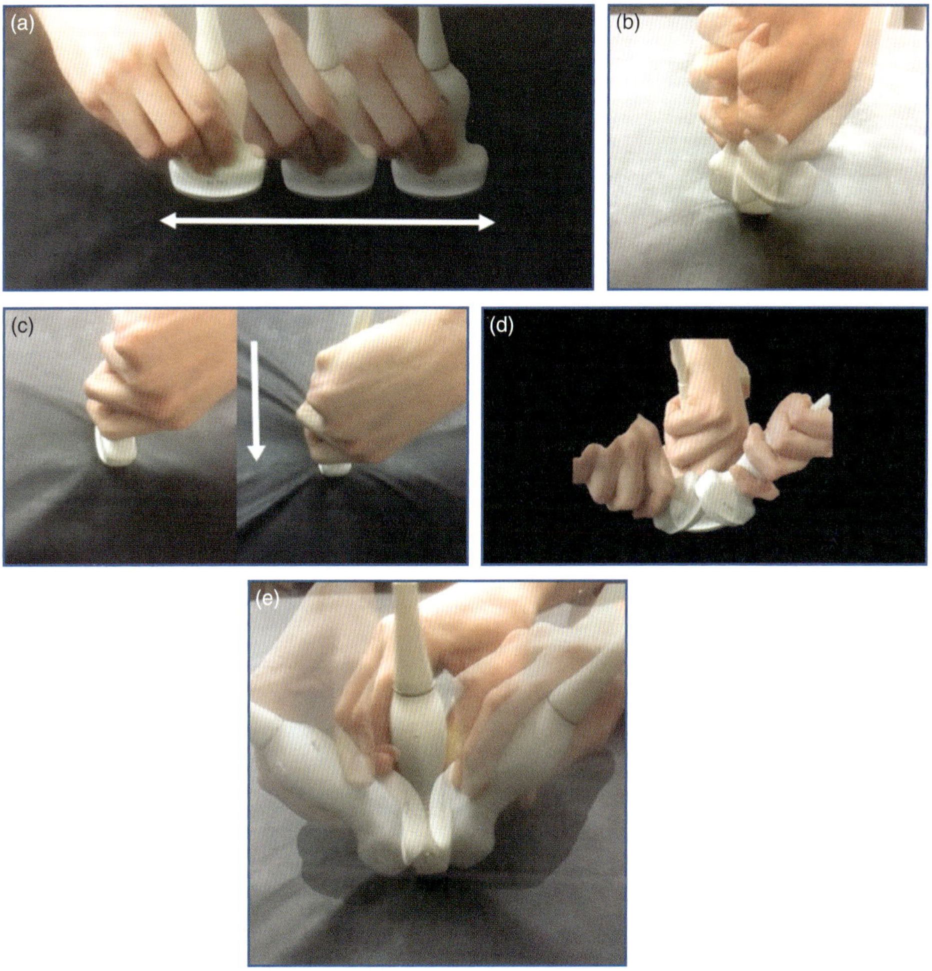

Fig. 16.18. Ultrasound movements: (a) sliding; (b) rotation; (c) pressure; (d) rocking; (e) fanning.

Fig. 16.19. Left parasternal long axis view. The right (RA) and left (LA) atria and the right (RV) and left (LV) ventricles are visible.

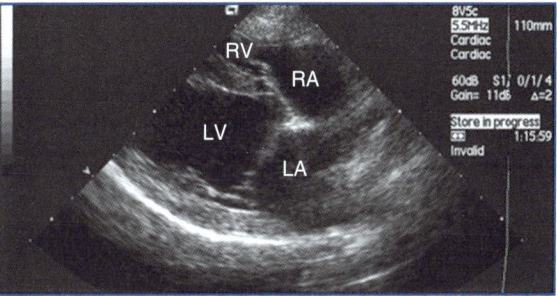

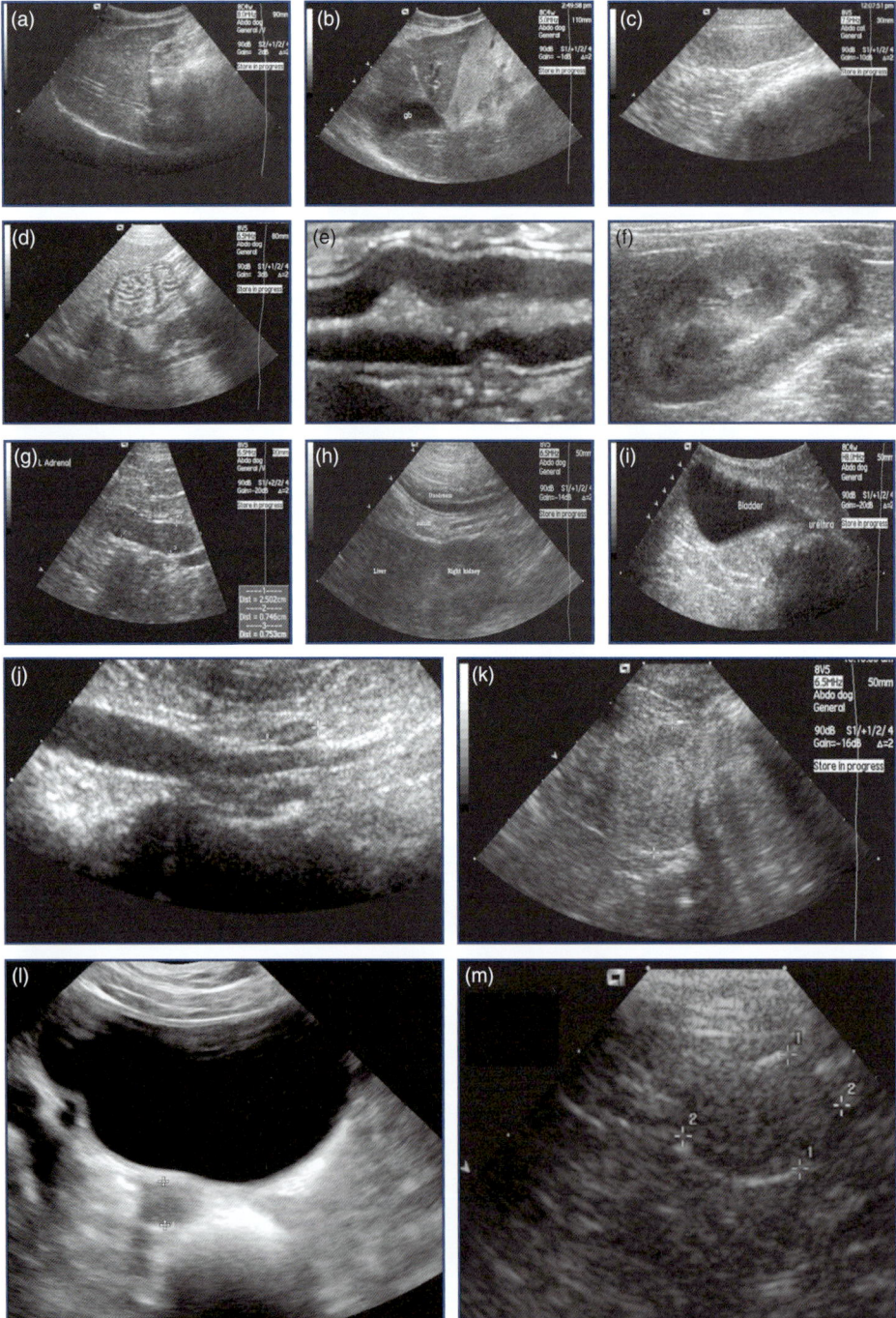

Fig. 16.20. (a) Normal liver. (b) Normal gallbladder (gb). (c) Normal spleen. (d) Normal stomach, short axis view. (e) Normal descending duodenum. (f) Normal kidney. (g) Left adrenal. (h) Normal right lobe of the pancreas. (i) Urinary bladder. (j) Normal medial iliac lymph node (between calipers). (k) Normal prostate (between calipers). (l) Normal transverse image of the uterus (between calipers). (m) Normal ovary (between calipers).

Clinical Skills Sheet

16.42. Imaging BVA/KC hips

Task:

Set up the equipment and 'patient' to achieve a hip score radiograph for the BVA/KC Hip Dysplasia Scoring Scheme[1] (British Veterinary Association/Kennel Club).

Ascertain the anatomical landmarks you would use to help centre and collimate[2] the primary beam appropriately.

Method
Select medium-sized or large cassette (dependent on size of dog). 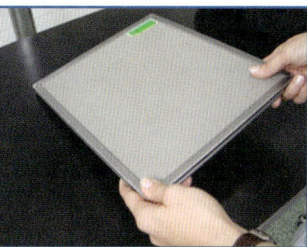
Place cassette on the table the correct way up. This is **very** important – one side is smooth; the other will have some kind of hinge or opening device on it and that is the side that goes on to the table.
Select a 'grid' that fits your cassette – place this on top of the cassette. The grid is a thin metal sheet which also needs to have the correct side facing up. It may have 'tube side' written on it; this is the side you should be able to see. If the grid is in your table, place the cassette under the table in the appropriate slot. 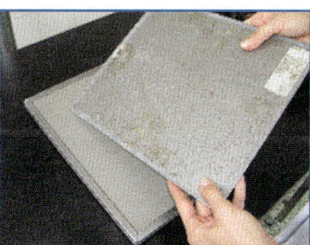 (A grid is used when the body area to be X-rayed is deeper than 10 cm approx. This helps to reduce X-ray 'scatter' and produce a clearer radiograph.)
You are now going to label the radiograph correctly: • Place a left/right marker on top of the cassette/grid – *specifying which is the animal's left or right side*. • Cut a 5 cm long piece of X-rite tape from the X-rite tape dispensing box . • With a biro (press heavily as you write), on the *grey strip* area of the X-rite tape write the Kennel Club number and date only. • Labels should be placed *within* the **primary beam**.
Place the dog in dorsal recumbency (on its back) on to the table. (You can use a white plastic trough. These troughs are radiolucent, meaning they will not show up on the radiograph if accidentally incorporated in the view.)
Sandbags are now placed over each thoracic limb to stabilize dog.

Method
Both pelvic limbs are extended caudally and tied securely in place. They are tied either to the table legs or to special 'fixing areas' on the X-ray table. An additional tie (often Velcro, sometimes masking tape) is used to strap the pelvic limbs together just above the stifles. 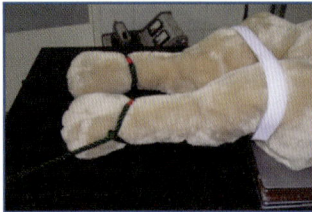 You must ensure that the patellae are facing directly upwards towards the ceiling by rotating the pelvic limbs medially.
Sometimes a small foam wedge is placed between stifles (optional) to keep the limbs parallel.
Your 'patient' should now look like this (the additional sandbag on the toes of the pelvic limbs is optional – it depends on your patient). 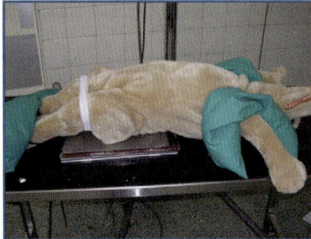
Ensure there is no rotation about the longitudinal axis of the dog's body.
With the dog positioned correctly over the cassette, the X-ray machine tube head is positioned over the area of interest, with the patellae to be included in the view. Centre the primary beam on the midline, level with the greater trochanters greater trochanter 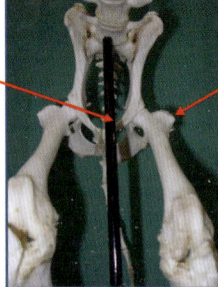
Collimate the primary beam to include both patella and lateral skin edges.
If not all of the above criteria are met, the radiograph will be returned to the veterinary surgeon responsible and the view will have to be re-done, involving re-anaesthetizing the patient and all of the explanations to your client, so it is a critical view to get right!

[1] BVA/KC hip dysplasia scoring scheme

This is a scheme run by the British Veterinary Association and the Kennel Club to try to reduce the physically disabling and sometimes terminally fatal genetically inherited condition of hip dysplasia.

- Any dog over **1 year** of age can be hip scored; they do ***not*** have to be KC registered.
- The radiographs of the dog are submitted to a panel of experts who give each hip a 'score' out of 53.

- The higher the score, the more severe is the level of dysplasia in that hip.
- The two scores are combined to give one total score out of 106. **The lower the score, the less affected are the hips**.
- This leads to a '**breed mean score**'. Each breed has an average score which, if this system is working, each year when these tables are drawn up (and people are *not* breeding from dogs with higher hip scores), the breed mean score should *reduce*.
- Sadly German Shepherd Dogs went from a BMS of 12 in 2006 to 19 in 2007.

[2] **Collimate**

This term means to alter the light emitting downwards from the X-ray head to include only the actual area that you want in your finished radiograph. This is switched on by depressing a button on the X-ray tube head and altering the size of the light by rotating two small dials on the tube head. This 'light' shows the margins of the collimation and thus the margins of the **Primary Beam**.

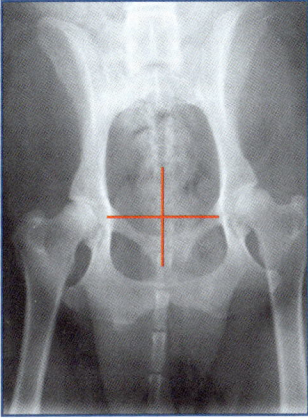

Note: for radiographs of the hips being sent for BVA/KC hip scoring, the patella should also be included within the collimation on the finished radiograph.

© RVC

Clinical Skills Sheet

16.43. Imaging caudo-cranial stifle

Task:

Set up the equipment and patient to achieve a caudo-cranial radiograph of the right stifle.

Ascertain the anatomical landmarks and where you would collimate the primary beam appropriately.

Method
Select a small cassette (or larger if required). 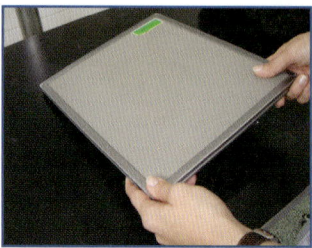
Place cassette on the table the correct way up. This is **very** important – one side is smooth and the other will have some kind of hinge or opening device on it. The smooth side faces upwards.
You will not need to use a grid for this view as the stifle is almost certainly going to be less than 10 cm thick (*see SS 16.42 Imaging BVA/KC hips, for further information on grids*).
You are now going to label the radiograph correctly: • Place a left/right marker on top of the cassette – *specifying which is the animal's left or right side.* • Cut a 5 cm long piece of X-rite tape from the X-rite tape dispensing box. • With a biro (press heavily as you write), on the *grey strip* area of the X-rite tape write the animal's details, usually its ID number, but this can be its name and the date. • Labels are placed *within* the primary beam.
Place the dog in *ventral* recumbency (on its chest) *either* into a large plastic trough *or* with sandbags placed at each side to stabilize the dog.
Place a sandbag or foam wedge under the *left* inguinal region to prevent rotation of the right stifle. This will have the effect of placing the patella *on to* the cassette. 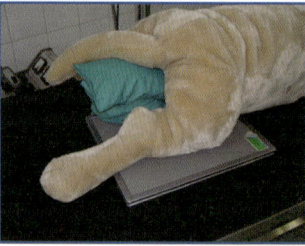

Method
Extend the right pelvic limb caudally and secure in place with a sandbag placed over the hock. Ensure that the cassette is positioned under the stifle. 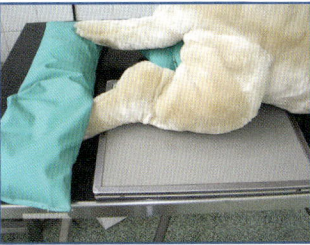
Because the dog's stifle will be further down the table, the tube head may not be centred over the area of interest. If this is the case, reposition the tube head to enable you to collimate.
Centre the primary beam in level with the femoral condyles, midway between skin edges. 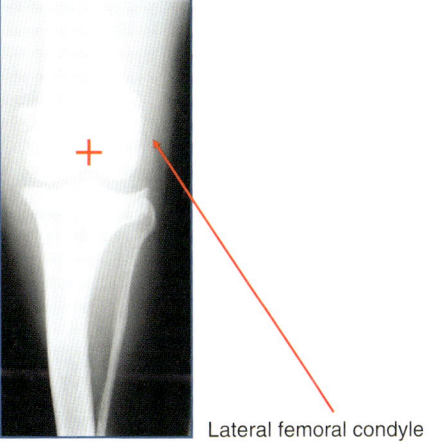 Lateral femoral condyle

Method

Collimate the primary beam to mid-shaft femur to mid-lateral skin edges.

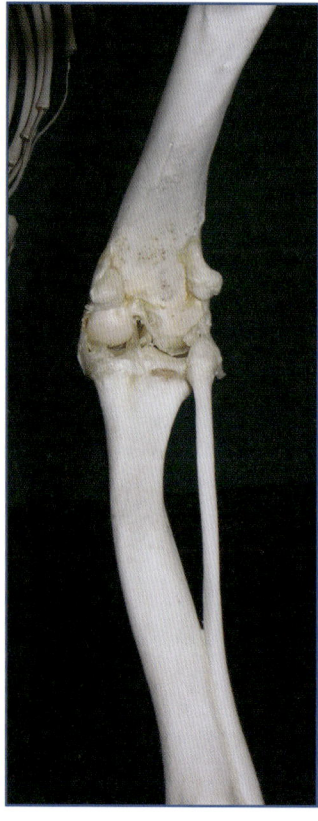

© RVC

Clinical Skills Sheet

16.44. Ultrasound (U/S) set-up

Method
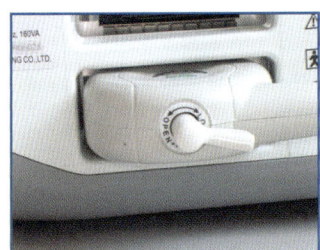 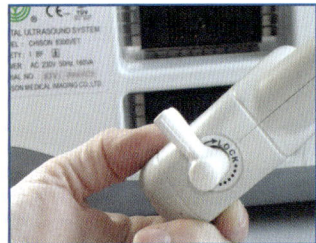
Ensure transducer (probe) is plugged into machine and locked into position.
Open the U/S keyboard flap … 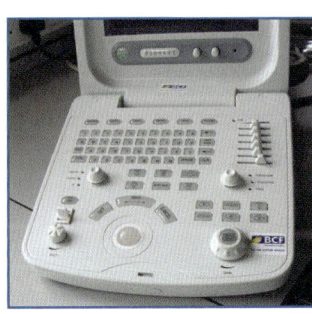 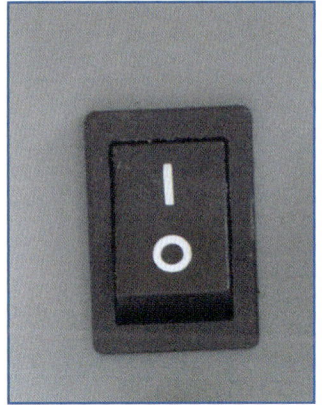
… switch on at mains and turn on machine (button at back).
If you wish to enter patient information, press **PATIENT** button and use keyboard with the tracker ball as a 'mouse' and **SET** button as 'left click'.
Select scanning mode (**ABDOMEN, OB/GYN, CARDIAC** or **SMALL PARTS** for this probe). 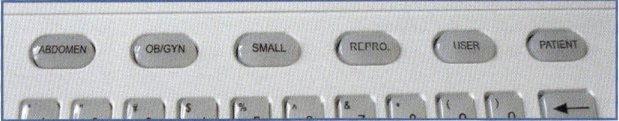
Choose how you would like the image to appear (choose B for 2 dimensional greyscale image). 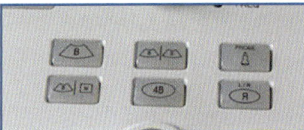

Method

Place transducer (probe) cable around your neck.

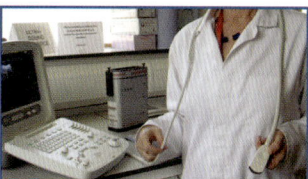

The probe can be used with either water or U/S gel as the transmission facilitator. (Use water for the phantoms – it's easier to clean out.)

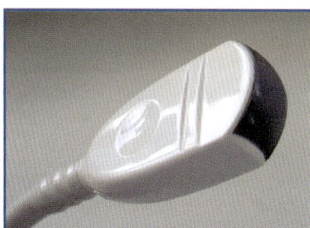
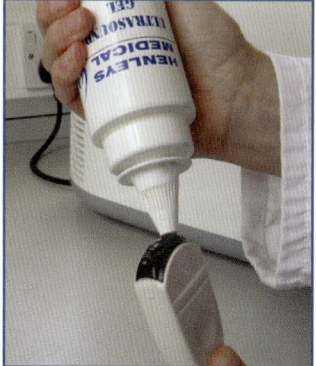

To use the phantom: pour 0.5–1cm water into the well. Manipulate the probe gently on the horizontal surface until you see a triangle or circle (depending on where the probe is positioned) on the U/S screen.

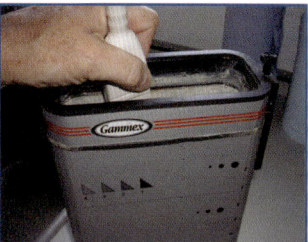

For example, with the probe above the diagrammatic triangles:

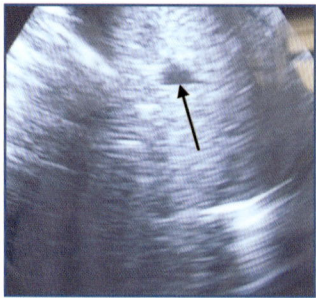
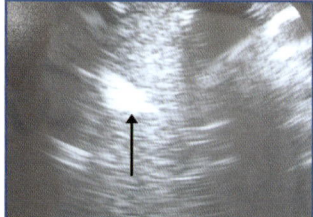

In the left-hand picture you can see the darkest triangle; in the right-hand picture the lightest triangle.

Method

To alter the quality of the image, use a combination of buttons (**DEPTH/ZOOM, FOCUS, GAIN**) and sliders (**TGC GAIN**).

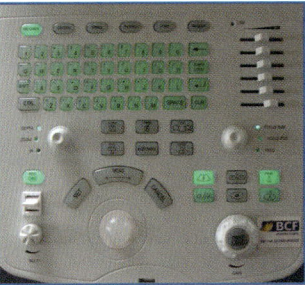

Measuring images:

Press **MEASURE** to bring up caliper. Position by using the tracker ball and press **SET** to fix. Position second caliper and press **SET** to measure distance. To remove measurements press 'clear' on the keyboard.

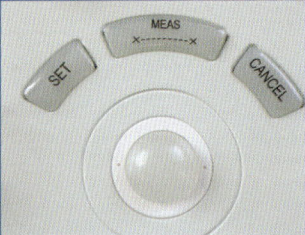

Wipe the probe head clean with tissue and return the head to its dock when you have finished.

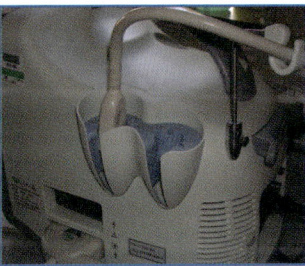

© RVC

17 Equine Radiography – Example Tarsus

Renate Weller and Alana Cyman
The Royal Veterinary College, London

Learning objectives

By the end of this chapter, students should be able to:

- Confidently name the anatomical landmarks of the tarsus.
- Position and acquire images in a safe manner for the standard radiographic views of the tarsus.

Clinical skills sheets (SS)

Three clinical skills sheets will be used in this chapter and these can be found at pages 275–290. Reference will be made to each skills sheet at the relevant section within the chapter. The details of the clinical skills sheets used are as follows:

SS 17.45 Radiographic help sheet: understanding radiographic projections

SS 17.46 Radiographic projections of the foot

SS 17.47 Radiographic projections of the tarsus

17.1 Radiation Safety

Before any exposure is taken, there are a few safety points that need to be addressed:

- Before any personnel can assist in helping to acquire the images you must ask if they are over the age of 18 and if there is any possibility that they could be pregnant.
- Correct personal protective equipment (PPE) must be worn, therefore a lead gown and thyroid protector are required. Always make sure that lead gowns are fastened correctly, leaving no open gaps on the sides.
- To avoid any exposure use a secure stable, preferably with brick walls, and section off the area you intend to use by placing a sign so that people are aware that this is now a radiation controlled area.
- Make sure all equipment is in working order and place your X-ray machine on the stand.
- Never hand hold the plate or x-ray machine; use holders and stands.

Terminology used in radiology positions (Fig. 17.1)

A 'standard set' of radiographs of the equine tarsus and other areas of the limb would be made up of four projections:

- **Lateromedial** – highlights the dorsal and palmar (plantar) aspects of the limb.
- **Dorsopalmar (plantar)** – highlights the lateral and medial aspects of the limb.
- **Dorsolateral-palmaro(plantaro)medial oblique (DLPMO)** – highlights dorsomedial and palmaro (plantaro) lateral structures.
- **Dorsomedial-palmaro(plantaro)lateral oblique (DMPLO)** – highlights dorsolateral and palmaro (plantaro) medial structures.

SS 17.45 for equine radiography help sheet

SS 17.47 for radiographic images of the tarsus

© CAB International 2018. *Veterinary Clinical Skills Manual* (eds N. Coombes and A. Silva-Fletcher)

Tarsus anatomy reminder

Knowledge of anatomy is important in order to take the best possible radiographs with the least number of exposures. Ensure that you know the basic anatomical structures and where to find them.

SS 17.46 for radiographic images of the equine foot

Make sure you set up your X-ray generator before attempting any plate positioning. Once confident with positioning, you can instruct your plate holder into the correct position. Always be aware of where your plate holder is standing and always keep them in a safe position.

When taking a tarsal radiograph, always remember to desensitize the horse's leg before positioning the plate. The plate must be parallel to the camera head and have a film focal distance of 1 m.

17.2 Tarsal Radiographic Views

Before setting up, it is important to look at conformation of a horse's hind legs as they commonly stand 'toe out' behind.

Spend time positioning the horse to make sure the animal is standing square and with even weight-bearing through all limbs and the cannon bone vertical in all directions.

Sedation may be required, to make radiographing easier and to avoid constant repositioning.

17.2.1 Lateromedial view

You will need:

- A medium-sized plate positioned close to the leg.
- A radiographic left or right marker placed dorsally on the plate.

1. Position the x-ray machine lateral to the leg, 90 degree to the sagittal plane
2. The tarsal joints slope proximodistally from lateral to medial; For the x-ray beam to go through the joints you can either centre the beam on the distal end of the tibia (the lateral malleolus sticks out and

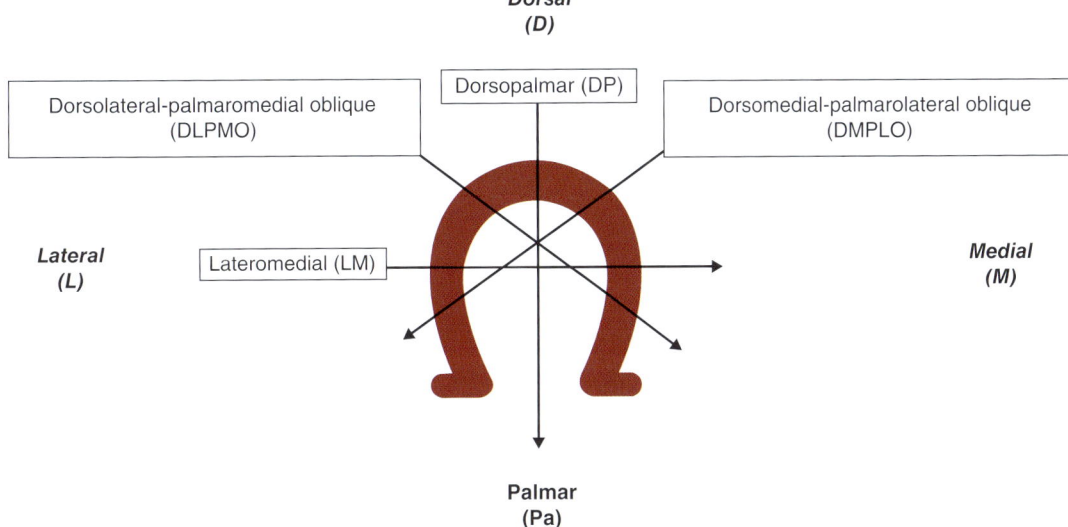

Fig. 17.1. Standard terminology for radiographic projections; views are named after the point of entry and the point of exit of the x-ray beam using anatomical nomenclature.

can easily be palpated) and use a horizontal beam or alternatively you can centre on the distal intertarsal joint and angle the x-ray beam about 5 degrees downward.

3. Collimate around the tarsus making sure to include the proximal end of the calcaneus and the proximal metatarsus.

17.2.2 Dorsoplantar view

You will need:

- A medium-sized plate positioned at the plantar aspect of the tarsus.
- A radiographic left or right marker positioned on the lateral side of the horse's limb.

1. Position the x-ray machine dorsal to the tarsus.
2. Center on the distal intertarsal joint.
3. Use a horizontal beam.
4. Collimate to include the proximal calcaneus and the proximal metatarsus.

17.2.3 Dorsolateral–plantaromedial oblique view

You will need:

- A medium-sized plate positioned on the plantaromedial part of the hock.
- A radiographic left or right marker positioned on the lateral side of the horse's limb.

1. Position x-ray machine on the dorsolateral aspect of the tarsus at a 45 degree angle to the dorsoplantar view.
2. Center on the distal intertarsal joint calcaneus and the proximal metatarsus.

3. Use a horizontal beam.
4. Collimate to include the proximal metatarsus.

17.2.4 Dorsomedial–plantarolateral oblique View

You will need:

- A medium-sized plate positioned on the plantarolateral aspect of the tarsus.
- A radiographic left or right marker positioned on the lateral side of the horse's limb.

1. Position x-ray machine on the plantarolateral aspect of the tarsus at a 45 degree angle to the lateromedial.
2. Centre on the distal intertarsal joint.
3. Use a horizontal beam.
4. Collimate to include the proximal calcaneus and the proximal metatarsus.

17.3 Providing Students with the Opportunity for Practice

A station can be set up using a fibreglass horse, a decommissioned X-ray generator, X-ray stand and an X-ray plate and plate holder. This can be useful when practising for positioning, getting familiar with how the equipment works and practising plate holding. Using a fibreglass horse is ideal as you can take as long as you like positioning without the concern of the horse moving or any pressures of the horse waking up. Equally, when positioning the plate it is good practice on how to work safely around the horse, minimizing risk of injury.

Clinical Skills Sheet

17.45. Radiographic help sheet: understanding radiographic projections

This is a simple technique to help you understand which areas you will see when you have taken a radiograph.
Visualize where the X-ray beam enters and exits the structure and what you will see will be on either side of this beam. The red arrows symbolise the x-ray beam, the blue box the leg and the yellow circles point out the highlighted aspects.
For a dorsopalmar projection: the lateral (L) aspect and the medial (M) aspect will be seen.

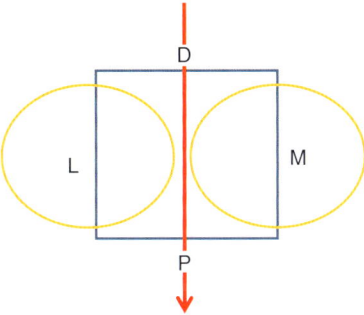

For a lateromedial projection: the dorsal (D) and palmar (P) aspects will be seen.

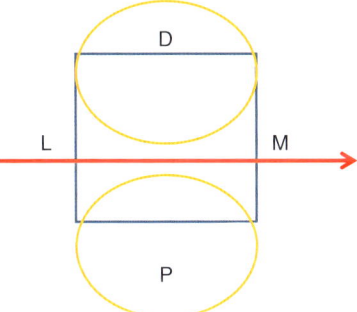

For a DMPLO: the dorsolateral aspect and palmaromedial aspect will be highlighted.

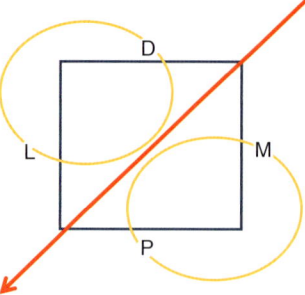

For a DLPMO: the dorsomedial aspect and the palmarolateral aspect will be highlighted.

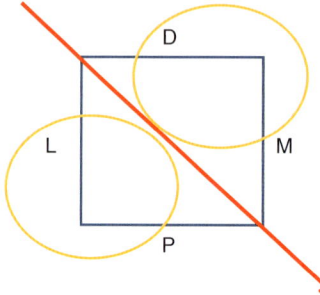

Clinical practice point:
So if you wanted to visualize a structure on the lateropalmar aspect, a DLPMO would be appropriate.

© RVC

Clinical Skills Sheet

17.46. Radiographic projections of the foot

Radiographic projections are named by the point of entrance of the X-ray beam into a structure, followed by where it exits.

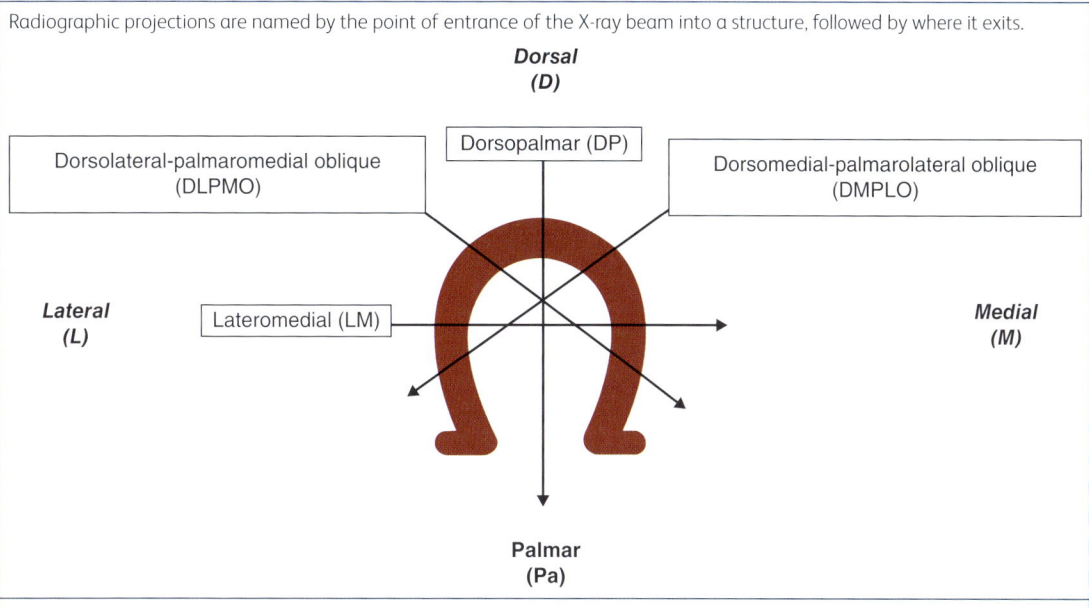

Equipment you need:
- Farriery kit for shoe removal and hoof preparation.
- Play dough or other material to pack frog grooves.
- Portable X-ray machine.
- Flat wooden blocks to raise feet for dorsopalmar (DP) and lateromedial (LM) projections.
- Block (tunnel or Hickman block) for oblique projections.
- Lead gowns, thyroid protectors, gloves.

In a live horse you would use wooden blocks but you can practise without them on the model horse.

Lateromedial (LM) projection

Used to assess:
- Dorsopalmar foot conformation, hoof–pastern axis.
- Pedal bone rotation/sinking.
- DIP joint.
- Navicular bone.

Position both front feet on blocks; position the foot you are radiographing at the edge of the block.

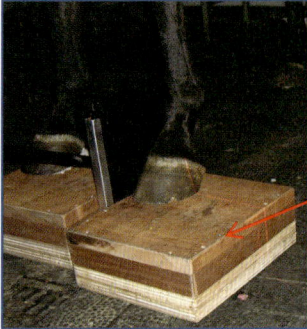

Wooden block

Position the X-ray machine lateral to the foot, align the beam parallel to the bulbs of the heel.

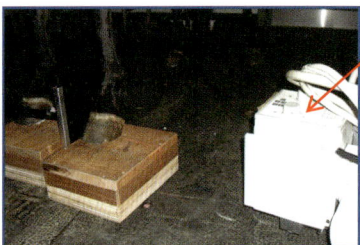

X-ray machine

Place the plate on the medial side as close as possible to the foot using a long-handled plate holder, making sure it is perpendicular to the X-ray beam/machine.

Centre (red cross) the X-ray beam about 1 cm below the coronet, halfway between the dorsal hoof wall and the heel.

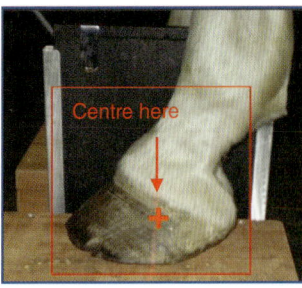

Centre here

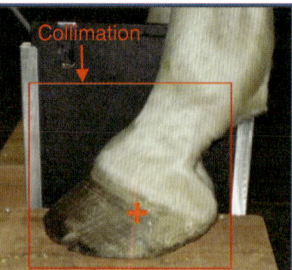

Collimation

Collimate (red box) around the foot up to mid pastern region, making sure you can see all four borders of the collimated area on the plate.

Lateromedial (LM) projection

Radiographic anatomy of the foot in a lateromedial projection.

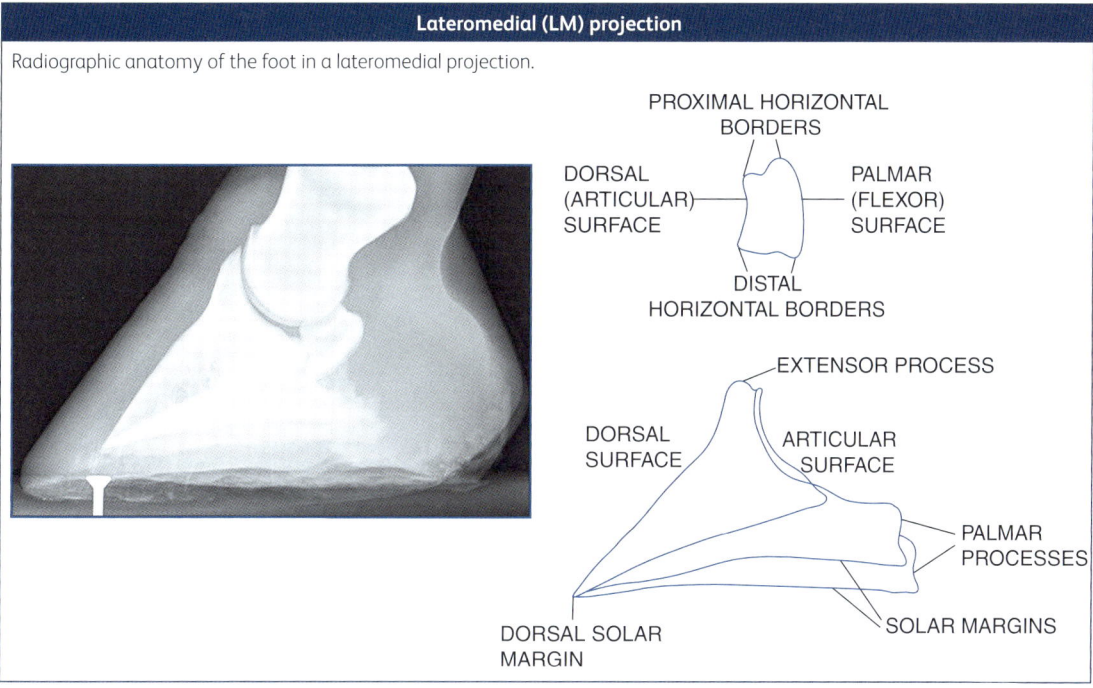

Dorsopalmar (DP) projection

Used to assess:
- Mediolateral foot balance.
- Ossifying collateral cartilages.
- Integrity of P3.

Position both feet on to separate blocks; this allows for centring of the X-ray beam on the DIP joint. Make sure the foot of interest is as close to the back of the block as possible.

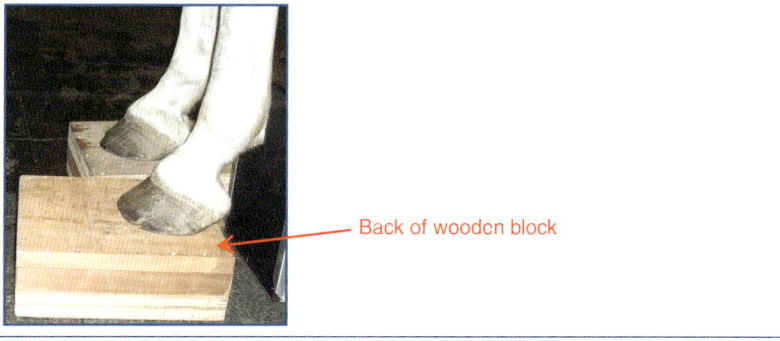

Dorsopalmar (DP) projection

Position the X-ray machine in front of the foot. The plate is positioned palmar to the foot in close contact with the foot, using a long-handled plate holder.

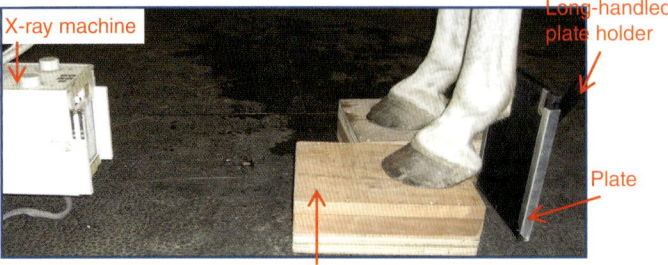

Centre (red cross) the horizontal X-ray beam about 1cm distal to the coronet.

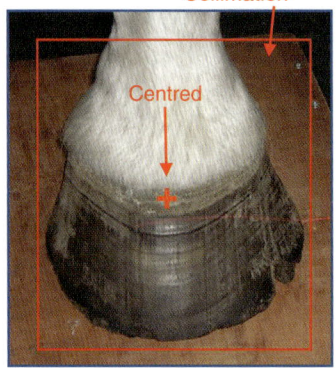

Collimate around the foot up to mid pastern region (red box), making sure you can see all four borders of the collimated area on the plate.

Radiographic anatomy of the foot in a dorsopalmar projection.

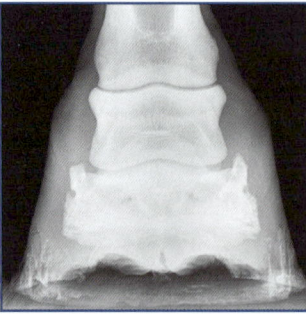

Dorsoproximal–palmarodistal oblique projections

As standard, this projection is performed twice and centres on different areas so that you can image the

- Navicular bone.
- Distal phalanx (P3).

It is then taken a third time centring on the navicular bone but using a different angle to visualize the navicular bone so that the other border can be assessed.

The horse stands on a tunnel block (*a tunnel block is where the plate sits inside the block*).

The X-ray machine is positioned in front of the horse and in a proximodistal direction.

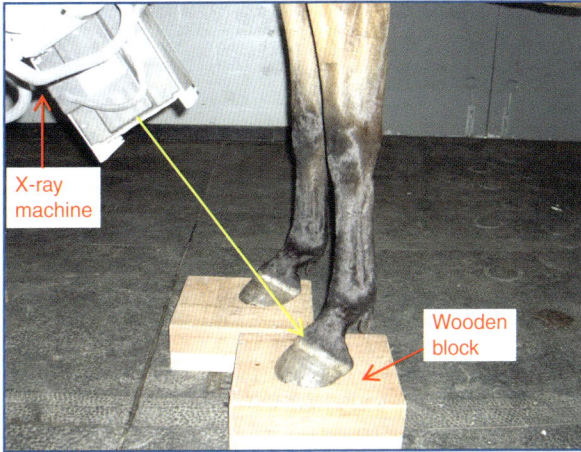

1st projection. Using a 60 degree angle:

- Centre X-ray beam on navicular bone.
- Collimate around the navicular bone.

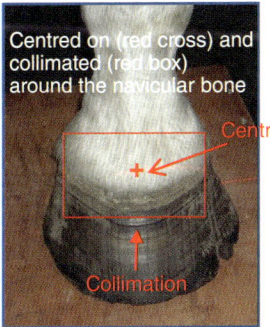

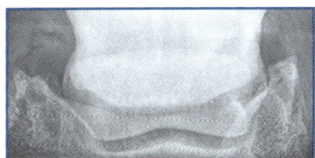

Radiographic anatomy of the navicular bone in a dorsoproximal–palmarodistal projection.

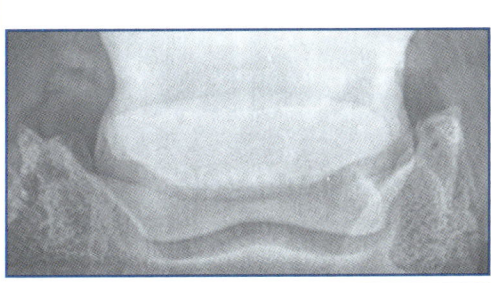

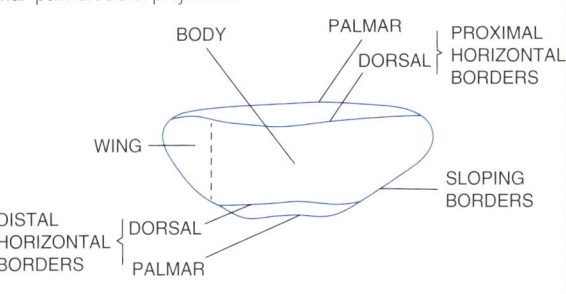

Dorsoproximal–palmarodistal oblique projections

2nd projection. Using a 60 degree angle:
- Centre X-ray beam on distal phalanx.
- Collimate around the distal phalanx.

Centred on(red cross) and
collimated (red box) around
the distal phalanx

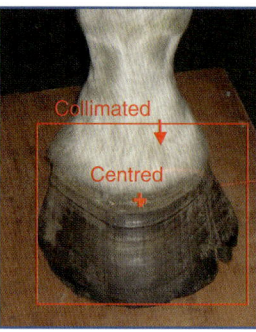
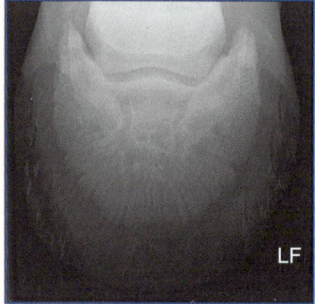

Both these projections are called dorso-60°-proximal palmarodistal oblique (60°DP) projections; they just centre on either the navicular bone or the distal phalanx.

Radiographic anatomy of the foot in a dorsoproximal–palmarodistal oblique projection.

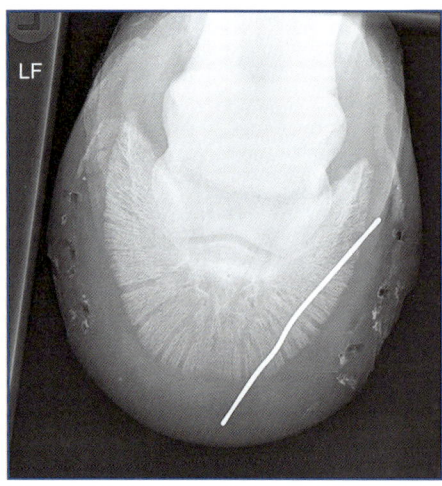
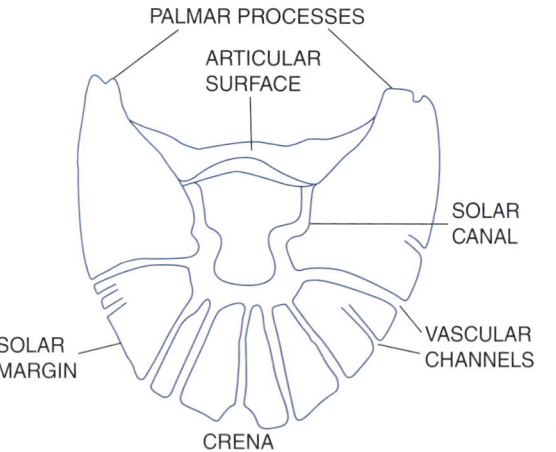

Dorsoproximal–palmarodistal oblique projections

3rd projection. Using a 45 degree angle:
- Centre X-ray beam on navicular bone.
- Collimate around the navicular bone.

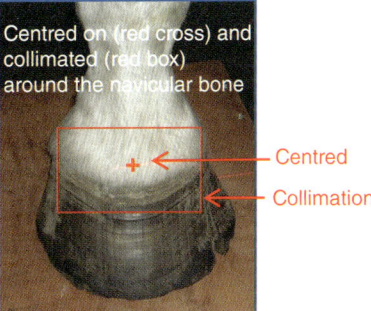

This uses the same method, just using a different angle. This is called a dorso-45°-proximal palmarodistal oblique (45°DP) projection.

Why the use of the different angles?
The different angles allow the different borders of the navicular bone to be assessed.
- The 60°allows the distal border of the navicular bone to be assessed.
- The 45° allows the proximal border of the navicular bone to be assessed.

Alternative to the method shown above, another method can be used, using a different type of block.
The same projection is achieved using a Hickman block instead of a tunnel block.
The foot rests in the Hickman block and is horizontal to the X-ray beam, negating the need to angle the X-ray machine.

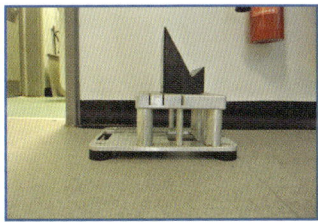

Palmaro-45°-proximal palmarodistal oblique projection

This projection is often referred to as the *flexor view* or the *skyline view*.
Used to assess:
- navicular bone.
- palmar processes of the third phalanx.

More specifically:
- flexor cortex of the navicular bone.
- corticomedullary junction of the navicular bone.

Palmaro-45°-proximal palmarodistal oblique projection

Place the foot on a tunnel block.

Position the foot as far back underneath the horse as possible whilst still keeping the foot weight-bearing.

This will help to avoid superimposing the proximal sesamoid bones and the proximal and middle phalanx over the navicular bone.

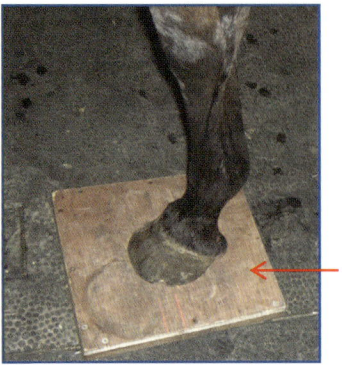

Wooden block

The X-ray machine is positioned on the palmar aspect of the leg under the abdomen of the horse.

It facilitates positioning of the X-ray tube when the foot is placed slightly pointing away from the horse.

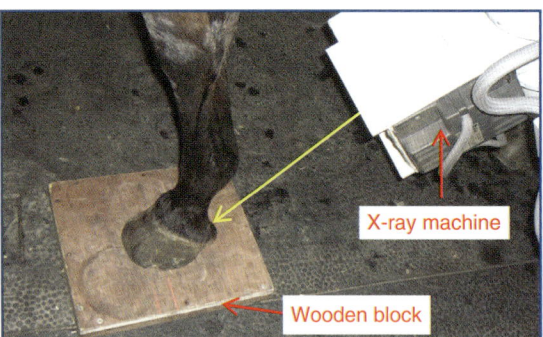

X-ray machine

Wooden block

Angle the X-ray beam in a proximodistal direction at 45 degrees.

Centre (red cross) the X-ray beam just proximal to the heel bulbs.

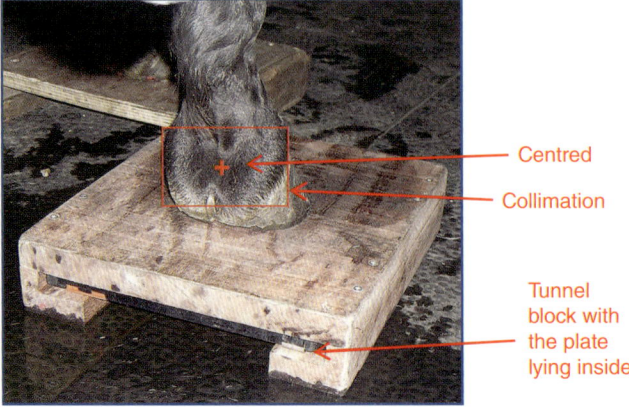

Centred

Collimation

Tunnel block with the plate lying inside

Collimate (red box) tightly around the navicular bone to reduce scatter.

Palmaro-45°-proximal palmarodistal oblique projection

Radiographic anatomy of the navicular bone in a palmaroproximal–palmarodistal oblique projection.

DORSAL (ARTICULAR) SURFACE

PALMAR (FLEXOR) SURFACE

Instructions written by: R.Weller, Dr Med.Vet PhD MRCVS MScVetEd. FHEA and J.Mullard MRCVS
Images: R. Weller, Dr Med.Vet PhD MRCVS MScVetEd. FHEA + EDI Rotation Handbook

© RVC

Clinical Skills Sheet

17.47. Radiographic projections of the tarsus

Radiographic projections are named by the point of entrance of the X-ray beam into a structure, followed by where it exits.
Remember that when referring to the hind limbs we use the term plantar instead of palmar.

Dorsal
(D)

Dorsopalmar (DP)

| Dorsolateral-palmaromedial oblique (DLPMO) | | Dorsomedial-palmaromedial oblique (DMPLO) |

Lateral **(L)**   Lateromedial (LM)   **Medial** **(M)**

Palmar
(Pa)

The tarsus is commonly called the hock.

Standard tarsus series includes the following projections:
- Lateromedial (LM).
- Dorsoplantar (DP).
- Dorso 45°-lateral- plantaromedial oblique (DLPMO) projection.
- Plantaro-45°-lateral dorsomedial oblique (PLDMO) projection.

Additional projections:
- Flexed LM projection (useful for evaluating the caudal aspect of the distal tibia).
- Flexed DP projection of the calcaneus and sustentaculum tali.

Lateromedial projection
This is particularly useful for evaluating the: • medial trochlear ridge of the talus. • calcaneus. • dorsal aspects of the proximal intertarsal, distal intertarsal and tarsometatarsal joints.
Position the X-ray machine lateral to the tarsus. As many horses have a tendency to stand 'toe out', it is important that the lateromedial view is lateral to the axis of the *limb* and not the horse. *'Toe out' means standing with the toe facing out (like a ballerina).*

Lateromedial projection

The intertarsal joints are angled approximately 5–10 degrees proximolateral to distomedially. This means that we need to angle the X-ray beam.

Angle the X-ray beam distally by about 8 degrees and centre about 10 cm distal to the point of the hock.

Alternatively:

Centre the X-ray beam on the lateral malleolus of the tibia (which is easily palpable). This will result in an angled beam at the level of the intertarsal joints, due to the diverging nature of the X-ray beam.

Position the plate on the medial side of the tarsus, as close as possible to the horse and aligned perpendicular to the X-ray beam.

Radiographic anatomy of the tarsus on a lateromedial projection.
Note that the chestnut is visible on the plantar aspect (yellow arrow)

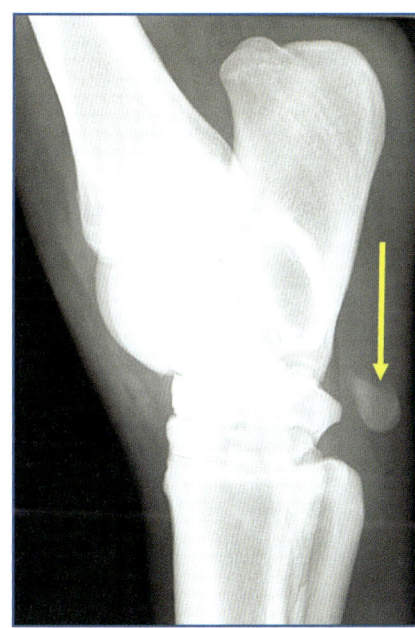
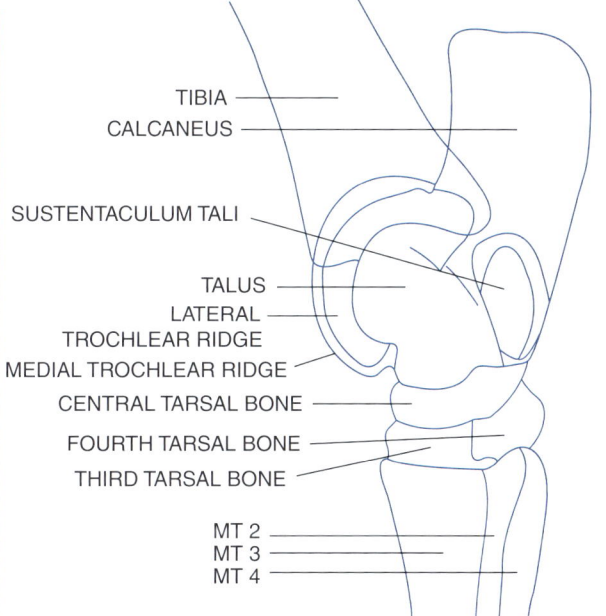

TIBIA
CALCANEUS
SUSTENTACULUM TALI
TALUS
LATERAL TROCHLEAR RIDGE
MEDIAL TROCHLEAR RIDGE
CENTRAL TARSAL BONE
FOURTH TARSAL BONE
THIRD TARSAL BONE
MT 2
MT 3
MT 4

On a truly lateromedial radiograph the trochlear ridges and the second and fourth tarsal bones are not superimposed, because:
- the medial trochlear ridge is larger and projects more dorsally than the lateral trochlear ridge; and
- the head of the fourth metatarsal bone is larger than the head of the second and is positioned in a more plantar location.

Dorsoplantar projection

This is particularly useful for evaluating:
- the medial aspects of the proximal intertarsal, distal intertarsal and tarsometatarsal joints.

Position the X-ray machine dorsal to the tarsus.

A true dorsoplantar view will need to take into account the 'toe out' nature of the hind limb of the majority of horses (they stand with their toe pointing out).

Centre on the central tarsal bone. Depending on the angulation of the tarsus, use a horizontal beam or angle the beam distally accordingly.

Position the plate on the plantar side of the tarsus, as close as possible to the horse and aligned perpendicular to the X-ray beam.

Radiographic anatomy of the tarsus on a dorsoplantar projection.

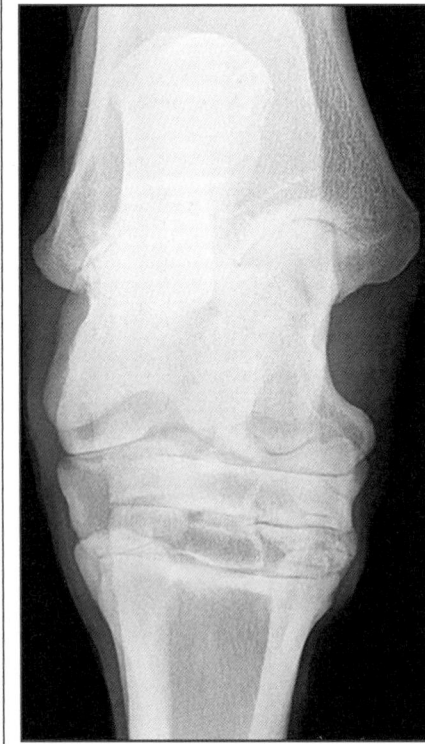
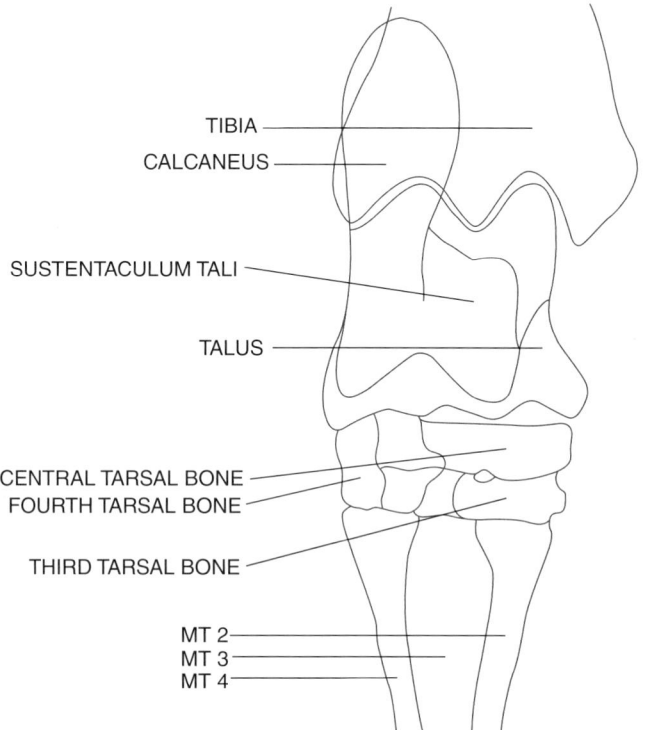

TIBIA

CALCANEUS

SUSTENTACULUM TALI

TALUS

CENTRAL TARSAL BONE
FOURTH TARSAL BONE

THIRD TARSAL BONE

MT 2
MT 3
MT 4

Dorsolateral-palmaromedial oblique projection DLPMO

This is useful for evaluating the:

- Dorsomedial aspects of the proximal intertarsal, distal intertarsal and tarsometatarsal joints.
- Calcaneus.
- Fourth tarsal bone and the fourth metatarsal (splint) bone.

Position the X-ray machine dorsolateral to the tarsus at an angle of 45 degrees to the lateromedial view.

Centre on the central tarsal bone, use a horizontal beam.

Position the plate perpendicular to X-ray beam on the plantaromedial aspect of the tarsus.

Radiographic anatomy of the tarsus on a dorsolateral-palmaromedial projection DLPMO.
In a well positioned DLPMO, the dorsal opening of the tarsal canal should be clearly visible (yellow arrow).

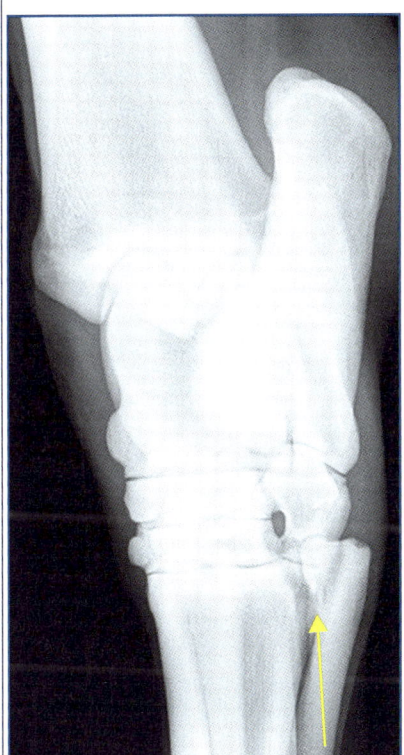
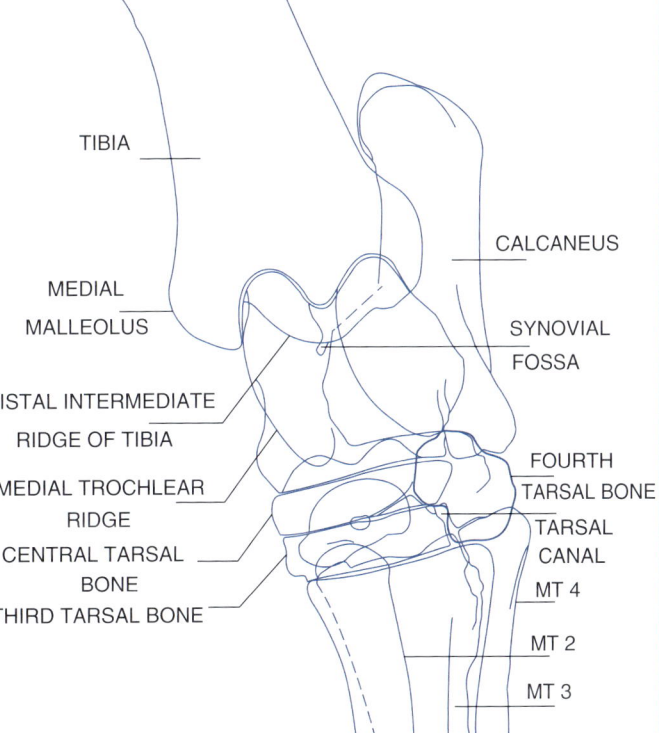

TIBIA

CALCANEUS

MEDIAL
MALLEOLUS

SYNOVIAL
FOSSA

DISTAL INTERMEDIATE
RIDGE OF TIBIA

FOURTH
TARSAL BONE

MEDIAL TROCHLEAR
RIDGE

TARSAL
CANAL

CENTRAL TARSAL
BONE

MT 4

THIRD TARSAL BONE

MT 2

MT 3

Plantaro-45°-lateral dorsomedial oblique projection (PLDMO)

This is the reverse way of taking a DMPLO. It is easier to take it is this way as it easier to position the X-ray machine.

This is the view of choice for evaluation of:

- Lateral trochlear ridge of the talus.
- Sustentaculum tali of the calcaneus.

It also skylines:

- Second metatarsal bone.
- Dorsolateral aspects of the proximal intertarsal, distal intertarsal and tarsometatarsal joints.

Position the X-ray machine plantarolateral (or dorsomedial) to the tarsus at an angle of 45 degrees to the mediolateral axis.

Centre on central tarsal bone; use a horizontal beam.

Position the plate perpendicular to X-ray beam on the dorsomedial (palmarolateral) aspect of the tarsus.

Radiographic anatomy of the tarsus on a palmarolateral-dorsomedial projection PLDMO.

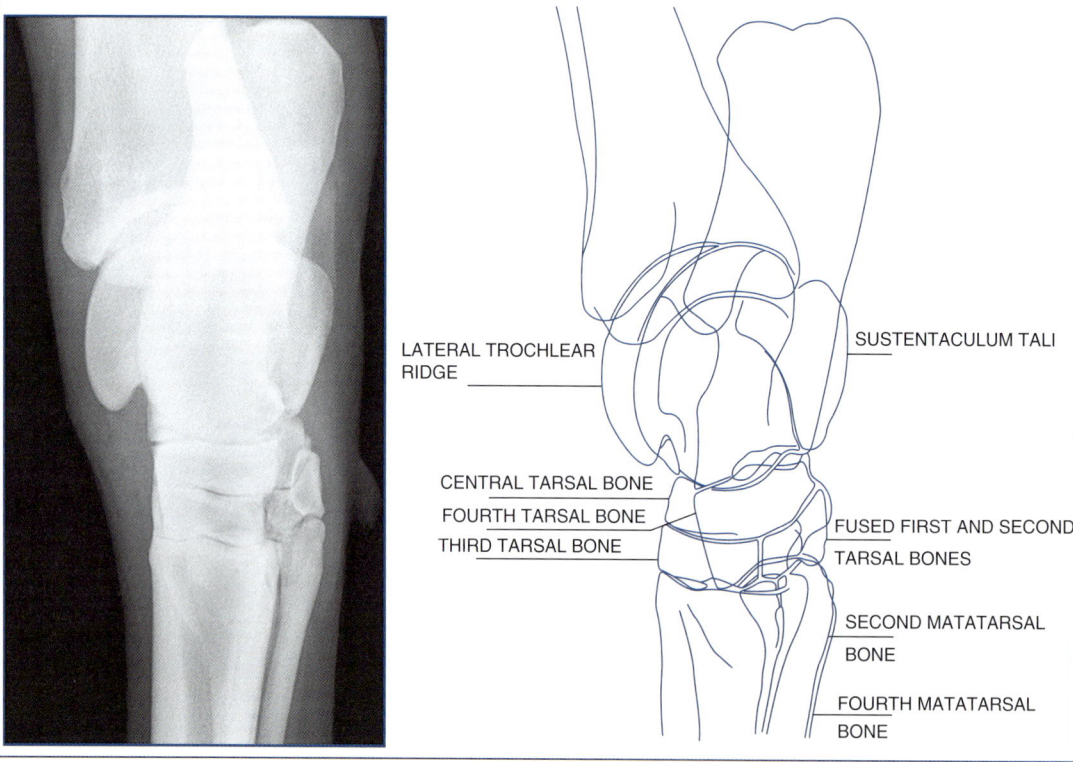

LATERAL TROCHLEAR RIDGE

SUSTENTACULUM TALI

CENTRAL TARSAL BONE

FOURTH TARSAL BONE

THIRD TARSAL BONE

FUSED FIRST AND SECOND TARSAL BONES

SECOND MATATARSAL BONE

FOURTH MATATARSAL BONE

Instructions written by: R. Weller, Dr Med.Vet PhD MRCVS MScVetEd. FHEA and J. Mullard MRCVS
Images: R. Weller, Dr Med.Vet PhD MRCVS MScVetEd. FHEA + EDI Rotation Handbook

© RVC

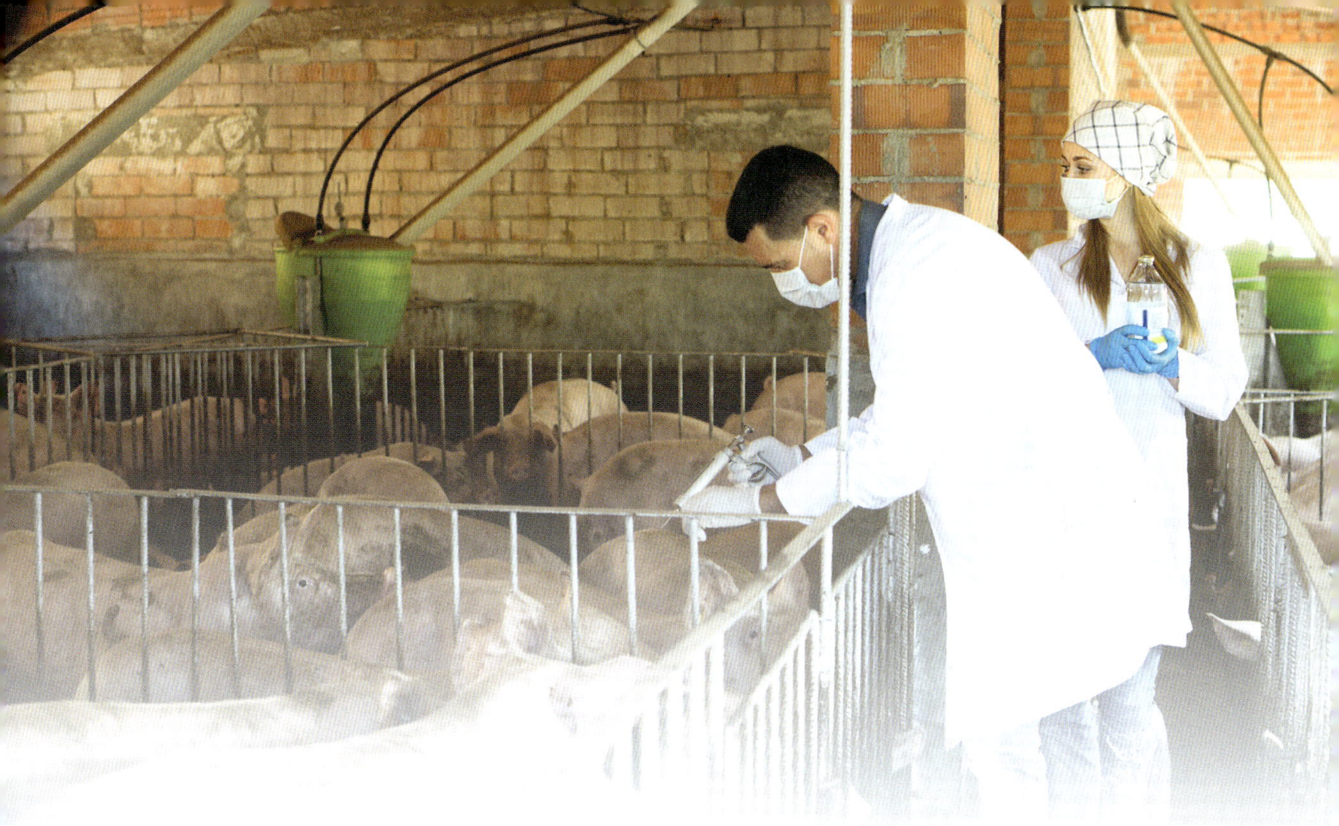

Section

7

Large Animal Skills

Section Editor: Isobel Vincent

Introduction

One of the most important skills related to dairy cow management is prevention of mastitis. Mastitis can cause considerable pain to the animal and impact on human and animal health and the farmer's profits. Therefore maintenance of udder health and advising all those who are working with dairy animals is an important skill for any veterinarian or veterinary nurse. The other large animal competences that are essential as Day One skills are related to giving injections, setting up fluid and/or drug treatments and introducing a nasogastric tube. These require specific skills and practising is essential on simulators and/or on live animals as much as possible until competence is reached. Another basic skill that is expected is equine shoe removal. Safe handling of the animal and the shoe removal process is an essential Day One skill that can be practised in the safe environment of the CSC lab.

The aim of this section is to provide that basic knowledge in large animal procedures. Within this section there are three chapters:

Chapter 18: Udder Health

Chapter 19: Equine Procedures

Chapter 20: Equine Foot Related Skills: Example Shoe Removal

Within each chapter you will find pictures and tips about how to conduct relevant basic Day One skills. Each chapter will also detail key points for each set of skills and point out the health and safety considerations, which are critical to good practice.

An overview of all the learning outcomes is presented below and the more detailed learning outcomes are presented under each chapter.

Learning objectives

After studying this section, students should be able to:

- Conduct the California Milk Test (CMT) and interpret the results.
- Perform an intravenous (IV) injection, place an intravenous catheter (IVC) and take a blood sample from a horse.

- Perform an intramuscular (IM) injection in a horse.
- Introduce a nasogastric tube on a simulator.
- Describe and demonstrate removal of a shoe in a safe manner.

What You Will Need

Clinical skills sheets

Eight clinical skills sheets will be used in this section. Reference will be made to each skills sheet at the relevant point within the chapter. Clinical skills sheets for the following accompany this section:

SS 18.48 Bovine sterile milk sampling method

SS 18.49 California Milk Test (CMT) sampling method

SS 19.50 Equine fluid therapy set-up

SS 19.51 Common sites for intramuscular injections

SS 19.52 Passing a nasogastric tube in a horse

SS 20.53 Shoe removal

SS 20.54 Paring the sole and trimming the hoof wall

A further skills sheet is used that has also been used in other chapters and cross-references are made in this section:

SS 9.18 Venepuncture techniques: blood collection by Vacutainer

Videos (V)

Three videos will be used in this section and reference will be made to each video at the relevant point within the chapter. Videos will be hyperlinked and the following accompany this section:

V 19.1 Equine jugular placement in a horse

V 19.2 Equine fluid therapy

V 20.1 Removing a horse shoe

18 Udder Health

John Fishwick and Isobel Vincent

The Royal Veterinary College, London

Learning objectives

By the end of this chapter, students should be able to:

- Obtain a sterile milk sample.
- Conduct the California Milk Test (CMT).
- Interpret the results from the CMT.
- Explain the purpose of doing a CMT.

Clinical skills sheets (SS)

Two clinical skills sheets will be used in this chapter and these can be found at pages 296–297. Reference will be made to each skills sheet at the relevant section within the chapter. The details of the clinical skills sheets used are as follows:

SS 18.48 Bovine sterile milk sampling method
SS 18.49 California Milk Test (CMT) sampling method

Introduction

Maintaining udder health and the quality of milk is essential not only for economic purposes but also for public health. Poor udder health can lead to subclinical and clinical mastitis. Mastitis is the most common disease of dairy animals and can lead to reduction or cessation in milk output, increased somatic cell and bacterial numbers in milk and antibiotic residues if treated for mastitis. Therefore knowledge about udder health and being able to do tests on milk samples to monitor inflammation and infection are essential.

18.1 Sterile Milk Sample

Obtaining a sterile milk sample is the first stage of the udder check. The udder is exposed to many microorganisms, due to contamination during milking from faeces and bedding, urine and any material from the cowshed. The teat canal is the primary physical barrier to invasion of any microorganisms to the udder. So examining the teats for any damage or injury is essential.

SS 18.48 for detailed guidance on how to obtain a sterile milk sample

Key points

- Obtaining a sterile milk sample is not the same as the California Milk Test.
- The focus is to clean the teat end, not the whole teat.
- Always remember to discard the first two to three squirts of milk into a bucket, not on the ground.
- Make sure to handle the sample bottle in a clean fashion.
- If at any point you feel the sample has been compromised, start again.
- Use teat-dip when you have finished.
- Do not forget to label your sample with farm name, cow number, quarter and the date.
- If you are sampling multiple teats, use a separate swab for each one.
- If you are sampling multiple teats, use a separate pot for each.

Once you have obtained a sterile milk sample, this may also be used in the California Milk Test.

293

© CAB International 2018. *Veterinary Clinical Skills Manual* (eds N. Coombes and A. Silva-Fletcher)

18.2 California Milk Test (CMT)

This is a test to measure the somatic cell count (SCC) in a milk sample: the higher the SCC, the greater is the chance of mastitis. To do the test, a CMT paddle and the CMT solution are required. Figure 18.1 gives a checklist for items that are required for the test. After adding the CMT solution to the milk sample, any signs of thickening are noted (Fig. 18.2).

SS 18.49 for a detailed procedure on how to do a CMT and how to interpret the clinical results

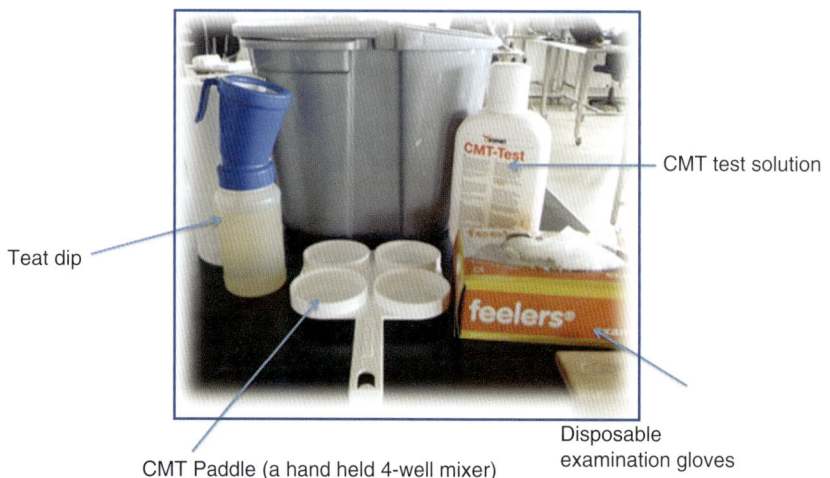

CMT test solution

Teat dip

Disposable examination gloves

CMT Paddle (a hand held 4-well mixer)

Fig. 18.1. The items required to do a California Milk Test.

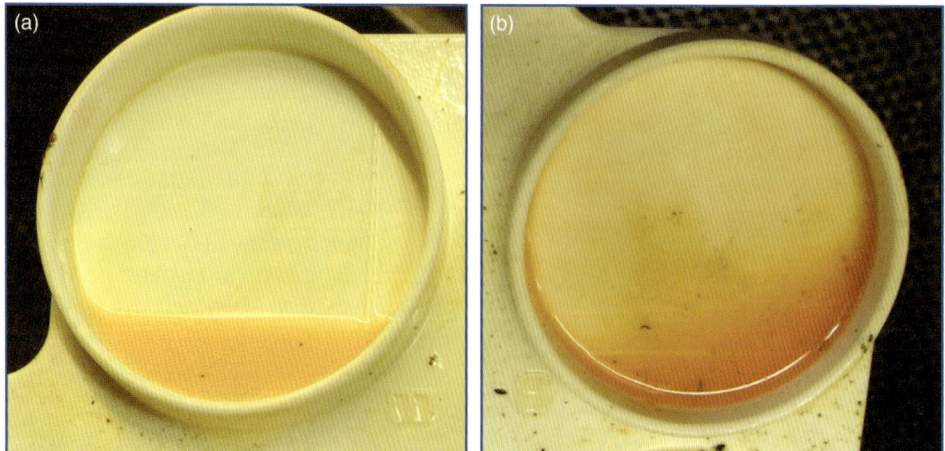

Fig. 18.2. After adding the CMT test solution to the milk sample, any signs of thickening are noted: (a) negative (no evidence of thickening or formation of precipitate); (b) trace (slight thickening that disappears with continued rotation).

Key points

- CMT is *not* the same as a sterile milk sample.
- Best results are obtained before milking.
- Gather all the equipment you will need prior to entering the stall.
- Make sure to expel stagnant milk from the teat prior to sampling, and use a bucket to do so. Never dispose of milk on to the parlour floor.
- Remember which teat applies to which well, to get accurate results.
- Do not forget to dip all four teats once you have completed sampling.

18.2.1 When might a CMT be useful?

Identifying infected quarters prior to sampling or treatment.

Clinical Skills Sheet

18.48. Bovine sterile milk sampling method

Method

*This is a general method for doing this task. As long as you are confident that you are obtaining a **sterile** sample, the method below can be varied.*

Equipment:
- Water/paper towels (if teat very soiled).
- Disposable examination gloves.
- Cotton wool + surgical spirit/sterile wipes.
- Sterile universal container (+spare).
- Indelible ink pen.
- Teat dip.

Procedure:
1. The teat should be visibly clean. If it is not, clean and **dry** it so that it is *visibly clean*. Clean water and disposable paper towels are acceptable.
2. Wear clean examination gloves.
3. Using cotton wool soaked in surgical spirit or suitable sterile wipes or swabs, clean the teat end and orifice thoroughly. NB: *You are only trying to get the teat end clean; do not clean the whole teat, as this just increases the chance of contaminating the teat end. After sterilizing the teat end, be careful not to touch the teat end with your hand.*
4. Look at the spirit-soaked cotton wool or swab after cleaning the teat end. If it is discoloured or there is any evidence of visible dirt, then repeat step 3 until it remains clean.
5. Take STERILE universal container.
6. Remove lid and ensure nothing touches the inside of the container or the inside of the lid at any stage (if it does, discard this container and start again). Ideally the lid should be held between the fingers of the same hand that holds the container, to prevent contamination.
7. Discard the first 2–3 squirts of milk into a bucket.
8. Without letting the teat end touch the container, strip out the milk so that it squirts into the container. Collect 2–3 ml.
9. Replace the lid, again without touching the inside of the lid or container.
10. If at any stage you suspect your sample has become contaminated, *start the whole procedure again.*
11. Label container clearly, using indelible ink pen, with the following information: Date, Name of Farm, Cow No., Quarter.
12. Use teat dip afterwards.
13. Refrigerate at 4°C. Do not freeze.

© RVC

Clinical Skills Sheet

18.49. California Milk Test (CMT) sampling method

Method

NB This is **not** the same thing as a **sterile** milk sample for bacteriology.

Equipment:
- Water/paper towels (if teats very soiled).
- Disposable examination gloves.
- CMT Paddle (a hand-held 4-well mixer).
- CMT Test Liquid + pipette.
- Teat dip.

Procedure:
1. The teats should be visibly clean but do *not* need to be sterilized. If they are not clean, use water and disposable paper towels. Make sure they are **dry** before sampling.
2. Wear clean examination gloves.
3. Discard the first 2–3 squirts of milk from each teat into a waste bucket.
4. Strip approx. 3 ml milk from each quarter into the corresponding well of the paddle, i.e. just enough to cover the base of the well. Make sure you know which well corresponds to which quarter, otherwise the results will be meaningless.
5. Tilt the paddle to pour off excess milk – use the line on the base of each well as a guide. Pour slowly to avoid any cross-contamination of the wells.
6. Add approx 3 ml of CMT liquid (i.e. about the same amount as the milk sample) to each well of the paddle.
7. Swirl the tray to mix the milk and CMT liquid. Observe each well whilst swirling for any indication of thickening of fluid or gel formation.
8. For each well note the result as Negative, Trace, 1+, 2+ or 3+ using the key below. Make sure you relate the result of each well to the quarter it refers to when stating or recording the result. (NB: The milk samples in CSC will be negative.)
9. Dispose of milk sample + CMT liquid into waste bucket and rinse paddle in clean water.
10. Use teat dip afterwards.

Interpretation of clinical results for CMT		
Interpretation and Grading of the CMT from Biggs: Mastitis in Cattle, Crowood Press, 2009		
Result	Description	Approx SCC (cells/ml)
Negative	Mixture remains free-running liquid with no evidence of thickening or formation of a precipitate despite continued rotation of the paddle	<200,000
T (Trace)	Slight thickening that tends to disappear with continued rotation of the paddle	200,000–500,000
1+ (Weak)	Significant thickening, but little or no tendency toward gel formation. Thickening may disappear after prolonged rotation of the paddle	400,000–1,500,000
2+ (Distinct)	Mixture thickens immediately. With continued rotation of the paddle, a gel accumulates in the centre of the well, leaving the outer edges exposed	800,000–5,000,000
3+ (Strong)	A very obvious thick gel forms, which needs to stick to the bottom of the paddle forming a distinct lump in the centre of the well	>5,000,000

© RVC

19 Equine Procedures

Imogen Johns

B and W Equine Vets, Breadstone Equine Hospital, Berkeley, UK

Learning objectives

By the end of this chapter, students should be able to:

- Know the locations for blood taking and intravenous (IV) injection in the horse.
- Understand the key differences between taking a blood sample and giving an IV injection.
- Describe how to perform each technique.
- Understand the indications for intravenous catheter (IVC) placement in the horse.
- Understand the procedure of IVC placement.
- Understand when an intramuscular (IM) injection might be required in the horse.
- Describe how to perform an IM injection.
- Understand the indications for passage of a nasogastric tube.
- Describe or perform the procedures on a simulator.

 Clinical skills sheets

Three clinical skills sheets will be used in this chapter, along with one from another chapter, and these can be found at pages 135–136 and 304–317. Reference will be made to each skills sheet at the relevant section within the chapter. The details of the clinical skills sheets used are as follows (in numerical order):

SS 9.18 Venepuncture: blood collection by Vacutainer

SS 19.50 Equine fluid therapy set-up

SS 19.51 Common sites for intramuscular injections

SS 19.52 Passing a nasogastric tube in a horse

 Videos

Two videos will be used in this chapter to demonstrate how to perform the clinical skills and these are:

V 19.1 Equine jugular placement in a horse

V 19.2 Equine fluid therapy

Introduction

The main equine procedures that are essential are giving intramuscular (IM) and/or intravenous (IV) injections, placing an intravenous catheter (IVC) for continuous treatment (drug or fluid administration) and introducing a nasogastric tube. Unlike with small animals, more assistance is necessary for these tasks and also a local anaesthetic may be used before certain procedures.

The methods described here are taught within the Royal Veterinary College clinical skills centre. You may not be able to try all these procedures in live animals but should be able to practise and explain how to do these tasks on simulators.

19.1 Taking Blood from a Horse and Giving an Intravenous Injection to a Horse

Taking a blood sample is a key part of the investigation of many disease processes and is sometimes done as part of routine health screening, pre-anaesthetic checks or drug testing in competition horses.

Giving an intravenous injection is an essential skill; many medications, including some antibiotics, sedatives

© CAB International 2018. *Veterinary Clinical Skills Manual* (eds N. Coombes and A. Silva-Fletcher)

19.1.1 Sites for blood taking

The jugular vein is the most common site for blood sampling in the horse. Although the left or right vein can be used, you will find it easier to take blood from the left vein if you are right-handed.

If smaller volumes of blood are to be taken (less than 10 ml), the transverse facial venous sinus can be used. This site can be useful if there is a problem with the jugular vein (a thrombus, for example) or the horse is behaving badly for the jugular sampling – sometimes horses are better behaved for the facial sinus sample. This sinus runs parallel to the facial crest; the site for venepuncture corresponds to the apex of a triangle formed by the intersection of the thumb and index finger below the facial crest and a line between the medial and lateral canthus of the eye.

Other sites that could be used include the cephalic vein or the lateral thoracic vein, but these are uncommonly used; the tail vein is *not* used in horses.

19.1.2 Sites for intravenous injection

The jugular vein is most frequently used for IV injections. The facial sinus is not appropriate for injections.

V 19.1 for equine jugular catheter placement in a horse

V 19.1 video.cabi.org/xpruj

19.1.3 Equipment required

- Depending on the size of the horse, a 1–1.5″ 20G needle is usually appropriate for both blood sampling and intravenous injection. An 18G needle can also be used, though horses will typically react more to the larger needles.

- Syringes, depending on the size of the sample required or medication to be injected.

- Surgical spirit to clean coat if obviously dirt contaminated.

- Hands should be clean but gloves do not need to be worn.

19.1.4 Blood sampling from jugular vein

Ensure that the horse is appropriately restrained by a competent handler. In most instances, no restraint beyond a head collar and lead rope are required, though some horses do not tolerate the procedure well (owners will often describe their horse as 'needle shy') and may need additional restraint, such as a nose twitch.

Stand to the side of the horse (left if you are taking from the left jugular vein). Locate the jugular vein in the jugular groove by holding off the vein approximately one-third of the way down the neck and observing the vein filling – it can be helpful to intermittently hold off and then release the vein if you are struggling to locate the vein. In horses that have a long-hair coat, it can sometimes be hard to locate the vein; using surgical spirit to wet the coat can help.

Once the vein has been located, keep the vein held off and distended, and gently slide the needle with the syringe attached into the jugular vein, parallel with the vein; the needle should be located in the top third of the vein. The lower down the vein you go (i.e. the closer to the shoulder), the more superficial the carotid artery is; as this vessel runs parallel to the jugular vein, this can result in inadvertent sampling of the carotid, causing a large haematoma. You will need to go through the skin and some subcutaneous tissue, but you do not want to go too deep and hit the carotid: an angle of approximately 20 degrees is usually sufficient. Advance the needle until it is at least halfway in; sometimes you will see some blood in the hub of the needle, but more commonly you will need to draw back on the syringe and see if there is blood in the syringe. If not, redirect your needle without coming out of the skin and try again.

You can also utilize a Vacutainer system to take blood: you will need a Vacutainer needle (similar gauge), a Vacutainer holder and Vacutainer blood tubes. The Vacutainer needle with the holder attached is placed into the vein as described previously, but blood will not drip from the needle. The Vacutainer blood tube is then attached to the needle and blood will flow spontaneously into the tube due to the vacuum. As long as the vacuum is intact, the tubes will fill to the required volume. The tube is then disconnected from the needle and the needle is removed.

SS 9.18 for blood collection by Vacutainer

19.1.5   Giving an IV injection in the jugular vein

The technique is very similar, though you should ensure that you are in the jugular and not the carotid artery by placing the needle into the vein first, without the syringe attached.

How do you know if you are in the vein or carotid artery?

- If the blood drips slowly from the hub of the needle, then you are in the vein.
- If the blood 'spurts' from the needle, then you are most likely in the carotid artery and you will need to re-direct the needle more superficially.

It is essential that medications of any type are not injected into the carotid artery, as this can result immediately in seizures and occasionally death of the animal. Pre-placing the needle is the easiest way to avoid this.

19.1.6   Taking a sample from the transverse facial venous sinus

Although the Vacutainer system can be used, it tends to be easier to use a needle and syringe. Locate the site for venepuncture as described in 19.1.1, then insert the needle with syringe attached at an angle of approximately 60 degrees, aiming towards the facial crest. Advance through skin and muscle and on to the bone surface – back off slightly and aspirate the sample.

19.2   Placing an Intravenous Catheter

This technique is not commonly performed in first-opinion equine practice, apart from where general anaesthesia is to be performed, or for euthanasia, where catheter placement is recommended. Most horses that require IV medication are given those medications via direct IV injection. Catheters are typically used in a hospital situation where ongoing IV medication or intravenous fluid therapy is required.

The most frequently used site for an IVC is the jugular vein, though the cephalic or lateral thoracic vein can also be used.

19.2.1   Equipment required

- Clippers.
- Surgical prep materials.
- Local anaesthetic, such as mepivicaine or lignocaine.
- Sterile gloves.
- Catheter. The gauge will depend on the size of the horse and what the catheter will be used for. Typically a 14-gauge catheter will be suitable for most horses, apart from small ponies and foals. Larger-bore catheters (12-gauge) can be used if high fluid flow rates are anticipated.
- Needle with suture material to secure catheter in vein.
- Superglue can be used for additional security.
- Extension set flushed with heparinized saline.

19.2.2   Preparation

A suitable site in the rostral third of the jugular vein is clipped and surgically prepped.

Local anaesthetic is injected subcutaneously halfway through the prep at the site of the catheter insertion and also the sites where the extension set is to be sutured in place.

Finish the prep and put on sterile gloves – this procedure should be done as a sterile procedure.

19.2.3   Method

Locate the catheter insertion site. If you have an assistant, ask them to raise the vein. If not, use the knuckle of the hand you are not placing the catheter with to raise the vein. Ideally this would be in the sterile prep area, but if not, remember this finger will no longer be sterile!

In some horses with thick skin you will need to make a small skin incision to get the catheter through the skin. If not, insert the tip of the catheter through the skin at an approximately 45 degree angle. You may feel a 'pop' when the catheter enters the vein, and blood should drip from the hub of the catheter.

Advance the catheter into the vein a small distance and then change the angle so that it is more parallel to the skin surface. Then advance the catheter off the stylet, ensuring that it goes smoothly into the vein. Blood should be dripping from the catheter.

Attach the extension set or a bung to the end of the catheter and flush the catheter. It should be easy to flush and blood should be aspirated if you draw back on the syringe.

Suture the catheter in place. Depending on the type of catheter you are using, there may be small holes on the side of the catheter to do this. Otherwise, place a suture around the hub of the catheter and then several more around the extension set.

 How long can the catheter remain in place?

Depending on the catheter material, if there are no complications the catheter can remain in place for 3 days to several weeks. Monitor for swelling, pain and discharge, or for a palpable thrombus or thickening in the vein, which could all suggest a septic thrombophlebitis. The catheter should be removed and submitted for culture if this occurs.

 V 19.1 for jugular catheter placement in a horse

V 19.1 video.cabi.org/xpruj

V 19.2 Equine fluid therapy

V 19.2 video.cabi.org/rqoxu

 SS 19.50 for how to set up equine fluid therapy bags and line

19.3 Giving an Intramuscular Injection

This technique is an essential technique to master; many medications, including vaccines, antibiotics and sedatives, are given or can be given via the IM route. Small volumes tend to be well tolerated by most horses, but larger volumes can be painful and thus correct restraint is essential.

19.3.1 Locations for IM injection

There are four main sites used for IM injections in the horse:

1. The neck musculature.
2. The gluteal muscles.
3. The pectoral muscles.
4. The semi-membranosus/semi-tendanosus.

For most routine injections, such as vaccinations, the neck is preferred as it is easy to do, the horses typically tolerate it well and restraint is easier. If repeated IM injections are required (for example, a horse is on a course of IM antibiotics), the volumes given may be large and thus rotating sites is recommended.

 SS 19.51 shows the common sites for IM injections

19.3.2 Equipment required

- Medication to be administered in syringe.
- Needles – for small volumes a 20G 1.5″ needle is sufficient; for larger volumes, a 19G or 18G 1.5″ needle should be used in adult horses.

19.3.3 Technique

Adequate restraint and a competent handler are essential, in particular if the gluteals or semi-membranosus/tendinosus are used.

For the neck:

The site for injection is a triangle with its base in front of the shoulder, the dorsal margin below the nuchal ligament and the ventral border dorsal to the cervical vertebra. The injection can be given on either side of the neck, but if you are right-handed it will usually be easiest to inject on the left side of the horse. The needle and syringe are inserted attached. Take a small neck twitch (in your left hand, pull and slightly twist the skin) and then slowly insert the needle to the hub next to the twitched area. Draw back on the syringe to ensure that there is no blood in the hub of the needle – this is an essential step to ensure that the medication is not given inadvertently into a vessel.

 For some medications, such as sedatives that can also be given via the IV route, this is not a major problem, but some drugs such as procaine penicillin *cannot* be given intravenously as the horse can have a severe reaction; thus, if there is blood in the hub of the needle, redirect the needle, draw back, make sure there is no blood and then inject.

For the gluteals:

The site for injection can easily be palpated on the dorsolateral aspect of the rump area. Do not go too close to midline or the hip. Many horses react to injections in this site, in particular the needle placement, so ensure that the horse is adequately restrained – the holder can take a neck twitch to aid this, or a nose twitch could be used. Stand on the side to be injected. For this technique it is usually best to have the needle off the syringe for placement, and then attach once the needle is placed. If you are injecting into the left gluteal, stand on the left side of the horse at approximately the level of the flank/stifle area. Stand close to the horse and firmly rub the area to be injected with your left hand, which is also holding the needle. Once the horse has become accustomed to this, locate the site to be injected and place the needle to the hub; the skin is quite thick in this area, so some force may be required. Some clinicians like to 'tap' the area with the fist several times before placing the needle. Once the needle has been placed, attach the syringe, draw back to ensure no blood is in the hub, and if there is none, inject.

Other sites:

The method is similar to that described above, in the locations described in SS 19.51.

19.4 Passing a Nasogastric (NG) Tube

The most frequent reason that a veterinary surgeon will perform this procedure is as part of the examination of a horse with colic, or abdominal pain. Oral fluids and medications can also be given via this route if needed.

19.4.1 Anatomical considerations

Diseases of the small (and sometimes large) intestine can result in fluid accumulation in the small intestine, due either to a physical obstruction or to a functional problem. This fluid can also accumulate in the stomach, if it cannot move distally in the gastrointestinal tract (GIT). Due to the muscular tone of the cardiac sphincter at the junction between the oesophagus and stomach, horses cannot vomit even if dramatic gastric distension is present. Passing a tube into the stomach via the nose (NG tube) is used to determine whether gastric distension is present and to relieve it if it is. Additionally, assuming no excess fluid is present, fluids can be administered via this route.

19.4.2 Equipment

- Nasogastric tube, size depending on size of horse.
- Two buckets; one with 2 l of water (or known volume).
- Plastic jug.
- Funnel.

19.4.3 Method

Adequate restraint is essential. The holder should stand on the opposite side of the horse to the person passing the NG tube. Although some horses tolerate this procedure, placement of a nose twitch is often helpful. Some tubes have marks on them which give you an idea of when the tube is in the nasopharynx and then in the stomach. If not, it can be helpful to place the end of the tube at the medial canthus of the eye and measure to the nostril, to give you an idea of how much tube will actually be in the horse before you reach the oesophagus. The tube is then passed through the ventral nasal meatus by ensuring that it is directed as medial and ventral as possible.

1. To do this, stand on the right side of the horse with the tube in your right hand. Do not stand in front of the horse, as the horse may strike at you with its front legs.

2. Placing the tube in a little water or using a small amount of K-Y jelly can help. Use your left thumb to direct the tube into the nostril, pressing it ventrally and medially. This is the part of the procedure that horses tend to react to most, as it is quite a 'snug' fit.

3. If you feel that you cannot pass the tube because it is physically being stopped by something and you are *not* at the nasopharynx yet, *do not* push further because you are most likely at the ethmoid turbinates; they are very vascular, and if you damage them a dramatic nose bleed can result. If you think this has occurred, pull the tube out a little and direct more ventrally and medially.

4. **Once the tube has reached the nasopharynx**, the tube is advanced until the horse swallows it. The tube cannot be forced into the oesophagus, but must be coordinated with a swallowing movement. The best way to determine whether the tube is in the oesophagus (rather than the trachea) is to look on the left side of the neck: in most cases you will be able to see the end of the tube moving down the neck. You should also be able to feel the end of the tube and/or feel the resistance to the tube as it moves down the muscular oesophagus. If it is in the trachea, the tube tends to be very easy to advance. Some horses will cough if the tube is in the trachea, but this is not a consistent sign so should not be relied on.

5. **Once in the oesophagus**, advance the tube into the stomach: you can use the mark on the stomach tube to help you determine whether the tube is in the stomach. Other ways to check are to listen for bubbles or smell for gastric contents. Even if there is a large volume of fluid in the stomach, it will typically not flow spontaneously and a siphon will need to be set up. A small volume of water is given, using the jug and the funnel, and allowed to run into the stomach via gravity. When the fluid is in the stomach, the tube is then lowered and the volume recorded. This should be performed two to three times to rule out fluid accumulation in the stomach (gastric reflux). Although you will see some vets 'sucking' on the tube to check for reflux, gastric contents can be inadvertently sucked into their mouth, with the potential for disease transmission; thus this is not the preferred technique.

6. If no reflux is obtained (less than 2 l net), then fluids can be administered as required. Usually a maximum of 6–8 l for a 500–600 kg horse is given.

 SS 19.52 for passing a nasogastric tube

Clinical Skills Sheet

19.50. Equine fluid therapy set-up

Task:

How to set up multiple fluid bags using transfer sets.

Method
Please note: this sheet is not the definitive version of all to do with equine fluid therapy. Also it does not discuss health and safety concerns to do with working in and around large animals.
You have worked out your calculation and decided your horse needs 20 l over 24 h at a drip rate of 2 drops per second. (For more details of how to work out an equine fluid rate, see CSC calculation sheet and on the CSC website.)
Now collect all your equipment together: • 4 × 5 l bags of fluid (Isolec). • Equine fluid line (STAT large animal i.v. set). • 2 transfer sets. • 2 drip stands (variable height ones).
Wash your hands.
Check the dates on the fluid bags and the general condition of fluid – not cloudy or contaminated and seals not broken.
Set up the drip stands at different heights next to each other.
Remove the outer plastic coverings from the four fluid bags.
Hang two bags on the higher drip stand, two bags on the lower drip stand (or use a ceiling-suspended gyro hanger if in a stable where there is one).
Open the equine fluid line packaging. There is a patient label on the drip chamber that can be completed at this point. 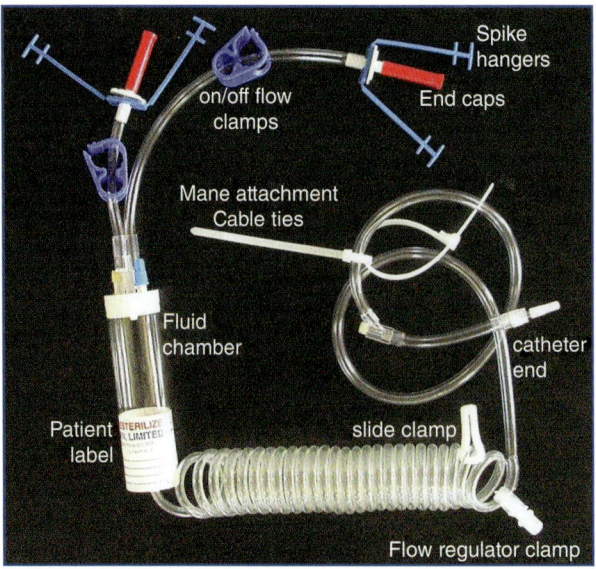

Method

Close the two on/off flow clamps on the upper Y tube lines (blue clips) to prevent fluid coming through the line when first attached.

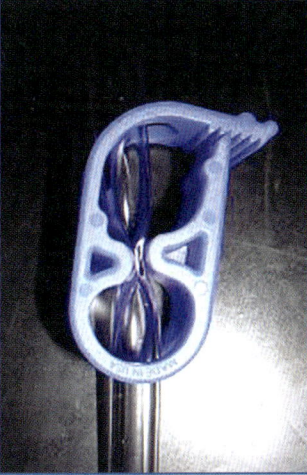

Close the lower slide clamp (below the spiral part of the tubing)

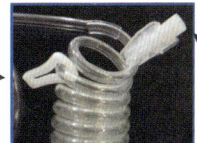

Close the screw flow regulator clamp tightly

Open the packaging of the two transfer sets, closing the (blue) on/off flow clamps.

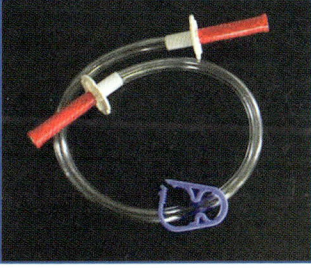

Snap the outlet port caps off the two lower fluid bags.

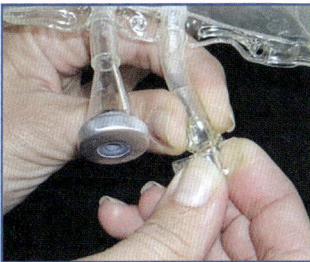

Method
Taking care not to break sterility, remove the red spike caps from the fluid line and push the spikes into the two lower fluid bag ports.   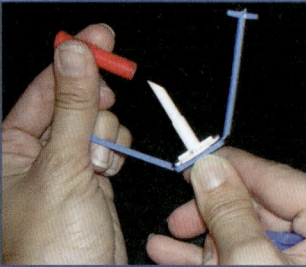
Attach the two blue spike hangers into the fluid bag holes as shown.   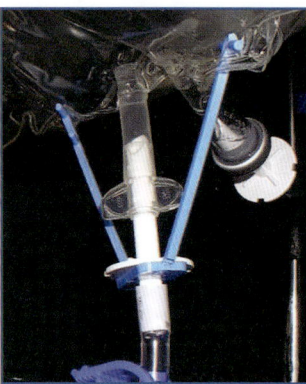

Method

Take one of the transfer sets, remove the protective spike cover (taking care not to break sterility) and insert one end into the UPPER fluid bag port and the other end into the INJECTION PORT of the lower bag. Repeat with the other transfer set.

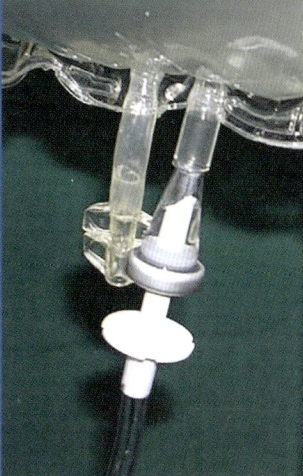

All bags are now connected.

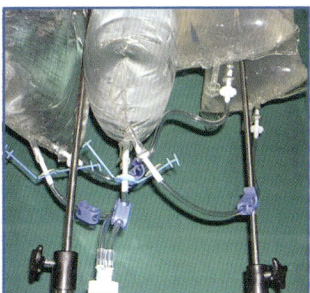

Method
Open the blue clips on the Y-part of the fluid line and squeeze the drip chamber, allowing the air to release into the fluid bag until the chamber is half full of fluid. 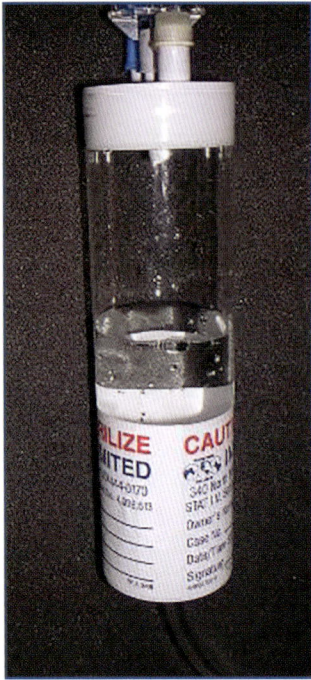
Open the lower slide clamp and unscrew the regulator clamp to allow fluid to run through the line *in a controlled manner* to get rid of any air bubbles.
Then close the slide clamp once you have set your drip rate using the screw regulator (this can be a bit tricky).
You can either open all four blue on/off flow clamps (two on the Y connector, two on the transfer sets) *before* you attach your now ready fluid line to the intravenous catheter placed in your horse, or afterwards – *as long as you remember to do so* !

© RVC

Clinical Skills Sheet

19.51. Common injection sites for intramuscular injections

Task:

Locate and be familiar with the common injection sites in the horse for intramuscular injections.

Common injection sites for intramuscular (IM) injections: • Neck. • Hamstrings. • Pectorals. • Gluteals.
Injection site: These are common injection sites because they are large muscle masses that are actively used by the horse. This promotes drug absorption and decreases the chance of swelling and pain at the injection site. The site should allow the needle to be placed deep in the muscle without danger of hitting bone, ligaments, nerves, or blood vessels.
Clinical practice point: The handler should stand on the same side of the horse as the person injecting so that both are kept safe should the horse act up. *Take extra care with 'needle-shy' horses: a twitch may be needed to relax the horse.*
How to give the IM injection • Remove the needle from the syringe. • Quickly and decisively insert the needle perpendicular to the skin. A fast stab is less painful for the patient. The entire length of the needle, up to the hub, should be inserted into the muscle. • Attach the syringe to the needle. • Always aspirate back before injecting anything: **NO blood = safe to administer the medication.**   **If there is blood = STOP:** **you must remove the needle and redirect the injection.** • Slowly administer the medication. • Properly dispose of the needle and syringe in a safe medical waste container. This technique can be performed with the syringe attached but always make sure to aspirate before injecting. When inserting the needle, there are different methods: • Pinch the skin next to the injection site, and insert the needle   *Or* • Holding the needle between your thumb and forefinger, tap the horse vigorously 2–3 times with the side of your palm at the injection site and, without breaking your rhythm, rotate your hand and insert the needle. ***Be bold with the injection; remember their skin is tough and you want to get through the skin to inject into the muscle.***

Common sites for IM injections:

Neck

Inject into the muscle inside of the triangle. Avoiding the nuchal ligament dorsally, cervical vertebrae ventrally and scapula caudally.

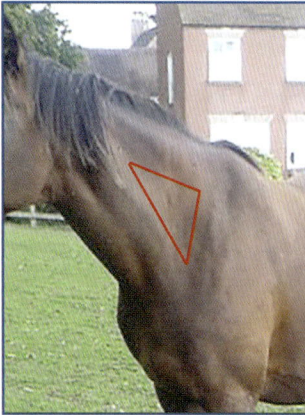

Pectorals

Note that this muscle group is prone to becoming sore easily. It is best to stand close to the shoulder, facing forward, and reach around to the chest.

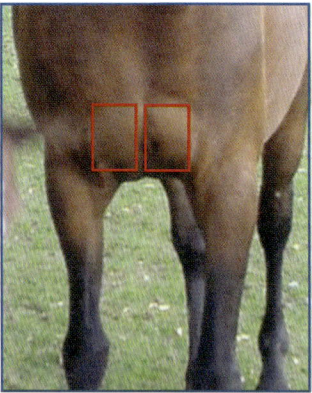

Hamstrings (semi-tendinosus/semi-membranosus)

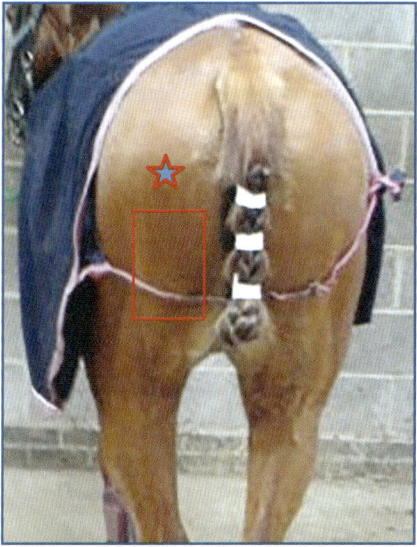

To find this injection site, locate the bony protrusion that makes up the point of the buttocks (red star) (tuber ischii).

Drop about 2.5 cm below the tuber ischii and inject into the large muscle mass along the back of the leg.

Be sure that you are injecting into the muscle mass rather than in the crevice between the semi-tendinosus and the adjoining muscle mass.

Clinical practice point:

Did you know?

The hamstrings are the preferred injection site in foals because it is one of the larger muscles on a foal's body.

Gluteals

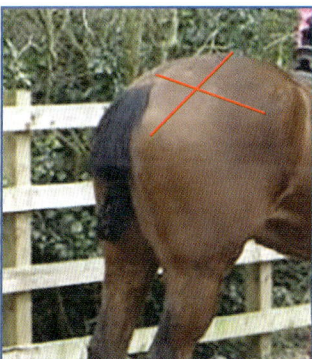

To locate the injection site find the:

- intersection of a line between the tail head and the point of the hip and a line between the top of the croup and the point of the buttocks.

The disadvantage to this site is that it has very poor drainage and thus would heal slowly if a needle abscess developed at the injection site.

> **Clinical practice point:**
> In a horse receiving a lot of medication, such as a course of IM antibiotic injections whilst in hospital, the injection sites used are rotated so that the horse is less likely to get sore.
>
> A commonly used procedure is 'right at night' so that the horse is injected in the right-hand side (either neck or gluteals) in the evening and then the left-hand side (either neck or gluteals) in the morning.

Instructions written by: J. Mullard MRCVS
Images: J. Mullard

© RVC

Clinical Skills Sheet

19.52. Passing a nasogastric tube in a horse

Passing a nasogastric tube (NGT) is essential in colic work-ups, to determine if there is reflux and for emptying the stomach if there is reflux.

This simulator will help you get used to the feel and handling of the nasogastric tube, passing it into the ventral meatus and into the oesophagus, and practising the technique of getting reflux out.

It is obviously only a simulator but this is a great way to practise as it is a skill that students do not often get a chance to practise in live horses, due to the emergency context and the owner's wishes.

These instructions are for use with the following simulator.

You will need a colleague to perform this task with.

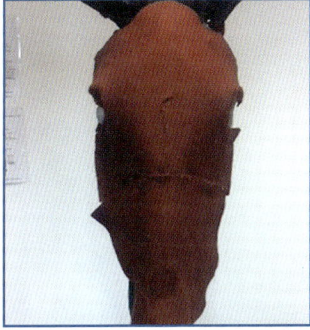

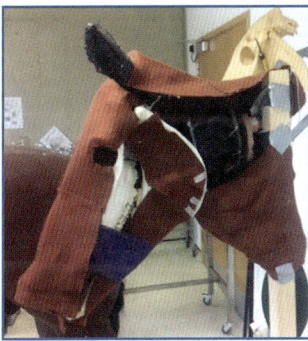

Do not attempt to open the jaw on the simulator, as it is held closed. A live horse will often toss their head around and may have their mouth open.

Clinical practice point:

Tubing a horse in real-life colic:

Tubing is used in an emergency situation to check if there is reflux. If there is, it allows emptying of the reflux (as horses cannot vomit).

Refluxing a horse relieves discomfort and pressure. If the reflux is left to build up, it can cause the stomach to rupture – this is fatal for the horse.

Common problems:

- Misdirecting the tube into the false nostril, or the nostril instead of the ventral meatus.
- Making contact with the ethmoids (turbinate bones) and causing a nose bleed.
- Placing the tube into the trachea instead of the oesophagus.

Other uses for tubing:

Not only is tubing used in emergency situations; it can also be used therapeutically to deliver oral fluids, which are often required if dealing with an impaction or, if the horse has been sedated for a long period of time, they are often given fluids as the sedation can affect gut motility.

Practical tips:

- The tube is like an unruly snake. The easiest way to stay in control of it is to put it around your neck, so that it is kept out of the way and is made easy to handle.
- Some veterinary surgeons place lubricant (K-Y Jelly, or their own saliva) on the end of the tube before inserting it.
- The horse's head position is important when passing the tube: their head should be bent in towards their chest to help faciliate tube placement and swallowing of the tube.
- Some veterinary surgeons put measurements on the tube so that they know when they should be in the stomach: they measure it on the outside of the horse and mark on the tube the level of the 14th rib.
- Always get someone to hold the horse when you are placing a nasogastric tube.

Refresher of meatus anatomy:

A meatus is a natural body opening, or canal. In the horse there are the dorsal, middle and ventral nasal meatus. The ventral meatus travels caudally to exit the skull just between the hamuli of the pterygoid bones.

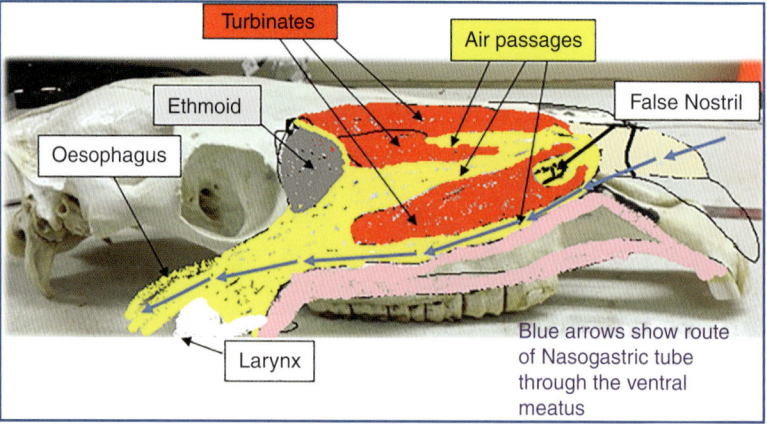

Get your equipment ready.

You will need:

- A colleague.
- Nasogastric tube (blue end is the mouthpiece for you; the other end of the tube is for the horse).
- Bucket.
- Simulator horse.

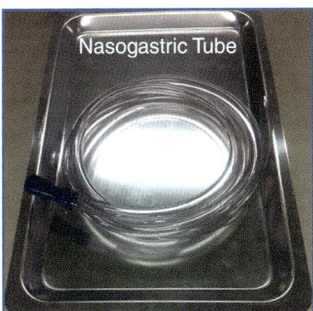 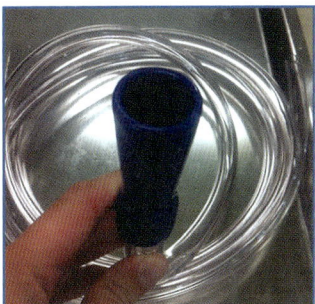

Insert the end of the tube into the horse's nostril and progress it slowly, aiming **ventrally and medially** (downwards and inwards) so that the tube enters the ventral meatus.

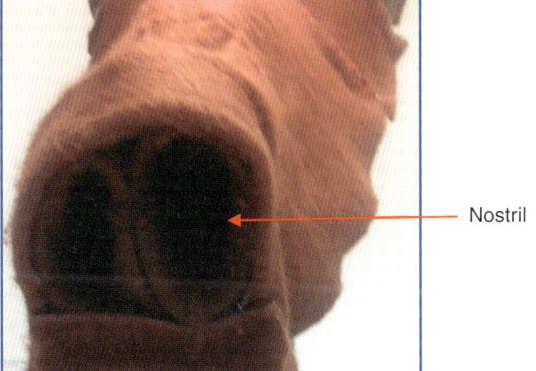

Nostril

If the tube won't advance, **STOP!**

- You have either gone up the nostril and not into the ventral meatus.
- or the false nostril/nasal diverticulum (in the simulator these are blind-ending tubes). } See Anatomy diagram

If you experience a grating feeling, this is because the tube is directed incorrectly and you are touching the side of the simulator. *Pull out the tube and redirect it more ventrally and medially.*

This is similar to the 'grating' felt when attempting to pass an NGT in a live horse and the tube is incorrectly directed into the dorsal or middle meatus and hits the turbinate bones, which then causes a nosebleed.

Once you have inserted the tube ventrally and medially you will find it advances upwards until you reach an obstruction or soft resistance if you try to gently advance it further. You have reached the pharynx.

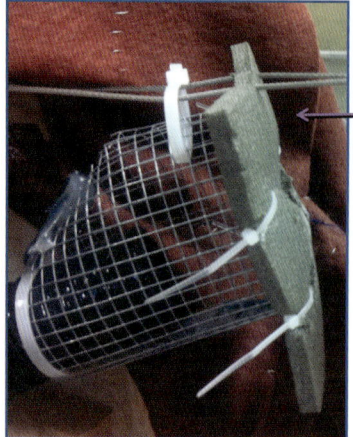

Pharynx; it is the green foam in the simulator

In the live horse (and the simulator) you have to wait at this point until the horse swallows the tube into the oesophagus.

With the simulator:

- Your colleague pulls the tube through the X cut in the green foam and then passes the nasogastric tube into the oesophagus (top hole, black tube).
- The student passing the nasogastric tube blows into the mouthpiece of the tube (to help advance the tube down the oesophagus) whilst advancing the tube up the ventral meatus and down the oesophagus.

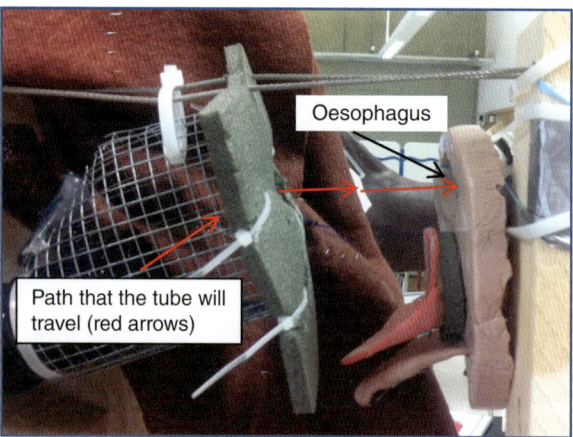

Oesophagus

Path that the tube will travel (red arrows)

You will reach the stomach. Now it is time to see if there is any reflux: keeping the blue end of the tube low, suck as hard as you can.

This sets up a siphon system, and the reflux (water in the simulator) will travel up the tube. When you can see the water in the tube, take it out of your mouth and point the tube at the bucket so that the reflux goes into the bucket.

Repeat this. You will find you get a little bit of reflux back to start with, and then it will flow freely (like a hosepipe): direct the reflux into the bucket.

To stop the simulator refluxing (so you do not cause a flood) just pull the tube back out of the stomach and oesophagus.

Now repeat the process but this time the facilitator puts the tube into the trachea.

Once you have finished with the simulator, make sure that you place the tube back into the bucket, and clear up if you have made any mess.

Clinical practice point:

When the tube enters the oesophagus in the live horse, the oesophagus closes around the tube and you have to apply positive pressure by blowing air down the tube to help advance it further along the oesophagus.

Clues that you are in the **oesophagus** in a live horse:

- Having to blow to advance the tube.
- The tube passed once the horse swallowed.
- You can see the tube advancing down the oesophagus by observing the neck area as it advances.

Clues that you are in the **stomach** in the live horse:

- You can hear gurgling noises.
- You can smell gastric odour.

If you have put the tube into the trachea by accident you will find you do not experience resistance or positive pressure, and the tube moves very freely. This is because the tracheal rings hold the trachea open and allow free passage of air.

If you are not sure whether you are in the trachea or not, if you put a very small amount of water down the tube the horse will cough if it is in the trachea.

The nasogastric tube is also used to give oral fluids. Using a pump or a funnel connected to the end of the tube, the fluid is poured down the tube and into the stomach.

Oral fluids are often given during the management of an impaction, or if the horse has undergone a long sedation.

Instructions written by: M. Bennett, C. Götschel, J. Mullard MRCVS
Model created by: M. Bennett, C. Götschel
Images: M. Bennett, C. Götschel and J. Mullard MRCVS

© RVC

Equine Foot Related Skills: Example Shoe Removal

Renate Weller and Peter Day
Royal Veterinary College, London

Learning objectives

By the end of this chapter, students should be able to:

- Confidently name the anatomical landmarks of the hoof.
- Recognize and name the tools used to remove a shoe.
- Demonstrate removal of a shoe in a manner safe for the horse, handler and clinician.

Clinical skills sheets (SS)

Two clinical skills sheets will be used in this chapter and these can be found at pages 321–328. Reference will be made to each skills sheet at the relevant section within the chapter. The details of the clinical skills sheets used are as follows:

SS 20.53 Shoe removal

SS 20.54 Paring the sole and trimming the hoof wall

Video (V)

One video will be used in this chapter to demonstrate how to perform the clinical skill and this is:

V 20.1 Removing a horse shoe

V 20.1 video.cabi.org/qpjuw

 Any equine clinician should be fully aware of the aetiopathogenesis, diagnosis, prognosis and treatment of foot disorders.

Introduction

Shoe removal is a very common procedure in equine practice and is hence an essential skill for every equine clinician. The foot is the most common site of front limb lameness in the horse. In order to be able to fully examine the solar surface of the hoof, shoe removal is essential. It is also usually required before radiography of a horse's foot and before surgery. Within this chapter, you will find information revising the anatomical landmarks of the hoof, what equipment is required to remove a shoe and how to remove a shoe safely for you, your patient and the horse handler.

20.1   Hoof Anatomy Reminder

Identification of anatomical structures with their correct anatomical and equestrian terms is essential in equine practice to be able to communicate with horse owners and also with farriers. Ensure that you know these basic anatomical structures and where to find them (Fig. 20.1).

20.2   Removing a Shoe from a Forelimb

Before any procedure, explain to the horse handler what is going to happen. Make sure the handler is

© CAB International 2018. *Veterinary Clinical Skills Manual* (eds N. Coombes and A. Silva-Fletcher)

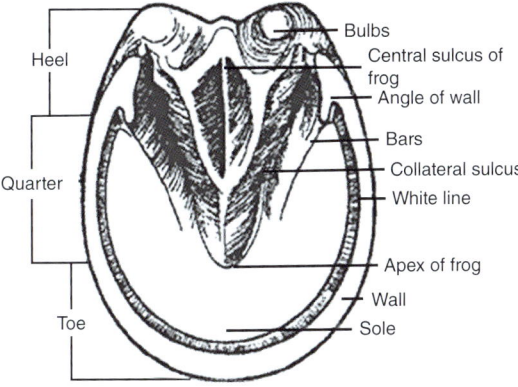

Fig. 20.1. Key anatomical features of the equine hoof.

confident in restraining the horse. Sedation is usually not necessary but may be required occasionally in unco-operative horses. Approach the horse in a safe manner and make sure you have gathered all the equipment beforehand.

 SS 20.53 gives full details about equine shoe removal, including the tools that are needed

Having referred to SS 20.53, you should now be able to remove the shoe from a horse's hoof. You should visit the Clinical Skills Centre to practise on the hoof model before moving on to the real thing.

 Remember, when examining a horse in a veterinary context, the hoof may be painful!

Try to practise approaching the horse and lifting fore and hind feet as much as possible so that you are confident in doing so before attempting any procedures. Do not forget the difference between lifting a fore and hind limb. With the hind limb hoof, rest the dorsal wall of the hoof on your thigh, supporting the limb in place with your arm closest to the horse.

20.3 Providing Students with the Opportunity to Practise Shoe Removal

Shoe removal is a non-invasive procedure and most horses do not find this stressful, hence students may practise this skill on live horses during extramural or intramural studies. Many students also find it useful to spend time with a farrier.

Before performing this skill on a live horse, students may find it useful to practise on cadaver legs or artificial feet first (Fig. 20.2). Ideally, cadaver legs are clamped in a hinged stand to allow the student to mimic holding the leg as for a live horse.

There is also a commercially available artificial leg, 'Blacksmith Buddy' (Fig. 20.3), which is hinged on a spring system and mimics the angle and resistance of a live horse.

Both models can be used for a whole series of foot-related skills, including paring out a hoof, searching for an abscess, applying a foot bandage and applying hoof testers.

 SS 20.54 gives more details on other equine skills, such as sole paring and hoof wall trimming

20.4 Examining for Shoe Removal

Similar to practising shoe removal, this skill can be examined on the live horse during extra- or intramural studies or as part of an objective structured clinical exam (OSCE, see Chapter 22 for more details). From a logistical point of view, especially when there are a large number of students to be examined within a tight timeframe, it is easiest to do this using cadaver legs. This allows a farrier to prepare an adequate number of feet with shoes in advance of the exam. Feet can be reused if a farrier is available during the exam to nail the removed shoes back on.

This means that the process of teaching, practising and demonstrating competence is unified for the students prior to graduation.

Fig. 20.2. Cadaver legs are ideally clamped in a hinged stand to allow the student to mimic holding the leg in the same way as with a live horse.

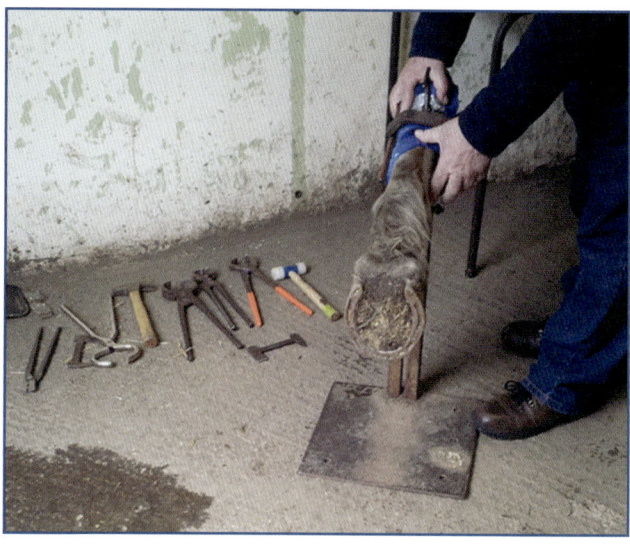

Fig. 20.3. 'Blacksmith Buddy'.

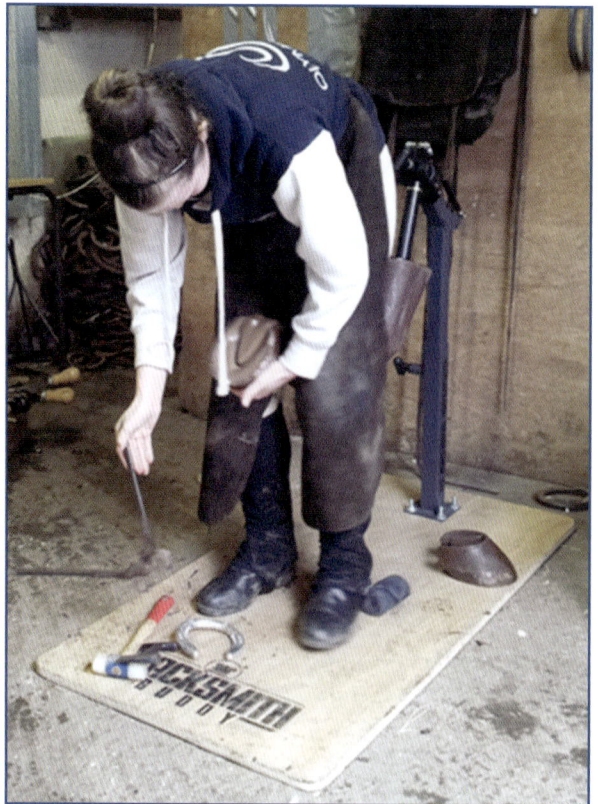

Clinical Skills Sheet

20.53. Shoe removal

Before you start, gather your equipment.
You will need:
- Apron/full chaps.
- Hoof pick.
- Buffer.
- Shoeing hammer (or plastic hammer).
- Protective glasses.
- Pincers.

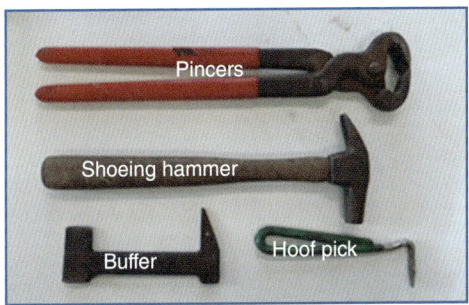

Note: equipment available from the CSC office.

Foot anatomy reminder

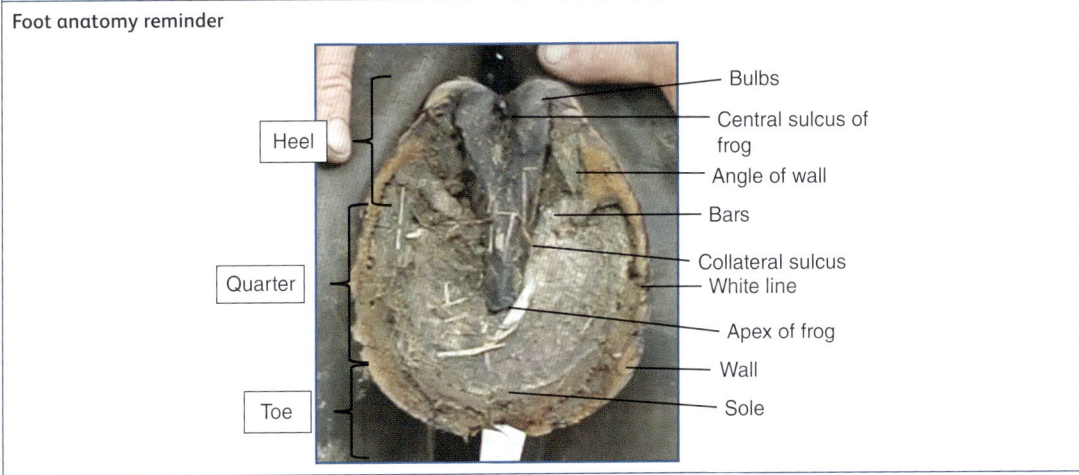

Clinical practice point:

Put on an apron or full chaps when applicable to a live horse.

Ensure the horse is adequately restrained and approach in a safe manner.

Pick up the horse's foot, using the same technique as to pick out a hoof (see instruction sheet on CSC website).

Forelimb:

Once raised, bring the horse's leg behind your adjacent knee to position the horse's leg between your knees, using both hands.

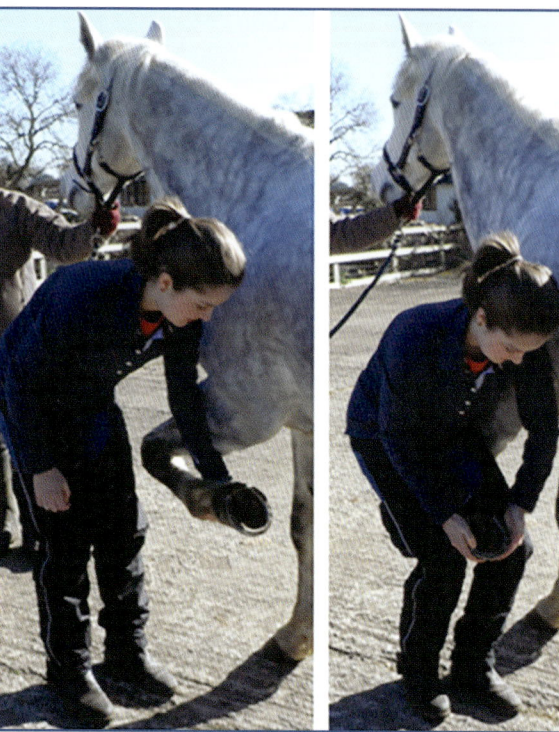
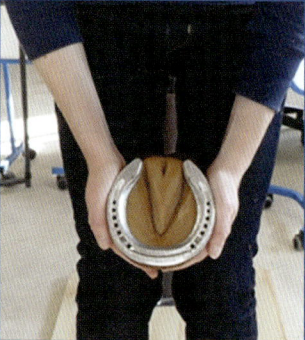

Ensure you have a stable and comfortable stance, with your knees bent.

Hind limb:

Once raised, rest the dorsal wall of the hoof on your thigh.

Use the hoof pick to remove any debris from the hoof, starting with the hoof pick nearest the heel and travelling down the collateral grooves.

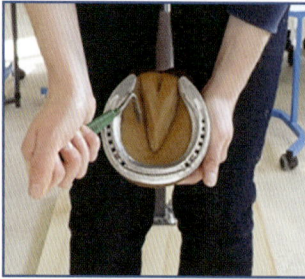

Note: care must be taken not to damage the frog.

Assess the number of nails in both sides of the shoe.

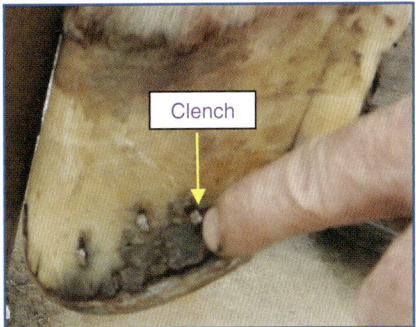

Nails are used to hammer the shoe on to the hoof. The nail goes through the insensitive tubular horn and then comes out through the hoof wall and the end is bent up. This bent-up nail is referred to as a clench.

Position the sharp flat edge of the buffer under the clench on the outer wall of the hoof and, using the shoeing hammer, raise the clench by hammering.

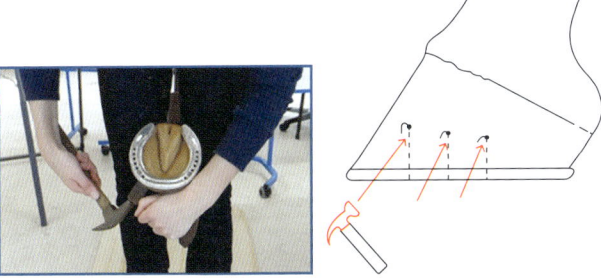

Repeat for all the clenches.

Starting at the heel, close the pincers under the shoe and prise downwards towards the toe.
This will begin to lift the shoe away from the heels.

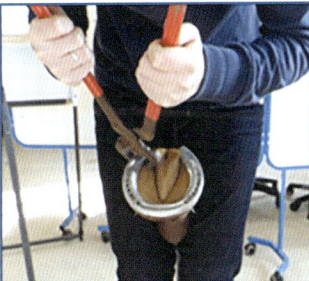

Continue in this manner, moving your pincers down towards the toe until all the nails on both sides of the shoe are lifted.

Once the heels and quarters are lifted, grasp the toe of the shoe with the pincers to remove the shoe.

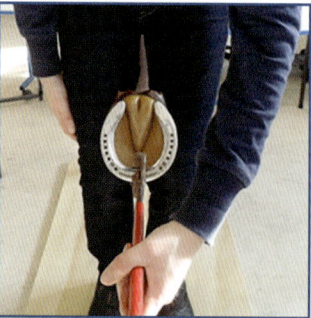

Remove shoe.

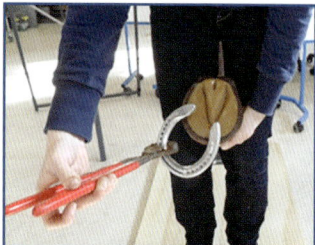

Make sure all nails are removed from the hoof and any loose nails are picked up from the floor and stored in a safe place.

Visually assess the hoof surface for any lesions or damage.

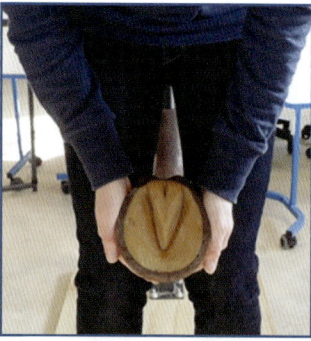

Instructions written by: J. Sharples and J. Mullard MRCVS
Images: J. Sharples and J. Mullard MRCVS

© RVC

Clinical Skills Sheet

20.54. Paring the sole and trimming the hoof wall

Paring the sole and trimming the hoof wall is part of routine foot care.

Routine trimming usually occurs every 4–6 weeks, but will depend on the condition of the horse's feet, whether they are shod or unshod and the type of work they are in.

Gather your equipment.

You will need:

- Apron/full chaps.
- Hoof pick.
- Hoof knife.
- Hoof nippers.
- Rasp.

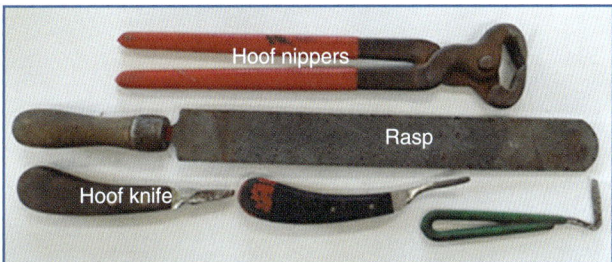

Note: equipment available from the CSC office. Please sign it in and out.

Clinical practice point:

Put on an apron or full chaps when applicable to a live horse.

Ensure the horse is adequately restrained and approach in a safe manner.

Remove the shoe as instructed in SS 20.53 (Shoe removal) if the horse is shod.

Foot Anatomy Reminder

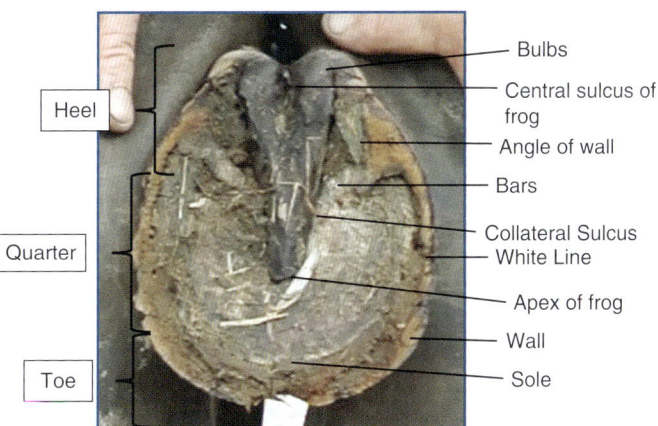

Remove any debris from the foot with a hoof pick and hoof knife.

Visually assess the:

- Frog.
- Heels.
- Sole.
- Hoof wall.
- White line.
- Foot concavity.
- Hoof symmetry.

Use the hoof knife to trim any loose or flaky horn on the bars or frog, taking care not to trim deeply as the frog bleeds easily. Keep the hoof knife flat and level to the sole; do not dig down!

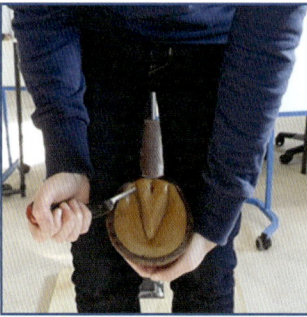

Pare any flakes on the sole away, continually testing the sole thickness by digital pressure (pushing the sole with your thumb, the sole should not flex under pressure).

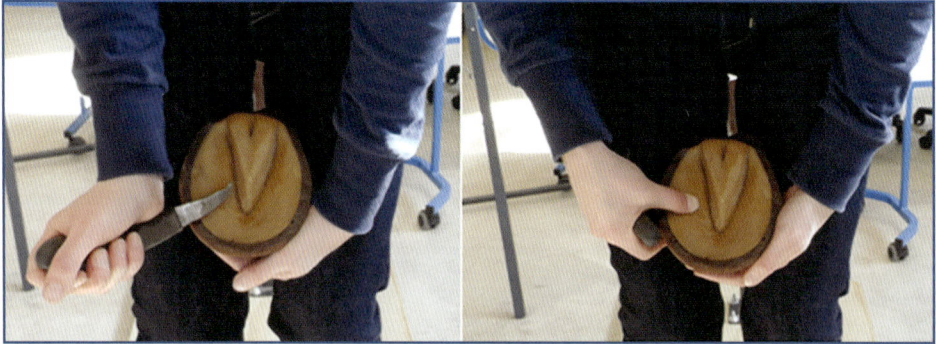

Starting at the toe, trim the hoof wall if needed with hoof nippers.

Trim the toe parallel to the solar surface.

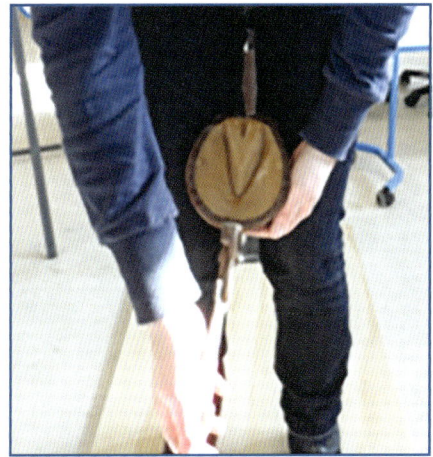 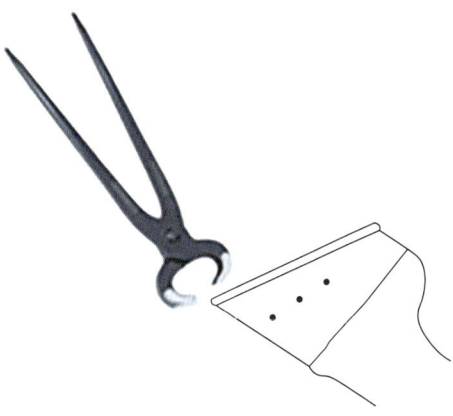

Note: do not trim the wall below the level of the sole.

Next, rasp the outside of the wall.

Hold the rasp handle in your dominant hand and use your non-dominant hand to hold the end of the rasp and with even pressure move in continuous circular motions.

Start from heel to toe, then across the quarters and toe.

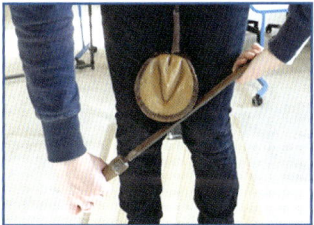

Note: always ensure you hold the rasp level.

Rasp the inside wall from toe to heel, have the rasp pointed towards you with the handle in the palm of your dominant hand.

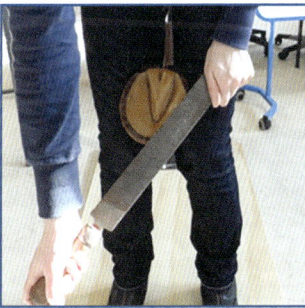

Do not rasp the frog, just the sole!

Finally, rasp the edge of the wall by running the file side of the rasp around the hoof to remove any sharp edges or rags.

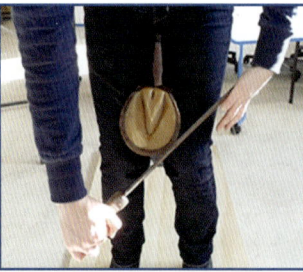

Assess the trimmed hoof for any alterations or changes that need to be done.

Instructions written by: J. Sharples and J. Mullard MRCVS
Images: J. Sharples and J. Mullard

© RVC

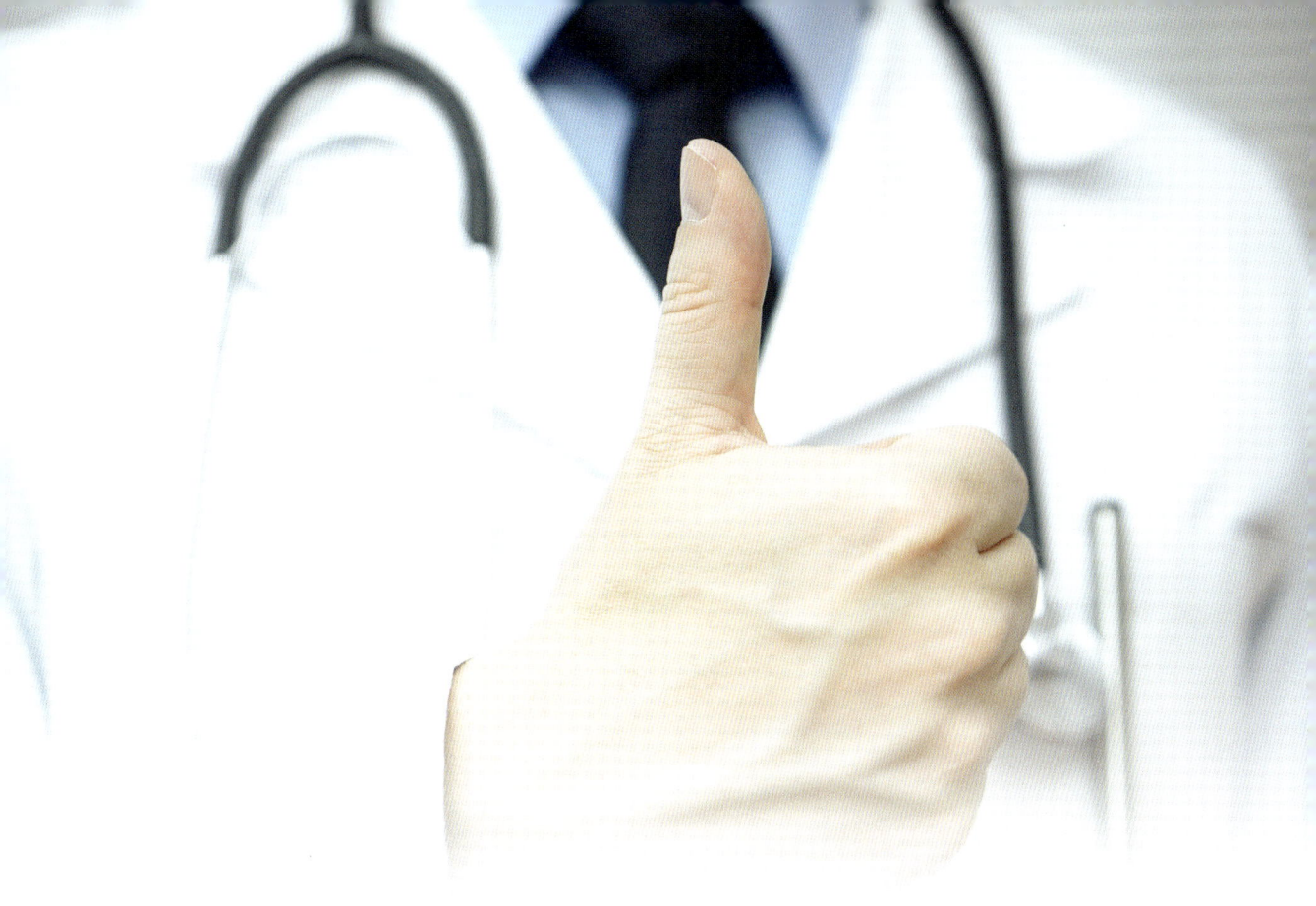

Section

8

Assessment of Clinical Skills

Section Editor: Nichola Coombes

Introduction

The assessment of a student's practical skill requires appropriate design of the examination and an objectively structured framework to ensure the accuracy and reliability of the outcomes during the examination. The assessment process should be structured as a series of 'steps' that are used to measure the ability of students to perform the different components of a clinical task. This process enables the assessor to make a reliable judgement regarding the different abilities and skills of the student. The use of a structured assessment also helps to make judgement of a student's performance more objective. The data generated by an assessment can be used to refine and improve the assessment tool and help to set standards of performance and criteria for pass/fail decisions. The assessments conducted in a CSC, which are known as objective structured clinical examinations (OSCE), were first introduced in the medical education sector in 1975 and at the RVC in 2004. OSCEs are now considered to be the gold standard for performance assessment. The two chapters in this section provide a full explanation of how OSCEs are designed, managed and used practically in the context of veterinary education.

Within this section there are two chapters as outlined below:

Chapter 21: Practical Assessments – Assessments in a Simulated Environment

Chapter 22: Objectively Structured Clinical Examinations – the Practicalities

Chapter 21 provides a full description of the basic concepts underpinning an OSCE. The authors explain how to develop an OSCE using itemized checklists and how performance during an examination may be weighted to derive a student's final score. Common errors that may arise in the writing of assessment checklists as well as other challenges and dilemmas are explored in detail. The outputs of OSCE assessment may generate a mountain of paperwork and today it is possible to purchase specific software that is designed to facilitate the recording and marking of a student's performance. A brief overview regarding commonly available OSCE software is described in this chapter. In addition, guidance is provided on how to determine the pass mark for any particular OSCE station. The experience of the RVC is presented as an example of standard setting and to make decisions regarding how many stations a student should pass to pass the whole OSCE exam.

Chapter 22 offers valuable practical guidelines and tips based on the author's 14 years' experience of designing and running OSCEs. Conducting an OSCE requires meticulous planning as once started the exam cannot be stopped until completion. So, all those involved in the examination process – from technical helpers and animal handlers to the assessors and the students – must follow strict guidelines on the day of the OSCE. The author describes all these processes and also offers 'don't do' points and valuable tips that may help the examination process to run smoothly. The practical management of an OSCE circuit and schedule requires precise timing; recorded announcements may be used to give information to examinees regarding the time available to perform the task as well as when to move between stations. The training of assessors and students should be included in preparation for an OSCE. Providing students with information about the format of the OSCE may reduce their anxiety regarding the examination process. Finally, a detailed 2-year timeline is provided to help educators plan and conduct an OSCE examination.

Practical Assessments – Assessments in a Simulated Environment

21

Stephen A. May and Ayona Silva-Fletcher
Royal Veterinary College, London

Introduction

Objective structured clinical examinations (OSCEs), for assessing the competences of medical students, were developed by R.M. Harden and his colleagues in the 1970s at Dundee Medical School in the UK. The OSCE is an assessment format in which the candidates circulate around a series of standard assessment stations and are assessed on their ability to perform each task by the use of a checklist that details the actions that they need to perform. In variants on this theme, the OSCE may include some knowledge-based assessments, such as analysis of a series of clinical findings or how to read a radiograph. However, the strength of the OSCE format is the assessment of practical procedures; knowledge-based elements can be more efficiently assessed in 'spot tests' or written assessments (Baillie *et al.*, 2014). In the veterinary sector, objective structured practical veterinary examinations (OSPVEs) have been established and this approach is considered a valid assessment tool for practical skills (Pead, 2008; May and Head, 2010). In this chapter we use the term OSCE to discuss OSPVE or veterinary OSCE. The chapter offers details on how to design and author OSCE (veterinary OSCE) stations, analyse checklists, conduct marking/grading, perform standard setting, discriminate between more and less able candidates and overcome bias.

21.1 Assessment Aligned with Day One Skills

Clinical success as a veterinary graduate depends on having not only a core of veterinary knowledge, but also a range of Day One (and subsequently Year 1) practical competences. These Day One competences are frequently determined by professional bodies to guide veterinary educational establishments in developing curricula that

meet their accreditation standards (AVMA, 2009; EAEVE, 2009; OIE, 2013 revised 2014; RCVS, 2003). Most veterinary educational establishments have gone on to develop their own Day One skills lists and guides based on national and regional needs for educator expertise, caseloads and facilities. In contrast to assessment of knowledge, historically, the assessment of practical skills in university veterinary programmes has been less developed, partly because of animal welfare considerations and variability between animal cases that has made standardization difficult. In the OSCE, for relevant stations, it is essential for validity and realism that animals are used. This means that for animal handling sections of an OSCE circuit, real animals must be used but for some aspects of practical assessment models, manikins and cadaver tissue can be used. Focused development of technical skills involving both formative and summative assessment is invaluable during the training of a veterinarian as a bridge between the classroom and the clinics. Then when presented with clinical cases in the workplace, in the final phase of their professional programmes, they are not hampered by a lack of basic practical skills and may focus on integration of the skills to resolve complex real-world challenges.

It is essential that those involved in authoring a station understand the underlying philosophy of the OSCE. The most important attribute that is being assessed is 'the doing' rather than 'the knowing' and thus the candidate's ability to perform 'the process' in front of an examiner as opposed to describing how they would undertake it in words. (Examiners must be alert to students who try to 'get away with' a description, and not credit this.) This was stated by Harden (1988, p.19), who described the OSCE of medical schools as 'an approach to the assessment of clinical competence in which the components of competence are assessed in a planned or structured way'. By definition the OSCE attempts to eliminate the subjectivity associated with many traditional types of assessment, and focuses on well defined areas for testing. As a resource-intensive

© CAB International 2018. *Veterinary Clinical Skills Manual* (eds N. Coombes and A. Silva-Fletcher)

assessment modality, it concentrates primarily on 'the doing' and leaves 'the knowing' to other well established forms of (predominantly) written assessment.

The competences must be clearly defined in both the skills teaching and the OSCE. The approach taken is to break high-level competences (for instance, basic surgery) down into different skills components, which may be tested independently in the OSCE as short practical procedures. For example, simulated consultations (or parts of consultations) using role play, choice of equipment, ability to use equipment, animal handling, as well as the decision and ability to put on protective clothing (health and safety and biosecurity) are all practical skills that can be teased out and tested objectively, as they are observed to have taken place.

Representing, as they do, staging posts in the development of overall clinical capability, it is essential that prospective authors know the expected outcomes for students at each stage of their course. OSCEs that are used to assess candidates in senior years will be different from those used to assess junior candidates. For example, in earlier years, OSCE stations may comprise mainly the animal-handling component of the task, while for later years clinical procedures will be the major focus. An individual OSCE station is intended to offer a short element from a real-life situation.

There are a number of approaches that can be adopted to authoring an OSCE, but for uniformity of design a template for the various assessment elements within a technique can be used. An example of a fully designed OSCE station grading sheet is given in Appendix 21.1. For those not familiar with the format, it will be useful to consult this document as it is necessary to know what is meant by a 'checklist' to fully grasp the concept and structure underpinning the OSCE.

Assessors fulfil their role in completing the itemized checklist and providing a global grade for each student. This is a subjective judgement of the overall performance of the candidate and in the examples discussed in this chapter it appears at the end of the checklist as 1 = bad fail, 2 = just fail, 3 = just pass, 4 = good pass. The subjective judgement for allocating an overall grade for a candidate must *not* take into account any particular failings recorded in the checklist; rather, it is essential the assessor judges the overall performance of the candidate on the OSCE station.

21.2 Blueprinting the Assessment

Blueprinting is a tool used in many professions to design examinations. The tool is used to identify content areas and their respective weightings in an examination. The blueprint also includes objectives and/or competences and the proportion of each type of question presented in the examination (i.e. multiple-choice question, short-answer question, OSCE station). A good guide for selecting which assessment method to use is Miller's cognitive and behaviour assessment pyramid (Fig. 21.1). The knowledge-based domains can be assessed using multiple-choice questions, short- and long-answer questions, extended matching questions and script concordance tests. To observe behaviours, OSCEs can be constructed and supported through a clinical skills centre and direct observations in real

Fig. 21.1. Miller's Assessment Pyramid, based on Miller (1990). EMQ, extended matching question; MCQ, multiple-choice question; OSCE, objective structured clinical examination; OSPVE, objective structured practical veterinary examination; SCT, Script Concordance test.

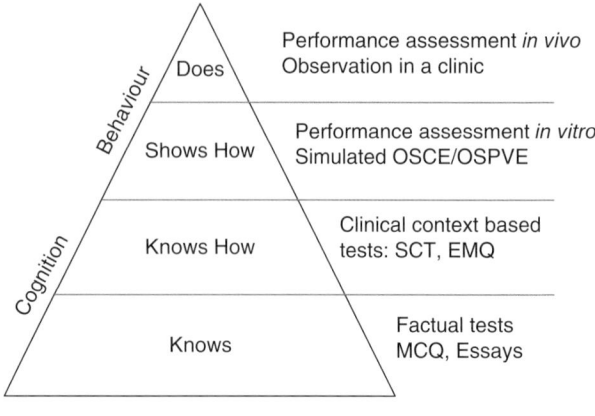

Based on Miller (1990)

clinical situations. The blueprint acts as a guideline for students, so that they understand how they are assessed, and it is also useful for internal and external examiners. At the end of an examination, the blueprint is helpful for evaluating the whole examination to see how well each content area has fulfilled its objectives and in particular how student performance matched the demands made over knowledge and professional skills.

Specific blueprinting of the OSCE will determine the number of stations and their content. The first stage of developing an OSCE involves deciding which practical skills to assess. Although the likely areas for assessment can be determined from curricular learning objectives, the assessment of many areas is not feasible using animals. Therefore, it may be more useful to decide what can be assessed using animals, models and manikins in the OSCE and then blueprint other parts of the overall assessment to complement the OSCE. Missing practical elements can subsequently be assessed in the workplace if it is not practical to assess these through OSCEs.

In order to adequately cover a full range of Day One skills, it is obviously necessary, for the veterinary OSCE, to use a range of large animal, small animal, surgery, laboratory and communications skills-related stations. Where there are skills that it is just not feasible to assess repeatedly using live animals, creative use of models and manikins can provide an adequate substitute. In many 'hybrid' stations, it is also possible to use a live animal for the initial animal-handling part of the procedure and then to move to a manikin or even a cadaver for an invasive treatment technique. Evidence suggests that for a summative OSCE, about 2 hours of assessment (18–20 stations) are necessary to assess a reasonable number of skills and to gain adequate reliability of the overall results (van der Vleuten and Schuwirth, 2005).

21.3 Item Development, Analysis and Further Refinement

The OSCE example in Appendix 21.1 is an original 'Assessment Checklist'. It lists specific actions that the candidate is expected to perform. This section expands on the analysis of this itemized checklist and presents a method for post-OSCE weighting of items. Weighting is where performance of a particular item will contribute to the overall mark by a factor greater than 1.

After an OSCE station has been used, an analysis can be performed to investigate not only each candidate's competence in performing the skill, but also the functioning of the station and the checklist itself. This will allow any subsequent revision of the station to be based on evidence obtained from the actual performance of the OSCE. This section concentrates on the performance of the items on the checklist and how each contributes to the ability of the assessment to discriminate between more able and less able candidates.

The major method for analysing the station functioning is to calculate the percentage of candidates performing each item on the checklist, each item usually comprising a single action on a line.

The item analysis provides evidence about which actions were trivial, being performed by almost all candidates, and these can either be omitted, or the checklist revised so that some lines include more than one action, i.e. actions were 'chunked' together (Box 21.1). Doing this would not affect the ability of the station to discriminate between capable and less capable candidates.

As well as revealing items that are non-discriminatory, item analysis assists one in making judgements concerning item weighting, as it indicates which actions are performed by only a proportion of candidates and these may be the actions that discriminate between the capable and less capable candidate. Should these less universally performed actions be deemed to be 'important' actions, by having a higher mark associated with them, i.e. weighting, it may improve the assessment's discriminatory power. Experience suggests that there should be no more than three or four such items, and a weighting mark of 3 or 4 is usually adequate. If there is an action that in the real situation would be extremely critical in such a case, this single item may be more heavily weighted with a value up to 4 marks. An example of this is when connecting the animal to an anaesthetic machine without having previously turned on the oxygen supply. This, in a real situation, may well lead to death of the animal, and an incorrect performance should, by way of not gaining marks, cause a candidate to fail the assessment.

The assessor ought to be informed where an action line is weighted, by having the mark printed on the assessment sheet next to the box that the assessor needs to shade in. Additionally, the presence of weighted items ought to be brought to the attention of the assessors in the assessors' information. However, there is hearsay evidence that knowledge of the weighting may influence the scoring of such items by some assessors. The final

Box 21.1. Chunking of items in a checklist.

With some stations chunking of items in a checklist may occur; for example, in preparing a blood smear and staining OCSE checklist where some actions may form part of a sequence of interactions:

Dispose of capillary tube AND glass slide in sharps bin [1]

To get the mark of 1, the student has to perform both actions.

As noted in the example above, there is an indication to the assessor about how many of the sub-actions are required to be performed by the candidate in order to achieve a score of 'has done' = 1 for that line.

This is an important consideration where actions have been chunked. Experience shows that there is much inter-assessor variation in what constitutes a 'has done' score where there are a number of actions on a single line and advice was not given. The assessors need to have this brought to their attention in the assessors' information *and* noted in the checklist, as shown in the example above.

Where items are chunked, one needs to consider the situation of formative OSCE, where feedback is given to students concerning their performance so that they may improve their skills. In this case, the assessor needs to be advised that each sub-action on a line is individually marked (with a tick or line) when it is performed and items/actions not performed are left unticked. Note that this is good practice for all actions but especially essential in this situation. Ticking the performed actions allows precise focused feedback to a candidate to be given about which sub-action has and which has not been performed, so that the candidate may subsequently practise to improve on their specific failings. If this sub-action recording is not performed by the assessor, then more general and less behaviour-focused feedback may be all that it is possible to give, which will be considerably less useful to the candidate.

The procedure of chunking the less discriminatory items helps limit the number of lines on the checklist, but it is considered advisable to initially author a complete checklist, which may, after being used and analysed, allow the evidence-based development of the least number of lines that are necessary, at the same time as retaining good discriminatory characteristics for the abilities of different candidates.

output from the station is a mark that includes the item weighting mark.

21.4 Alternative Methods of Performing a Task

For some tasks, there may be different ways, each perfectly acceptable, of performing them. It is necessary to label the alternative methods 'Method A' and 'Method B' and make these readily apparent to the assessor to record the candidate's action for either method, depending on the approach adopted by the candidate (Box 21.2). The method used by the candidate must be readily identifiable by the assessor without asking the candidate what is being performed, i.e. the assessment checklist needs to be written to allow a clear distinction to be made concerning which method is being used, so that it can be assessed as relevant.

The different methods may have a different number of actions/items on the checklist. In order to accommodate this there needs to be a different item weighting so that whichever method is used, the candidate receives the same final score for a correct performance. The assessor needs to be advised about this and that the method not used should be recorded as having scored 0 for each item. However, using the software Clinquest, marketed by Speedwell UK Ltd, a non-coded section may be compensated for during the Optical Mark Reading process.

21.5 Order in Which Actions are Performed

When authoring an assessment checklist, it is likely that the actions will have been ordered within the checklist in what seems to be the most logical order for them to

---

Box 21.2. Example of an OSCE that uses Methods A or B.

An example of this is shown on the checklist below, taken from an OSCE which assesses the candidate's ability to take a fine-needle aspirate from the popliteal lymph node or space of a dog model.

Two techniques are acceptable for obtaining the sample

EITHER A (5–15)

5. attaches needle to syringe and guards point until required for use	1.0	0.0
6. holds syringe and inserts needle into lymph node	1.0	0.0
7. applies negative pressure via the plunger without adjusting their hand position	1.0	0.0
8. applies 1–5 ml of suction with the syringe	1.0	0.0
9. releases negative pressure – volume of air in syringe to zero	1.0	0.0
10. redirects the needle within the node	1.0	0.0
11. re-applied 1–5 ml pressure within syringe (or moves needle with pressure ON)	1.0	0.0
12. does NOT remove needle from node whilst relocating needle	1.0	0.0
13. releases negative pressure within syringe – volume of air in syringe ~ zero	1.0	0.0

If negative pressure released and syringe does NOT return to zero, examiner say "Assume that the volume of air in syringe is back to zero and you may evacuate the syringe in situ"

14. withdraws the needle from the lymph node	1.0	0.0
15. removes the needle from the syringe	1.0	0.0

OR B(16–20)

16. The needle is detached or never attached to the syringe	2.2	0.0
17. holds the needle plastic area in their fingers	2.2	0.0
18. inserts the needle into the lymph node	2.2	0.0
19. redirects the needle several times within the node	2.2	0.0
20. removes the needle from the lymph node only once	2.2	0.0

In the example, each item in Method B is weighted to 2.2 marks. Completing this section completely will give the same mark that would be obtained from completing Method A.

---

be performed. However, where there is no sequential dependency, one must not expect candidates to perform the actions/items in the order that they appear on the checklist, and this difference in order of performance is rarely of any importance. Assessors, unless otherwise informed, should accept and record the actions in whatever order they are performed (it may be necessary to advise them about this). Hopefully, when each action is performed, the assessor records it with a tick on the appropriate line on the checklist. However, there are some instances where one action must precede another. The format that is adopted for this sequential coding is to use the symbol ► at the start of the line. This is taken to indicate that this action must be preceded by the one that is noted on the line above it. This is

an agreed format for signalling that actions must be performed in the indicated sequence. For absolute clarity it is better to use the symbol on both lines:

• at the end of the preceding line A; ►

• ► B, at the start of the next line.

This indicates most clearly the exact sequence that A leads to the actions on line B.

For example, in an OSCE where an anaesthetic machine is being checked ready for use (see Appendix 21.1), the order for most actions is not important, but certain actions must be performed in sequence (Fig. 21.2).

Item 11 must precede item 12, 12 precede 13, and 13 precede 14. The scoring that we use is that if the first item is not immediately followed by the second item,

11. Checks contents pressure on 'in use' cylinder	1.0	0.0
12. ▶ Turns on oxygen flow meter	1.0	0.0
13. ▶ Watches bobbin moving over the range	1.0	0.0
14. ▶ States/confirms notes that bobbin is free and rotating	1.0	0.0

Fig. 21.2. Example of anaesthetic machine uses, with items 11–14.

then neither item is scored as having been performed correctly, as their performance is linked, hence both (or all three in the example above) items are scored as 0.

The assessors' instructions should include all details about the order of performance of items.

21.6   Precise Terminology to Stop a 'Scattergun' Approach

It is important that the checklist has been authored in such a way that candidates who really do not know how to perform the task are not credited with having performed actions at random, i.e. some candidates may not know how to perform a particular task, but rather, on seeing the equipment available, adopt a scattergun or 'grapeshot' approach in which every possible action is completed so that some correct actions have been undertaken. A checklist should be authored in such a way that one can differentiate this approach from a more precise, structured and knowledgeable one. For example, in the situation of assembling an anaesthetic system, the wording that may overcome this potential problem could be:

'assembles T-piece correctly without fitting pieces together randomly'.

21.7   Percentage of Students Performing Each Item

The illustration in Fig. 21.3 is a section from a checklist detailing a horse-handling OSCE. Each item (line) has added to it a hand-written number. These are the calculated percentages of candidates performing that item, i.e. the action on that line.

21.7.1   Universal performance

The numerical values show that some items in Fig. 21.3 are performed by almost all candidates, for example

more than 98% for items 20, 21, 22, yet others are performed by only a small proportion of candidates, e.g. 47% for item 23.

Where more than 95% of students perform an action (e.g. items 20, 21 and 22) the item is suitable for either omitting totally or chunking these actions together on to one line. This will reduce the length of the checklist without affecting the discriminatory ability of the station.

Chunking may also be done for more trivial items or those considered to be of lesser importance. Such examples are items 27 and 29. However, chunking may be difficult here as they are time-separated actions. One possible wording to combine these that might appear on this checklist is:

'27. Asks horse to trot, and after 28; subsequently to walk (Tick as done – both required).
28. Trots back in straight line'

(Note: it is advisable to inform assessors about this and that both actions in item 27 are necessary for score = 1.)

Referring back to the illustrated mark sheet in Fig. 21.3, items 20, 21, 22 may also be considered to fall into the category of being items of lesser importance, although the evidence from the data of the percentage performing the task is that a few candidates do not do these actions, so that they may well need to be included.

21.7.2   Items performed by few candidates

These are potentially discriminatory items. Note item 23 in Fig. 21.3, which only about half of the candidates performed. This action may be considered a safety issue/welfare procedure when leading a horse and so may be important enough to be weighted; we have found that a weighting mark of +3 is usually adequate. For this checklist, item 23 was not the only action with a low percentage of candidate performance; other items also showed a low percentage of candidates performing them (not shown here) and they also were considered for weighting. An item that is

20. lines the horse up in the direction of travel	100	1.0	0.0	6
21. instructs the horse to trot on - verbal/clicking/gentle pull on lead rope (may perform few strides of walk first)	98	1.0	0.0	7 8
22. maintains position beside left shoulder of horse	98	1.0	0.0	9
23. extends lead rope to provide some slack - approx 18"	47	1.0	0.0	10
24. at the predetermined point (prior to turning) asks horse for walk	85	1.0	0.0	11
25. makes a right turn in walk	85	1.0	0.0	12
26. Stays on outside of circle	91	1.0	0.0	13
27. asks horse for trot	96	1.0	0.0	14
28. trots back in straight line	85	1.0	0.0	15
29. asks for walk	100	1.0	0.0	16
As necessary direct the candidate to place the horse back in the stall	–			17

Fig. 21.3. Section from horse-handling checklist.

deemed to be critical may be weighted with a value up to +4 or more marks; such an item might be turning on the oxygen supply prior to connecting an animal to an anaesthetic machine. This large weighting mark is in place of a red line item. This is extensively discussed in the next section.

21.8   Red Line Actions

Red line actions are actions that when performed (or not performed) in the correct manner or order are deemed to be critical steps in the activity, and the term red line is used to suggest an immediate cessation or fail at that assessment. There is the particular problem associated with situations within an OSCE where an action might in the real situation be likely to cause the death of the animal. A similar situation, especially when live animals are used, is where the candidate does not correctly perform important health and safety actions and so exposes themself or other staff to potentially dangerous situations. It is accepted that these situations present a dilemma in running and assessing an OSCE. These actions may be deemed to be so important as to warrant being a red line action; however, since OSCEs were introduced in 2004 at RVC, we have adopted the practice that there should not be any individual action, however important, to be considered as 'red line'. Despite this, it is accepted that there is a real problem when immediate safety issues occur.

There may need to be a different approach to the safety consideration of potential red line actions between formative and summative OSCE. Formative OSCE should be considered a 'safe' place where all actions, however incorrect, may be performed by a candidate, and corrected in a non-threatening manner, so giving the candidates the chance to learn from their errors.

Where there is a potential safety problem (for example, the candidate having very long nails which might injure an animal being handled; or dangly earrings or other jewellery which may easily get caught by an animal; or placing themselves in a potentially dangerous location or position) one should aim, at least in formative OSCE, to attempt to overcome these potential problems and so allow the candidate to benefit totally from the OSCE. In a summative OSCE this may be impossible and the only recourse is to terminate the actions of the candidate at this station. Naturally, the actions already performed should be scored as = 1 and those not attempted should be scored as 0. The candidate will be likely to fail, as most of the actions will not have been attempted. In the case of inappropriate attire, it may be that the attire of the candidate will not be suitable for them to attend other stations also. Naturally, prior warnings to candidates about dress are given in order to avoid failing at a number of assessment stations. (Students learn from the formative OSCE to take this seriously so it is usually not a problem in summative OSCE.)

In the case of the candidate putting themselves into a dangerous location, a spoken warning to the candidate may suffice. There should be a note present in the checklist, such as:

'Performed task without causing any distress to the animal. Performed task without placing themselves in position of danger.'

These items may be weighted, if deemed necessary, in various different situations, or in summative OSCE. If a candidate has performed most actions correctly and so gained a high objective mark, unless the important items are weighted it is likely that they will pass the OSCE. The subjective grade given by the assessor, even if a bad fail is given, will not ensure that the candidate fails in such an instance. This is shown in the section on standard setting later in this chapter, and in the graph that details the linear regression approach to setting the pass–fail mark (see Fig. 21.10) and in the graph labelled Sheep Foot Trim (see Fig. 21.8).

21.9 Common Errors in Writing Assessment Checklists

There are a number of common errors that occur when authoring an OSCE. It is a not infrequent problem for a single author to write the assessment checklist in the form of their 'telling/teaching' approach. It may be that teachers have difficulty in wording the assessment checklist in the format that is questioning the actions of 'the candidate'. The checklist wording should read:

'The candidate: Calculates ..., or selects ..., or holds ..., or carries ..., or uses ... or does not ...'.

An example of a checklist which shows poor wording and should be avoided is illustrated in Figure 21.4.

The wording in Fig. 21.4 demonstrates many common errors, including the use of the word 'correct', which means the assessor has to make a judgement about something that they may not know anything

about (even though the correct value is noted in this example). It could be reworded so that 'The candidate':

'1. Calculates the weight of pethidine required which is ...' (may be different on different days)

If this OSCE is assessing the ability of candidates to calculate the required dose for an animal and the volume to administer, these values are factual and those candidates who undertake the OSCE early in the series may pass the calculation details and the correct value to their peers who attend the OSCE later, so that the later candidates who have been primed are not really being assessed in their ability. For this reason, it is good practice, where there is repeated use over a few days of such an OSCE and where a calculation is required to be performed, to have available a number of different animal weights. This will result in different drug volumes being required. The syringe choice need not be different, but the stated absolute value may be different for OSCEs run on different days.

A frequent error that is seen is using the word 'appropriate' without any explanation. (In the example in Fig. 21.4, the term 'appropriate' is explained as 1 ml syringe, 23–25 G 3/8 needle.) This error frequently occurs when describing 'appropriate clothing'. Clothing that one assessor may judge as appropriate may be deemed by another assessor to be incorrect. Where there is a definable 'correct', it should be defined so that there is no room for uncertainty. The author must give precise details in the checklist and explain these as necessary in the assessors' information. Usually, simple rewording can eliminate all these errors.

Whilst the form of the wording is not a serious error where the assessors can interpret the likely meaning, it does suggest that the author has not taken into account fully that the OSCE is assessing the actions of 'the candidate'.

The example that is illustrated in Fig. 21.4 may have been developed from teaching notes, which is a good technique, but these often require substantial rewording to convert them into an objective assessment.

Say "Please Begin"

1. Calculate the correct mg of pethidine: 15 mg
2. Calculate the correct volume of pethidine to be administered: 50 mg/ml – 0.30 ml
3. Select an appropriate syringe size: 1 ml
4. Select an appropriate size needle: 23–25 G 3/8 inch length

Fig. 21.4. Example of poor wording in a checklist.

21.10 Challenges and Dilemmas

Accepted situations where there may be a dilemma include the following:

1. Connection of a patient (model dog) to an anaesthetic machine without previously having turned on the oxygen supply. In the example in Fig. 21.5, item 21 is weighted so that a correct procedure is rewarded by a high mark. An incorrect procedure will mean that the candidate obtains lower marks and so will be likely to fail the assessment. The grade given by the assessor must not take into account this incorrect single action.

2. Inability to obtain a blood sample. If obtaining a blood sample is considered to be really important, remembering that a model vein is being used, this step should be weighted so that obtaining a sample gives a mark of more than 1 (say, = 3). However, the subjective grade given by the assessor must still be determined by the overall performance of the candidate, not whether a sample was obtained or not.

3. Inability to turn a sheep. In this instance, one should also consider the difficulty for a disabled student. All students should receive the same information about requesting assistance from the assessor. Provided they perform all other aspects adequately, and either turn the sheep solo or do so with directed assistance, they should be graded according to their overall performance.

4. Handling small furry animals. There are a number of accepted procedures for picking up these animals and some of these may not be acceptable in some situations. However, provided the animal is handled in a manner that does not cause it distress or injury, the procedure should be allowed to continue and the grade given according to overall performance.

5. Candidates placing themselves or another staff member in a dangerous situation, or a candidate's actions causing distress or pain to an animal. This is potentially the most serious situation that can emerge,

even in a formative OSCE. In this situation, the assessor is obliged to intervene in the procedure. However, this is optional if this intervention can take place in a manner that directs the candidate to a more acceptable approach, or correct procedure, so that the OSCE can continue. The assessor correcting the candidate so that their performance is safe will benefit the candidate, especially when the candidate realizes that they have performed inadequately – perhaps in ignorance – and they will readily accept advice about how to accomplish the activity correctly. Stopping a formative OSCE fulfils no real function. Therefore, unless the OSCE is summative, this is the approach that is recommended.

21.11 Analysis of Marks

The OSCE produces a mountain of assessment papers. For example, a 20-station OSCE for 150 students will produce at least $20 \times 150 = 3000$ results sheets. It is obviously a major task to ensure that all papers are secure and that the results for each candidate are assigned correctly to them.

Several systems have been developed to capture and process data when conducting OSCE examinations. The following are some examples but there are more systems.

1. Clinquest (https://www.speedwellsoftware.com) can be used to create individual station or assessment sheets, with candidate responses interpreted by Speedwell's OSCE software Clinquest and Optical Mark Reading (OMR) technology.

2. eOSCE (https://eosce.ch) is an electronic system that can be run using iPads to create an efficient and entirely digital preparation, execution and analysis OSCE and is a paperless system, less erroneous and quicker to evaluate.

3. OSCEOnline (https://www.osceonline.com) has web, Android and iPad apps for conducting online paperless OSCEs.

If using a paper-based system such as Speedwell's Clinquest software, the assessment checklist details

Anaesthesia Lack Continued
The candidate

21. turns on Oxygen BEFORE (or within 10 seconds of) connection to the animal	4.0	0.0
22. connects the patient end of breathing system to ET tube of animal	1.0	0.0

Fig. 21.5. Example of connection of patient (model dog) to an anaesthetic machine.

are printed on to a prepared template purchased from Speedwell. The software codes each sheet for each candidate at each assessment station and conveniently the papers are printed in the sequence in which each candidate will appear at stations as they pass around the circuit. Subsequently, the assessment sheets are scanned using an Optical Mark Reader controlled by the Clinquest software. Marks can then be exported to Microsoft Excel to determine the pass mark for each station and for standard setting. Alternatively, if some of the more automated software (which uses an iPad instead of paper sheets for scoring) is used, the marks will be analysed directly by the software. The mark distribution is presented by a graphical representation of the number of candidates obtaining each mark (or % mark) and this can be performed using Excel Pivot Table software. Figure 21.6 shows the mark range for a station that has a skewed distribution. This most extreme example of skewed distribution of marks was obtained from the OSCE station for Equine Hoof Testing.

The graph in Fig. 21.6 illustrates that the marks obtained by the candidates are strongly skewed, with almost all candidates having performed all of the items on the checklist. As all candidates are obtaining near maximum marks, this station might not be considered to have an adequate mark range to allow it to be discriminatory. On the other hand, the result illustrated does suggest that all candidates are capable at performing this task, with a small number that could receive extra remedial help.

For some stations, it may be that there are items/actions which need to be performed that have been omitted from the checklist, and these may be the 'critical few' actions which would have separated the capable from the less capable candidates more completely.

The results from a different station illustrate the other extreme situation: an almost normal distribution of marks (Fig. 21.7).

From the graph illustrated in Fig. 21.7, it can be seen that many candidates perform the majority of the items, that almost none perform all items (maximum number of items = 20) and that a wide range of marks is obtained.

In practice, many stations have a mark distribution that is between these two extremes. The consequence of the non-normal distribution of the marks for most stations has prompted us to use the median value as the measure of central tendency in all analysis. The pass mark for each station is therefore the median value of the mark for the particular cohort of the students. These data can be used to give general written feedback to the whole year for each station. This will highlight to the student the areas in which they need more practise and their strengths as a whole year group.

21.12   Grade Mark Distribution

The global grade given by the examiner is also taken into account in the analysis of marks. In a similar manner to

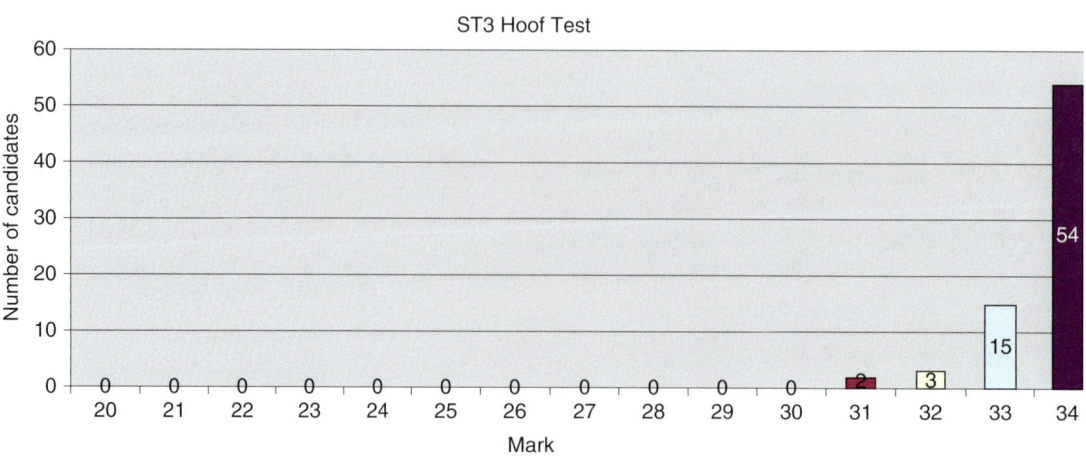

Fig. 21.6. Graph showing skewed distribution of marks from an OSCE station.

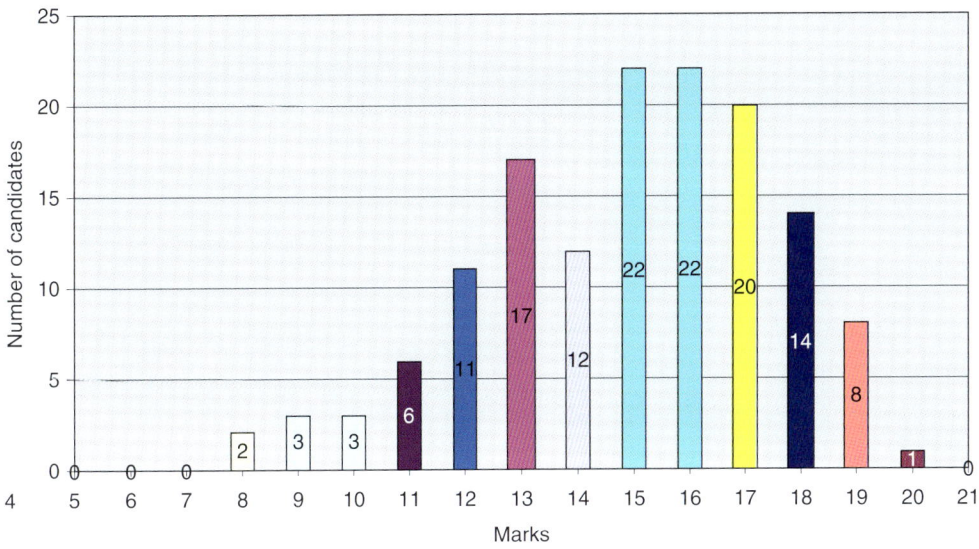

Fig. 21.7. Graph showing normal distribution of marks from an OSCE station.

the overall mark distribution, the mark distribution within each grade can be computed. Figure 21.8 shows how the marks associated with each grade are distributed and the extent of overlap of the marks for the different grades.

Although there is some overlap of the candidate's marks at a particular grade with those of another, the majority of marks within each grade do not overlap with those of a different grade. Additionally, there is good separation of the median mark value for each grade, which is indicated by the appropriately coloured dots. This station does discriminate well between capable and less capable candidates.

In an ideal situation there would not be any overlap of marks between grades. However, this is rarely achieved; there is almost always an element of overlap. The greater the overlap, the more uncertainty there is about how well the station discriminates between capable and less capable candidates. Another indication of the discrimination between grades is the number of marks separating the median mark for each grade. In the example in Fig. 21.8 these are well separated. However, not all stations may show such exemplary characteristics (Fig. 21.9).

As can be seen in the illustration from the assessment station in Fig. 21.9, there is extensive overlap of marks for candidates given different grades. The median marks for each grade are numerically close,

with the median mark for grades 1 and 2 being the same at 15 marks.

This station does need careful revision. One interpretation is that assessors are basing their subjective grade decision on some factor that is not being assessed in the objective checklist. This station results in a problem with setting the pass–fail cut score.

21.13 Standard Setting

One method for setting the pass/fail mark, using the marks and grades for all the candidates, from all assessors at a station, is described here. This is considered a better method than just using data from borderline candidates, an analysis known as the 'borderline groups method'. The latter limits the data used to a small proportion of the total number of candidates.

The method of choice is the linear regression method, especially where the student number is large (Wood et al., 2006). Graphically it may be represented as in the conceptual diagram in Fig. 21.10.

Figure 21.10 shows that there may be a discrepancy between the assessor's subjective judgement of whether the candidate merits a pass or a fail and the pass–fail situation that results from the checklist mark obtained by the objective scoring of whether a candidate has, or has not, performed an item on the checklist.

In Fig. 21.10, the assessor has graded one candidate as 'just pass' (grade 3) who is deemed to have failed as their objective mark is less than the calculated pass–fail mark. Additionally, two candidates graded as 'just fail' (grade 2) by the assessor actually pass, having obtained an objective mark greater than the pass–fail value.

The strength of this method is that the assessor's subjective judgement of the pass–fail boundary is made robust by it being aggregated into a boundary based on the individual judgements across all candidates. An assessor's decision of whether an individual candidate merits a particular grade, being a subjective judgement, may be influenced by various factors causing 'halo effects' that cloud an individual judgement. However, this method ensures that the checklist mark links the determined threshold back to actual performances. The halo effects mean that the discrepancy in the pass–fail result of a small number of candidates, as shown in the conceptual diagram, often occurs in practice.

An important feature of this standard setting process, after the OSCE has occurred, is that the assessor will not know the pass–fail mark boundary. For this reason, the assessors are advised not to utter any encouraging comments (e.g. 'Well done') as this might suggest to the candidate that they have done well, which may be contrary to the reality, even if the assessor gave them a subjective 'just pass' grade.

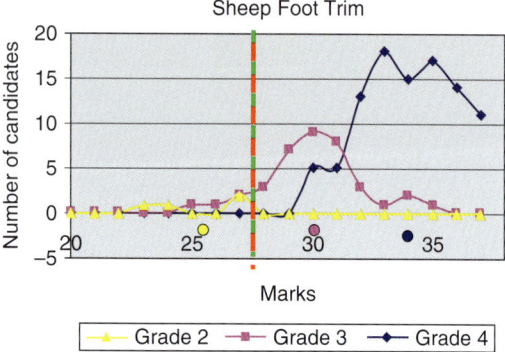

Fig. 21.8. Graph showing median mark and the subjective grade (2–4) distribution that candidates were given from an OSCE station. Grade 4 (good pass); Grade 3 (just pass); Grade 2 (just fail). In this illustration, there were no candidates graded as 1 (bad fail). Red/green line indicates pass mark of 27.7 marks; coloured circles (yellow, pink and blue) show median value of the marks at each grade.

Fig. 21.9. Graph showing median mark and the subjective grade (2–4) distribution that candidates were given from an OSCE station. Grade 4 (good pass); Grade 3 (just pass); Grade 2 (just fail); Grade 1 (bad fail). Median marks for each grade are shown by coloured dots.

21.14   Issues with Standard Setting

It must be accepted that the standard setting process is a subjective practice and there is no agreed best methodology (Boursicot *et al.*, 2004, 2006). However, it is considered that standards are best set in relation to examinees' performance (Cusimano and Rothman, 2004) and the linear regression method has been considered more robust than other methods (Wood *et al.*, 2006).

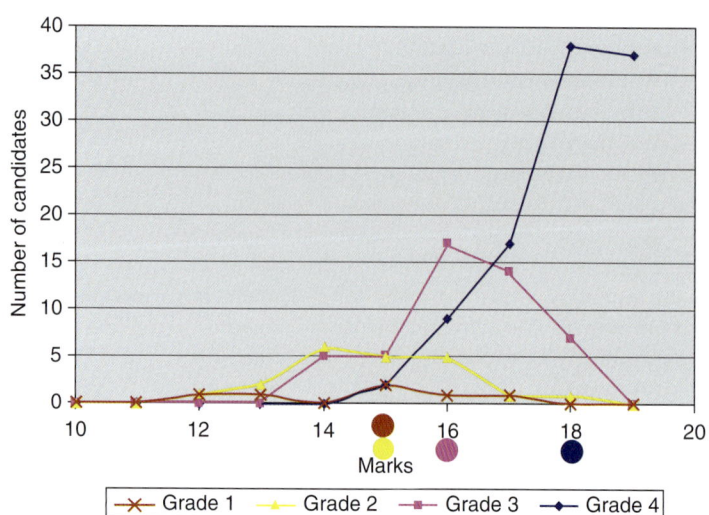

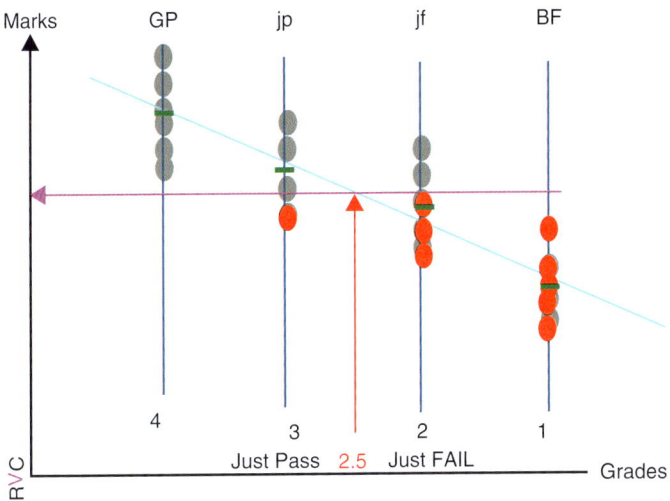

Fig. 21.10. Graph showing least-squares linear regression method for setting the pass/fail score. The marks are grouped according to their associated grade: bad fail (BF) = 1; just fail (jf) = 2; just pass (jp) = 3; good pass (GP) = 4. Single green line on each grade line is median mark for that grade. Light blue sloping line represents linear regression line through median value of each grade. Pass–fail transition lies midway between just fail of grade 2 and just pass of grade 3, being a grade of 2.5 (upward pointing arrow). Horizontal purple arrow is drawn at point of intersection of 2.5 line with regression line; this value represents the pass–fail mark. Those candidates with marks less than the pass–fail mark are deemed to have failed (red dots).

The linear regression method differs from other methods of standard setting by utilizing all the objective and subjective data from all the candidates to set the pass–fail threshold after the OSCE has taken place, and conforms to the best practice of setting the pass mark in relation to actual (rather than predicted) candidate performance.

The linear regression analysis depends on there being a linear relationship between the median of the objective marks at each grade and the subjective grade given by the assessor. In most OSCE stations, this close relationship does appear to apply. However, for some stations, this relationship does not occur and is an indication that a revision of the checklist is required.

21.15 Overcoming Bias

It must be remembered that the assessor's impression of the ability of a candidate is subjective, and while their professionalism and expectations about an activity may be used to set the pass–fail standard overall, their judgement about the ability of an individual candidate may have an unperceived element of bias. This bias may be a reflection of the ability of those candidates who attended the station immediately prior to the current candidate, as a contrast with those performing much less well (or so much better). Alternatively, characteristics of a particular type of candidate may influence the subjective grading by the assessor. It is well documented that there may be an assessor (or rater) bias, e.g. 'halo' and 'horns' effect (MacDougall *et al.*, 2008). It must also be remembered that assessors who have acted as teachers in the preceding year(s) know the candidates and this fact may unwittingly influence an assessor in making their subjective judgement of a candidate's ability, separately from the performance on the day.

In the standard setting procedure adopted here, the pass or fail status of any candidate is based on their performance of the activity. The objective mark that they achieve by performing each activity is noted on the checklist. The subjective grading by the assessor for each candidate is used to set the overall pass–fail standard. However, by using the data from all students and all assessors at a station, any bias effect that may affect the grading of an individual candidate is eliminated.

The next chapter offers details of practical considerations for organizing an OSCE.

References: AVMA (2009) *North American Veterinary Medical Education Consortium (NAVMEC) National Meeting 1: Report*, Las Vegas, Nevada, Feb 11–13, 2010. American Veterinary Medical Association, Schaumburg, Illinois. Available at: http://aavmc.org/data/files/navmec/navmecmeeting1report.pdf (accessed 18 November 2017).

Baillie, S., Warman, S. and Rhind, S. (2014) *A Guide to Assessment in Veterinary Medicine*, 2nd edn. School of Veterinary Sciences, University of Bristol. Available at: https://research-information.bristol.ac.uk/files/32763793/a_guide_to_assessment_in_veterinary_medical.pdf (accessed 18 November 2017).

Boursicot, K.A.M, Roberts, T.E. and Pell, G. (2004) *Standard Setting for Clinical Competence at Graduation from Medical School: Is it Possible to Achieve Consensus?* Association for the Study of Medical Education, Edinburgh, UK.

Boursicot, K.A.M, Roberts T.E. and Pell, G. (2006) Standard setting for clinical competence at graduation from medical school: a comparison of passing scores across five medical schools. *Advances in Health Sciences Education Theory and Practice* 11(2), 173–183.

Cusimano, M.D. and Rothman, A.I. (2004) Consistency of standards and stability of pass/fail decisions with examinee-based standard-setting methods in a small scale OSCE. *Academic Medicine* 79(10), Supplement S25–S27.

EAEVE (European Association of Establishments for Veterinary Education) (2009) *European System of Evaluation of Veterinary Training (ESEVT): Manual of Standard Operating Procedure*. European Association of Establishments for Veterinary Education (EAEVE), Zurich, and Federation of Veterinarians of Europe (FVE). Available at: http://www.eaeve.org/fileadmin/downloads/SOP/ESEVT__Uppsala__SOP_May_2016.pdf (accessed 17 October 2017).

Harden, R.M. (1988) What is an OSCE? *Medical Teacher* 10(1), 19–22.

MacDougall, K., Riley, S., Cameron, H. and McKinstry, B. (2008) Halos and horns in the assessment of undergraduate medical students: a consistency-based approach. *Journal of Applied Quantitative Methods* 3(2), 116–128.

May, S.A. and Head, S.D. (2010) Assessment of technical skills: best practices. *Journal of Veterinary Medical Education* 37(3), 258–265.

Miller, G.E. (1990) The assessment of clinical skills/competence/performance. *Academic Medicine* 65(9), Supplement S63–S67.

OIE (2013) *Veterinary Education Core Curriculum. OIE Guidelines*. Office International des Épizooties (World Organisation for Animal Health), Paris. Available at: http://www.oie.int/Veterinary_Education_Core_Curriculum.pdf (accessed 17 October 2017).

Pead, M.J. (2008) Assessment: Cinderella or Sleeping Beauty? Evolution of final examinations at the Royal Veterinary College. *Journal of Veterinary Medical Education* 35(4), 607–611.

RCVS (2014) *Day One Competences Statement*. Available at: https://www.rcvs.org.uk/document-library/day-one-competences-statement/ (accessed 17 October 2017).

van der Vleuten, C.P.M. and Schuwirth, L.W.T. (2005) Assessing professional competence: from methods to programmes. *Medical Education* 39, 309–317.

Wood, T.J., Humphrey-Murto, S.M. and Norman, G.R. (2006) Standard setting in a small scale OSCE: a comparison of the modified borderline-group method and the borderline regression method. *Advances in Health Science Education* 11, 115–122.

Appendix 21.1. Anaesthetic Machine Safety Marksheet

Station 12: Anaesthetic Machine Safety

Candidate Name: &CandName   **Candidate No:** &CandNo

Site: &Centre   **Date:** &Circuit   **Session Time:** &Session

Identify candidate by name and number. "Your name is ", "Your candidate number is... ". Check against the student page provided
Ask the candidate "Have you read the scenario?", "Do you understand what you have to do?" and then say "Please begin"

Say 'do tell me what you are doing while you perform these tasks' and 'please begin'

1. Checks that all cylinders are turned OFF.	1.0⬚ 0.0⬚
2. Uses ratchet key in correct position first time- not rotate !	1.0⬚ 0.0⬚
3. Turns on the reserve oxygen cylinder.	1.0⬚ 0.0⬚
4. Checks the contents- pressure adequate.	1.0⬚ 0.0⬚

If Candidate attempts to exchange oxygen cylinder say "you do not need to change the oxygen cylinder"

5. Turns on oxygen flow meter and checks that the rotameters rise so oxygen is flowing.	1.0⬚ 0.0⬚
6. Turns off spare cylinder.	1.0⬚ 0.0⬚
7. Uses Oxygen Flush/Rotameter to empty contents.	1.0⬚ 0.0⬚
8. Checks/listens to the oxygen supply failure alarm.	2.0⬚ 0.0⬚
9. Repeats check for second reserve cylinder. (ie sections 3, 4 and 6).	1.0⬚ 0.0⬚
10. Turns on 'in use' cylinder.	1.0⬚ 0.0⬚
11. Checks contents pressure on 'in use' cylinder.	1.0⬚ 0.0⬚
12. ▶ Turns on oxygen flow meter.	1.0⬚ 0.0⬚
13. ▶ Watches bobbin moving over the range.	1.0⬚ 0.0⬚
14 ▶ States/confirms notes that bobbin is free and rotating.	1.0⬚ 0.0⬚
15. Turns off flowmeters.	1.0⬚ 0.0⬚
16. Check - press emergency oxygen supply knob.	2.0⬚ 0.0⬚

Vaporisers:

17. Presses release Knob to rotate control.	1.0⬚ 0.0⬚
18. Checks that the vaporiser knob rotates easily.	1.0⬚ 0.0⬚
19. Checks level of Anaesthetic agent is at line through window.	1.0⬚ 0.0⬚
20. Says that anaesthetic agent needs to be added/picks up anaesthetic bottle.	1.0⬚ 0.0⬚

At this stage say 'you do not need to add any agent to the vaporiser'.

21. States the machine is ready for use. OR ask is the machine ready for use - confirms YES	1.0⬚ 0.0⬚
22. Does not make an incorrect statement in regards to the machine's safety.	1.0⬚ 0.0⬚

Examiners Global Score

GP - Good Pass, JP - Just Pass, JF - Just Fail, BF - Bad Fail	GP⬚ JP⬚ JF ⬚ BF⬚

Objectively Structured Clinical Examinations – the Practicalities

Nichola Coombes

The Royal Veterinary College, London

Introduction

This chapter is a narrative based on over 14 years of practical experience of conducting Objective Structured Clinical Examinations (OSCEs) at the Royal Veterinary College (RVC). It is a mixture of 'lessons learnt', mistakes to avoid and is interspersed with a personal view of how to run an OSCE. The emphasis is on what it takes to make the process 'work' – remembering that the format is unlike a traditional desk-based exam, yet has to be as reliable, despite the obvious difficulties involved in staging an exam involving 22 or more assessors, different species of animals, multiple support staff and stressed students. Running an OSCE is akin to putting on a theatrical play. You need certain key characters to make it run smoothly as well as the 'actors' (students), who need to have learnt their 'lines' (tasks). 'The show must go on' is pertinent to this sort of high-budget, high-stakes exam, for once the process has started the students must not be aware of the occasional chaos behind the scenes.

22.1   What is it?

There are swathes of information available to discuss the finer points of this exam; see Chapter 21 'Practical Assessments' for details regarding the pedagogical reasons for OSCEs, but here is a summary.

- **Objective** – because all candidates are assessed using exactly the same task and criteria, then it is objective (as opposed to subjective). The task is broken down into an itemized list or 'recipe' on the mark sheet as to how to perform that task. The student either does that element of the task, or does not (see OSCE mark sheet at the end of this chapter).

- **Structured** – so it can be assessed at each structured stage.

- **Clinical** – all candidates are assessed using exactly the same stations/questions and the application of theoretical knowledge in a clinical situation is measured.

- **Exam** – speaks for itself!

22.2   The OSCE Circuit

The students will have a series of smaller 'exams' called 'stations' run consecutively to make a 'circuit'. These are usually 5 minutes long, though other institutions may shorten this to 4 minutes or extend it to 10 minutes, but they must all be the same amount of time, or the circuit will not work.

The student performs a task for the allotted time, they exit the area, move on to the next station as the student who has performed that task exits and moves on to their next task, until they have all completed the circuit. If you have 12 stations, you could have 12 students taking the exam at a time, though in practice there will be at least one 'no candidate' slot within the circuit to allow a comfort break for the assessors. After all, a 12-station OSCE will be at least 1 h 20 minutes and assessors may require a break in that time. So, rather than stopping the exam (much to the assessor's embarrassment) it is easier to allow a break in the circuit. When there isn't a candidate, the assessor knows they have a few minutes to get a drink and use the bathroom if required. There are also 'rest stations' built into the circuit for the comfort of the student, so if there were 12 stations, we would add two rest stations into that circuit. Usually the circuit will require a rest station to allow the student to get changed into or out of theatre attire, or take off surgical gloves. This also enables

© CAB International 2018. *Veterinary Clinical Skills Manual* (eds N. Coombes and A. Silva-Fletcher)

the student to have a drink of water (which is provided in the station) and use the bathroom should they need to. It is also a useful point of contact for staff running the circuit to see if all is well with the student in the rest station, as stress can affect people in unusual ways. There have been tears, laughter, rigid quietness, excess sweating and low blood sugar to deal with.

There will be a scenario outside of each 'station' – either a room or a screened-off area – for the student to read for approximately 1 min before entering the station (Fig. 22.1). There is an automated timing system with verbal/visual prompts on a wall-mounted TV screen announcing to all involved what is happening. The RVC has the following audio prompts (Fig. 22.2):

- Please enter the station.
- 2 minutes (elapsed).
- 1 minute to go.
- Please exit the station and move on to the next station (at 5 minutes).

They then have 1 min to read the next scenario.

The scenario will also be inside the room for the student to refer to should they forget what they have to do, or it may have some pertinent information such as the name of a pet, or a calculation they need to perform. Exam nerves make the memory unreliable, we have found.

22.3　Justifying the Process

Once you have decided you want to run an OSCE to examine your students *and* have justified the whole process, actually doing it can be daunting. There are some immediate questions you need to ask and answer: How? What? Why? When? Where? Who?

22.3.1　How are the stations selected?

To do this you need to focus on what you want to assess. Is it a broad range of general skills, or very specific

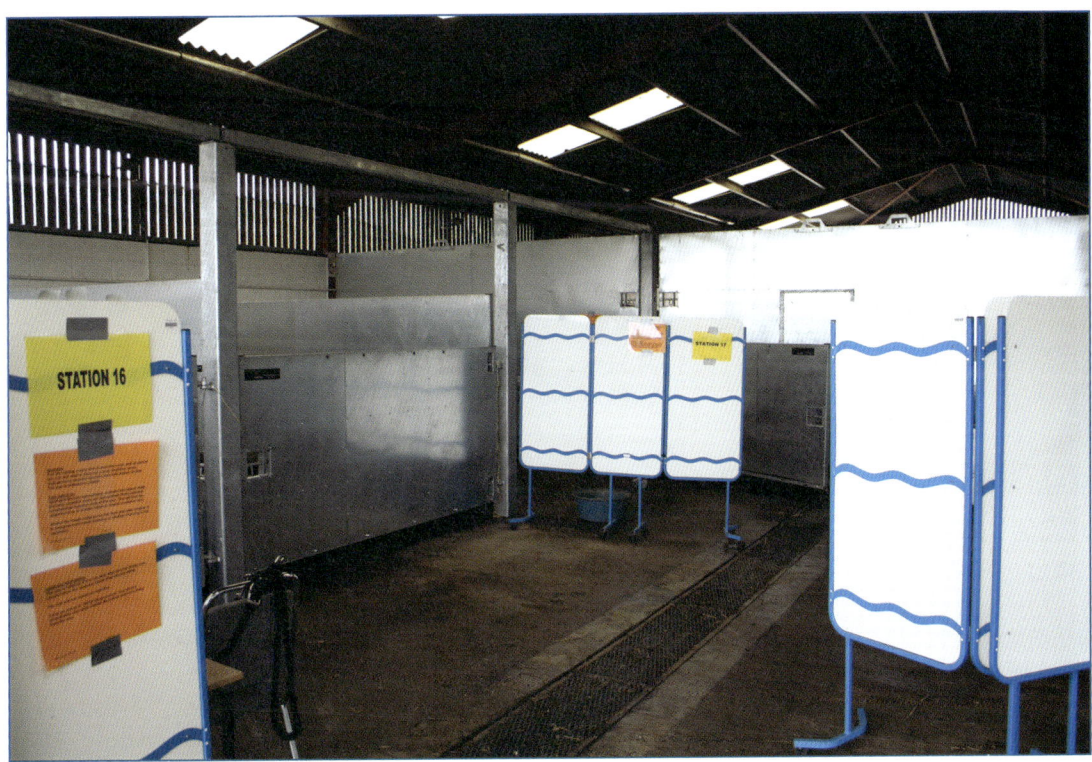

Fig. 22.1. The OSCE stations are screened off from each other in a barn and the scenario that the students read before entering the station is shown here (station 16).

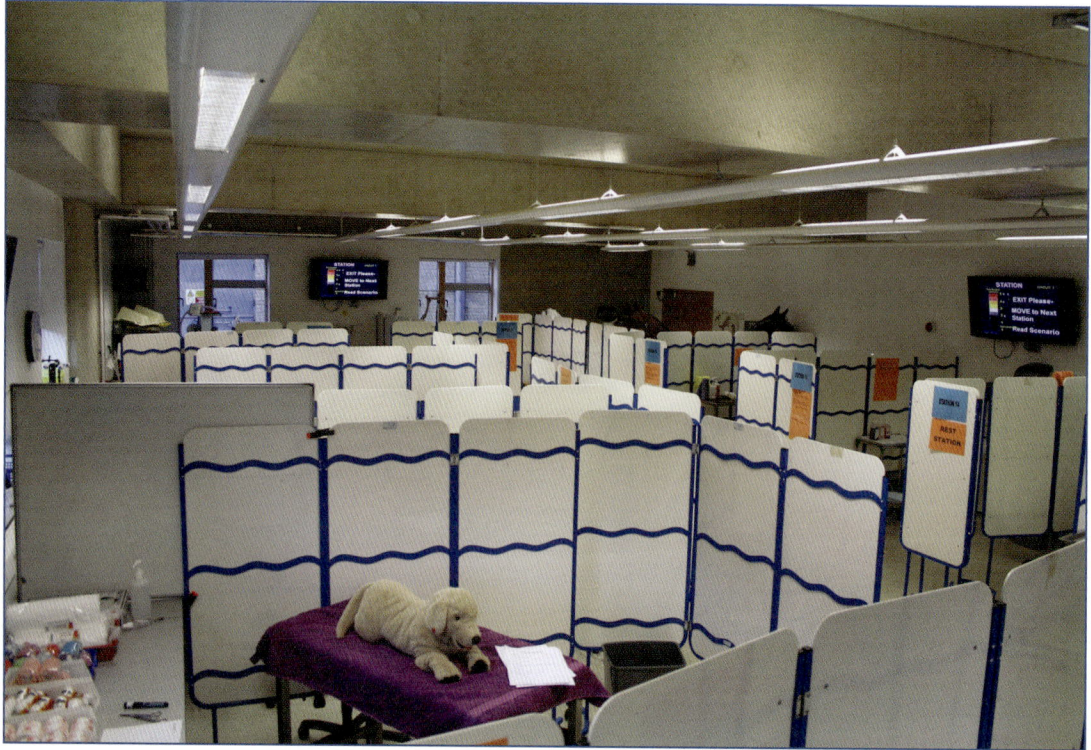

Fig. 22.2. The picture illustrates how screens separate the OSCE stations. The wall-mounted TV screens display the instructions.

to a course (e.g. microbiology lab-based tasks). There is no point in running an OSCE station for something you can test on a computer, or with paper and pen. Always justify why you need to have the student perform this task in front of you. If it can be assessed in another way, then do so. OSCEs are expensive, curriculum-time consuming and staff-time intensive to run. You have to be able to justify their expense for a practical skill that cannot be examined in another setting or manner.

22.3.2 How do we train and select the assessors?

Assessors can be sourced from a wide range of available staff. Usually once the exam format is embedded in the curriculum, all clinical staff are obligated to assess. It is usual to have staff relative to the skill from an aligned teaching/clinical area (e.g. surgeons assessing suturing) but as long as staff are 'competent' in that field, they do not necessarily need to be qualified to the highest level. It also needs to be said that just because a member of

staff has an apparently 'relevant' qualification, it does not mean that they are still relevant in that area. Staff who have a general veterinary qualification and have then gone on to specialize in a narrower clinical field may no longer be able to assess a more general veterinary skill that they have not performed since they graduated several decades ago.

The original remit for an OSCE was that a non-clinical staff member should be able to mark the student, so it was originally run with administrative staff assessing. After all, the students are either performing the task according to the mark sheet, or they are not. However, in practice this can cause considerable problems and so it is usual to have clinically trained vets, nurses and para-clinical staff as assessors. It also has to be remembered that students need to have confidence in their assessors. If they do not, they may challenge the results, whereas if they are marked by faculty who they know teach this skill or perform it, they are confident that they have been fairly marked.

OSCEs can be subjective, especially if verbal feedback is to be given, as is often the case in a formative exam. This feedback is hugely important to students and so it has to be given by someone who is not just filling in a mark sheet about the skill, but who *understands* the skill.

It is usual to run a 'formative' (practice) before their summative OSCE for the cohort being examined. In effect, this enables trainee assessors to be integrated into the circuit as well as allowing students to undertake a practice at the exams format.

During this formative, new assessors can either stand alongside experienced assessors for a period of time before marking for themselves, occasionally with the guidance of their mentor, or they have experienced the system for themselves as students. They may not be familiar with the mark sheet and so will have this explained to them by a relevant staff member.

22.3.3   How do we train our students in their approach to this exam?

This is an unusual exam format. Students who have always sat written exams with a script of questions to answer in an anonymous setting may struggle with the immediacy and intimacy of performing a task in front of another person who is not a peer and who may have taught them the task. Their assessor may be someone they have been taught by or someone they may not know at all. Some students really struggle with nerves in this setting. They say it is not realistic to be doing a task in this way. However, they will be judged at all stages in their veterinary career by people who are potentially a lot more critical: the animals' owners as well as their employer. If you are attending to an animal in a critical situation, with the owner present, it will be far more stressful. It can be difficult to convey this fact to a student struggling with exam nerves and who realizes that the qualification they want so desperately may depend on how well they perform.

This is why we make sure that all students have done a formative version of this exam. It is compulsory that they attend, but not that they pass. For the veterinary students (who undertake a 5-year course) the formative exam is set in the first half of their 4th year, so that if they cannot attend for illness reasons, they will be able to sit it the following year as a 5th-year student with that year's 4th-years – which is still 2 months before their final OSCE. It is also why they get a 1 min verbal feedback in the formative exam. This does not just cover how they performed the task, but also the

assessor may comment on other aspects of the exam format that they need to be aware of; for example, how they approached the exam and time management. If the student appears to have had a problem with one element of the task (such as a calculation) and took all of the time trying to get this correct, it may have benefitted them to start with the more practical side of the task; for example, if the task is to set up a drip line, then work out the drip rate and demonstrate sterile technique whilst doing so. They could at least assemble the drip set and fluid bag, then move on to the calculation. Doing something practical often helps if students are nervous; calculations can be difficult for some students. Or if you are the other way inclined, start with the calculation then move on to the practical part. Some students miss part of what they have been asked to do, so if they are told by the assessor to take a few more seconds reading the scenario through to work out exactly what has been asked of them, this will help them in the Finals OSCE.

22.3.4   What and why?

An OSCE is used to test a student usually because there is no other uniform way to examine multiple students demonstrating their ability to perform a defined practical task. The difficulty arises where assessors want to add elements to the exam that could be tested in other ways. The question needs to be asked when a new station is being authored, or an existing one changed: 'Could this be examined in a desk/computer-based exam format?' If it could, then it should. If it is a truly practical skill such as suturing, or a health exam on a horse, for example, then an OSCE is the correct place for it.

22.3.5   When?

Within a veterinary course there will be certain bench marks that will need confirming. These could be at a certain point, for example, as a measure of how well in general the students are doing with their practical skills prior to going out into local veterinary practices as students, right up to when they qualify and graduate as veterinary professionals. They can also be used if a postgraduate course is being run to assess the level of competence of the attendees.

22.3.6   Where?

This is very variable and depends on the available facilities and space. They could be out-sourced to another facility so that students from one educational centre will attend another just for these exams. Or they could be run on the campus of the attending students.

22.3.7 Who authors the stations?

Usually the authors are 'clinically relevant staff'. This is a widely sweeping term. In reality what we find is that there are always fundamental disciplines that need to be represented in any standard clinical OSCE: core disciplines such as anaesthesia, radiography, theatre practice, animal handling, laboratory skills, to name but a few. Every specialist might also assume that their specialism needs to be examined within this format. We have found that general practitioners are more able to focus on relevant 'Day One Skills' (RVC, 2017), that is, the basic skills that a new graduate would be expected to perform upon graduation. They are the clinicians who have to mentor new graduates at the very start of their careers. However, we have also found that a variety of staff have an idea for an OSCE. The author could be a world expert in their field, or a laboratory technician. The ideas may occur whilst taking part in an OSCE; they can be a fertile breeding ground for facility to say, 'This is good, but we should be examining this area'. Or if a new model is designed that enables us to test an element of a skill, this may lead to a new OSCE being written.

Often staff all agree that a skill needs examining, but in reality it is very difficult or impossible to do so. There could be unacceptable elements detrimental to animal welfare. A clinical exam performed on an animal once is acceptable, but to perform that on an animal several times may not be. A good example is cat restraint. There was an OSCE based around 'Safely handling a cat, remove from a cat basket, demonstrate how to restrain for blood sampling' – a very important skill that many students struggle with. However, you may get a live cat out of a basket once and perform this task on the cat, but you will not be able to do this 25 times in a row. So, even if you sourced multiple cats in multiple baskets in multiple rooms – is this acceptable? Or feasible practically? (See Chapter 15.)

Once an idea has been thought through and written into an OSCE format, it will then be sent to various members of staff to check that they agree with the principles. At this point any steps omitted will be added or superfluous ones removed as well as practically trialled on someone. We need to make sure that any OSCE is not one person's view of how that skill should be performed. It needs to be based on best practice and referenced to current literature as well as to RVC teaching material. We have had OSCEs based on a skill that we all thought was being taught, only to find out that it was not, or that it was done in a different way, or even that the formula used for a calculation was not the same as stated and examined in the OSCE. This has led to 'blueprinting' (see Chapter 21).

22.4 Infrastructure

We are very fortunate to have a dedicated Exams team and CSC team who jointly run these exams, as well as good support from the information technology (IT) and even catering teams to enable smooth running and on-the-spot problem solving with any potential issues that arise.

The CSC team's roles leading up to the exam include:

- Teaching the students clinical skills.
- Working out the layout for the stations.
- Authoring the OSCEs (for an example, see Appendix 22.1 below).
- Advising other clinical staff on authoring and 'how to'.
- Ordering the consumables and other equipment.
- Arranging any animals used.
- Liaising with other departments around the college.
- Physically setting up the exam (this can take up to a week).

The CSC team's roles on the day of the exam include:

- Staffing the clinical area and outside barn area to ensure that the stations technically run well.
- Maintaining stocks of consumables.
- Answering clinical queries from assessors.
- Assessing as required.
- Reassuring distressed students.
- Re-setting stations if complicated.
- Handling animals as needed.

The Exams team roles include:

- Organizing/printing the paperwork for the exam.
- Assigning the students to a time slot.

- Assigning the assessors to relevant stations.
- Gate-keeping the computer-based exam bank.
- Updating exams as required.
- Running the timing system within any specific clinical exam area.
- Organizing any special requirements for individual students.
- Hosting the external examiners.

22.5   Maps/Layout

As an OSCE generally involves multiple groups of people, it is very useful to draw a layout of where the stations will be and to walk around the area to make sure that the facilities you have can support the stations you have selected. Some stations need a sink, others a fixed lab bench or a separate room (radiography or communications skills, for example). Some need more space than others do, or to be set in a barn. This plan can then be distributed to the parties involved for others to make sure that the circuit will be effective. There is also a physical limitation to the number of stations that can be run within the space you have. Our lab facility can accommodate 12 stations, so if a 14-station OSCE is suggested as relevant, it cannot be accommodated unless additional space can be found in adjoining rooms, for example.

22.6   Consumables and Equipment

Each station will have its own unique set of equipment required (Box 22.1). This could be actual equipment (e.g. microscope, centrifuge or anaesthetic machine) or consumables (bandaging, cannulas, microscope slides) or even animals can be listed as 'equipment' required.

Some equipment will need ordering weeks in advance. Or if it is a model, or other piece of fundamental equipment, there needs to be a spare. It is also wise to over-order. If there are 100 students expected to use one syringe each, and they get nervous, drop one or possibly two, you could potentially use up to three per student, so 300 syringes would be needed. Use a 25% extra

factor and all should be well. If there are specific animals, their health status has to be accommodated; for example, an OSCE that involves sheep being 'tipped' for a clinical examination of a foot will need to have taken into account whether the ewes are pregnant, so running this in early spring would not be viable. Or if it was how to trim a sheep's claw, the sheep need to have claws that need trimming and enough sheep to allow one animal per four students.

22.7   Planning – Think Ahead

This is vital: without forethought, the OSCE will not work. Some stations need 6 months pre-planning (e.g. booking actors for communication skills stations, sourcing cadaver material) and farriers or other expert essential assessors need 3 months' notice.

Box 22.1. Equipment list for Hand Wash OSCE.

Equipment List

Please list all items required for the station, spares, or any station set-up that is important. Also quantities of equipment and if it is a 'distractor'

NB: Needs setting by a sink with a disposable hand-towel dispenser

- Ordinary tablet soap.
- Range of antibacterial handscrub solutions (to include Hibiscrub/povidone–iodine).
- Alcohol hand gel bottle.
- Paper towel mounted on wall in dispenser (elbow-operated).
- Normal hand towel.
- Foot-operated bin.
- Flip-top bin that requires user to lift the lid with hand.
- Clip board.
- Pencil.
- Chair for assessor.

Notes to assessor:

- Make sure pedal-top bin is closed after each student.
- Make sure there is adequate soap in dispensers and disposable towel in dispenser.

22.7.1 Do a visual 'map' of the set-up and 'route'

Depending on where your OSCE is set, certain stations do not work well together and others need to be sited in certain locations within a room or building. This has a cumulative effect as to where other stations can be sited and if certain stations can be run. For example, if running a suturing station, it makes sense if the one before it is a gloving/gowning station; if not, it needs to be a 'rest' station to make sure the student can be attired suitably in theatre wear. It is useful to walk around the room or setting physically, to pace it out and see if the stations chosen will 'work'.

Draw a map of the route, regardless of the amount of stations in the OSCE, to highlight the places where you could 'lose' a student or there may be issues with high traffic 'logjams' of students and they could get misdirected to the wrong part of the route.

22.7.2 Have a meeting with all the concerned parties

All of the different departments and staff involved in an OSCE need to meet prior to the exam to ensure that all parties know of their expected role, including who will be responsible for each element of the exam – practical set-up, ordering, sourcing staff, student liaison, etc.

22.7.3 Keep everyone in the 'loop'

OSCEs change rapidly – mark sheets, equipment lists, assessors, timings: make sure all of the people involved have the *latest* details.

22.7.4 Look after your staff and students

OSCEs can be a physically gruelling experience for examiners and staff running them. They can be running for up to 6 days spread over 2 weeks, with 12 sessions of 3 h, two per day. Make sure there are plenty of refreshments and occasional 'no-candidates' to allow for a trip to the bathroom for assessors. Spacing of 'rest stations' for students should *ideally* be placed with no more than six 'active' stations in between them. Students are stressed and with any more than this we see more upset students who struggle to continue.

22.8 A Timeline to Run a Veterinary OSCE

This is a guide as to how long it can take to arrive at the end point of putting on an OSCE, with the least drama and with taking into consideration the students, the animals, the staff involved in the practical set-up, writing the exams and assessing on the day. For this purpose, the following is the author's timeline for the 5th year's final OSCE exam run each year in early April. This has 26 stations (20 live, 6 rests) and runs over 5 or 6 days, involving 240 students and up to 200 assessors. It may surprise you to realize that this exam will have been thought of at least 20 months *before* it occurs.

22.8.1 Timeline

This timeline uses the situation of preparing for the April 2017 Finals exam, so it starts in April 2015.

> **April 2015** *(2 years before)*
> Finals OSCE for current cohort

- Following this exam, a post-OSCE meeting is attended by the Exams team/CSC team and any other interested parties. General feedback by the teams is discussed as well as looking at any written feedback given by assessors regarding how well a station has run, if mark points need changing, or scenarios need to be re-worded. Quite often, a different set of students will elicit a different set of 'issues'.

June 2015 *(22/23 months before)*
- Anything learnt from the April 2015 OSCE finals is put into place or followed up.

July 2015 *(21 months before)*
- Stations suggested for 4th year formative in November 2015 (these are the students that will be taking the 2017 exam). The CSC team and the Exams team look at suitable stations, spotting 'gaps' or potential for new stations, then request relevant staff to write them, or the CSC team do this.

August 2015 *(20 months before)*
- New stations written or old stations revised.

> **September 2015** *(19 months before)*
> Re-sit Finals OSCEs from April 2015 exams

October 2015 *(18 months before)*

- Any revisions or new stations *must* be complete by now to give time to get into OSCE software format, as they will need trialling in the Formative 4th year exam run in November 2015.

> **November 2015** *(17 months before)*
> Formative exam for the cohort taking the April 2017 finals exam

- This formative allows new stations to be trialled and new assessors to be 'trained'. This has more rest stations than the real OSCE, but still takes over 2.5 h to complete, with stations based in the barns and the CSC in the same way the Finals will be. They have 1 min verbal feedback from the assessor to the student to highlight any potential areas to be addressed at each station.

December 2015 *(16 months before)*

- Post-formative OSCE meeting – always a good idea; any feedback from students given to staff, assessors, Exams team, actors from the communication skills stations, can occur here to make improvements for future exams. If stations need slight re-wording of a scenario, if too many mark-points, etc., this needs to be done quite near to the finish of the exam or it gets 'forgotten'. (What went well, what not so well – these points are actioned over the next few months.)

December 2015–April 2016 *(16–12 months before)*

- Continue re-writing stations. It can take a considerable time to get the original authors to do this and to be checked by other staff. The Exams team then needs to put any changes into the software.

> **April 2016 Finals run** *(12 months before)*
> Same post-OSCE meeting, which may have repercussions for April 2017 exam to make things run smoothly

September 2016 *(7 months to go)*

- Re-sit for students who failed April 2016 exam. Post-OSCE meeting may have influence on April 2017 exam to make sure all runs smoothly, any points actioned.

October 2016 *(6 months to go)*

- Assessors assigned to exam timetable by Exams team; this always has to be with at least 6 months'

notice to give clinicians time as they are rota'd on in 6-month blocks.

> **November 2016** *(5 months to go)*
> Formative OSCE run for cohort taking the April 2018 OSCE Finals

November 2016 *(5 months to go)*

- Put together a list of OSCE stations, liaise with Exams team about viability of stations, any feedback from the external examiners to consider also.

December 2016 *(4 months to go)*

- Email the 5th year BVetMeds to remind them to plan their revision ready for the exam in April.

January 2017 *(3 months to go)*

- Re-email BVM5 in similar email to make sure the Christmas spirit has not made them forget to plan their revision. These students will get regular emails from the CSC team regarding the exam. We set up an email 'count-down to OSCEs' which makes students focus on their revision and the feedback from them is positive about this, even though they say 'it freaks me out'!

- Once the station list has been finalized, certain stations known to need more time to organize are looked at first.

- Book the communication skills actors. This may have been done earlier in the year when booking for other OSCE's running, but by now the scenarios will be known and they may be gender specific or require a certain 'type' of actor, e.g. 'elderly farmer'.

- Order any required cadaver material.

- Book the farrier/blacksmith.

- If certain models are required that take 6 weeks or more to make/deliver, order those.

- Ascertain if animals are available (if sheep foot trim station used, this may need up to 6 months' notice to make sure their feet need trimming in April and are not trimmed just before exam), as discussed earlier.

February 2017 *(2 months to go)*

- Draw up OSCE 'maps' for the station layout in CSC/barns. Walk around CSC lab to make sure that stations that have particular requirements are sited in the right place; e.g. if it needs a sink, if it needs its own room (communications skills, radiography).

March 2017 *(1 month to go)*

- Double check that stations are sited in the right place.
- Check that actors for communications skills have the scenarios.
- Expect visits from assessors to check how to do some tasks and to discuss the OSCE logistics in general.
- Expect more students in the CSC daily drop-in sessions.
- Answer emails from worried students or see them in person.
- Check all is well with the animals required.
- OSCE timing system checked by IT.
- Consumables ordered.
- Check equipment lists are up to date, print off and laminate ready for checking off when the station is set up.
- Arrange porterage for heavy items if needed to be moved to the outside stations.
- Organize which staff are working which days, whether they will be inside or outside. Try to give everybody a break at some point (we have four CSC staff).

The week before

- Close the CSC for the whole week.
- Porters bring OSCE screens over from storage (Monday).
- Set up the exam inside (Monday/Tuesday/Wednesday).
- Set up the exam outside in the barns (Friday).
- Double check all the equipment is available plus spares.
- Double check the stations.
- Meet with the assessors in groups, do demonstrations of the skill if required.

- OSCE assessors' meeting for them to check their stations (Thursday pm/Friday pm).

The Monday morning of the 6-day exam (before the exam starts)

- Answer last-minute queries from assessors.
- Sort out the animals for outside stations, water/hay.
- Help round up sheep/cows if needed.
- Make sure all assessors know the layout of the building/barn (toilets, tea availability).
- Meet the communications skills actors, make sure all is well.
- Set up 'last minute' stations – get bloods out for blood smear, set up milk for sterile milk or CMT station, make sure O_2 switched on.
- Check and check again everything OSCE!
- Step into stations to assess if required.

22.9   To Conclude

An OSCE is a labour-intensive exam format for assessing students uniformly when run well. Run badly it is potential chaos and hugely stressful and so would be deleted from the curriculum in the favour of 'spot tests' or simply the hope that the students writing about a practical task is enough. It is unlikely to be so. It is hoped that this chapter outlines for you the practicalities of putting on an OSCE and enables you to do it for your own establishment.

Reference: RVC (2017) *Bachelor of Veterinary Medicine Day One Skills Handbook.* Available at: http://www.live.ac.uk/Media/LIVE/PDFs/day_one_handbook.pdf (accessed 3 October 2017).

Appendix 22.1. An example scenario and the relevant OSCE mark-sheet.

Title for OSCE: Hand washing

This Station tests the student's ability to:

Perform a clinical hand wash.

This is a 5 minute station *(Note: This is the part that the student will see outside the station)*

Scenario:

You have just finished handling a patient and must now demonstrate the appropriate hand hygiene before handling another patient.

Your task is to:

Carry out the full hand washing procedure to ensure thorough cleaning of your hands. Ensure the actions carried out can be clearly seen by the examiner.

Additional Information:

This is not the same as scrubbing up for surgery.

	Method	Marks
1	Remove hand and wrist jewellery (plain wedding band may be worn)	2
2	Nails are natural (not false), short, clean & unvarnished	1
3	Turn on the taps – to produce a steady flow of comfortable temperature of water	1
4	Wet hands and wrists thoroughly	1
5	Depress soap dispenser pump and apply 2-3 pumps of antiseptic hand wash (e.g. Hibiscrub) onto free hand	2
6	Step 1 : Grasp wrist of left/right hand with right/left hand and rub rotationally	1
7	Repeat for other wrist	1
8	Step 2: Rub hands together – palm to palm	1
9	Step 3: Place the palm of the right hand over the back of the left hand and rub together	1
10	Repeat with left palm over back of the right hand	1
11	Step 4: Interlace the fingers of both hands and rub together	1
12	Step 5: Interlock fingers of both hands – backs of fingers touching opposing palms – rub together	1
13	Repeat on the other side, i.e. so left hand is uppermost.	1
14	Step 6: Clasp the left thumb in the right hand and rotationally rub together	1
15	Repeat for the right thumb	1
16	Step 7: Using fingers of the right hand held together, place in the left palm and rub backwards and forwards	1
17	Repeat for the other hand	1
18	Rinse both hands and wrists thoroughly under the running water	1
19	Does NOT wash wrists after completing hand wash steps 1 – 7 (can rinse them off with hands, but must not now be washing them anew)	3
20	Completed hand wash has taken at least 60 seconds	2
21	Turn off taps with the elbows (or use a paper towel if appropriate for the taps)	3
22	Dry hands sufficiently using **disposable** paper towel	3
23	Dispose of used paper towel into foot-operated bin ONLY	3

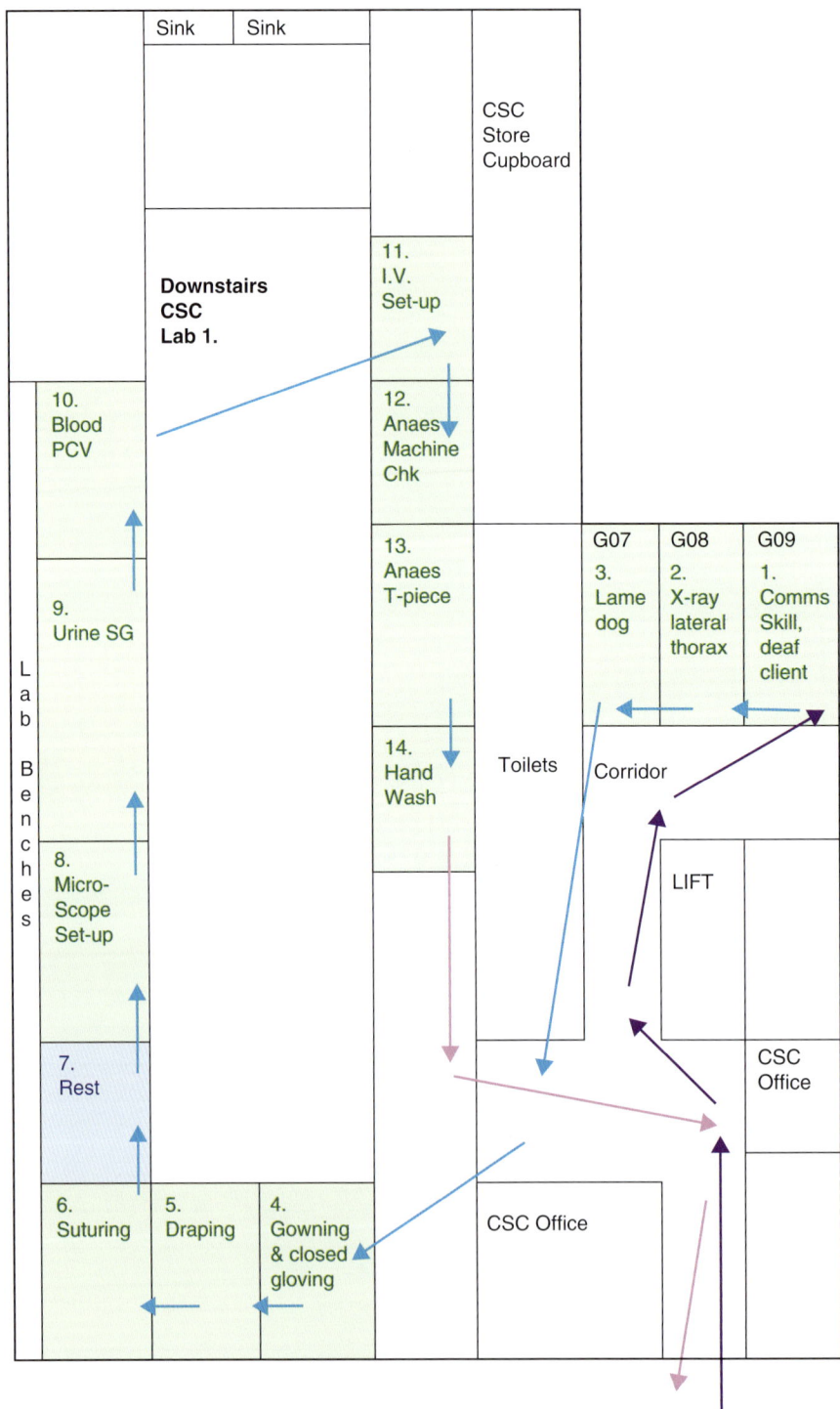

Fig. 22.3. Clinical skills centre layout for a 14-station OSCE circuit.

Section 9

Moving Forward

Section Editor: Ayona Silva-Fletcher

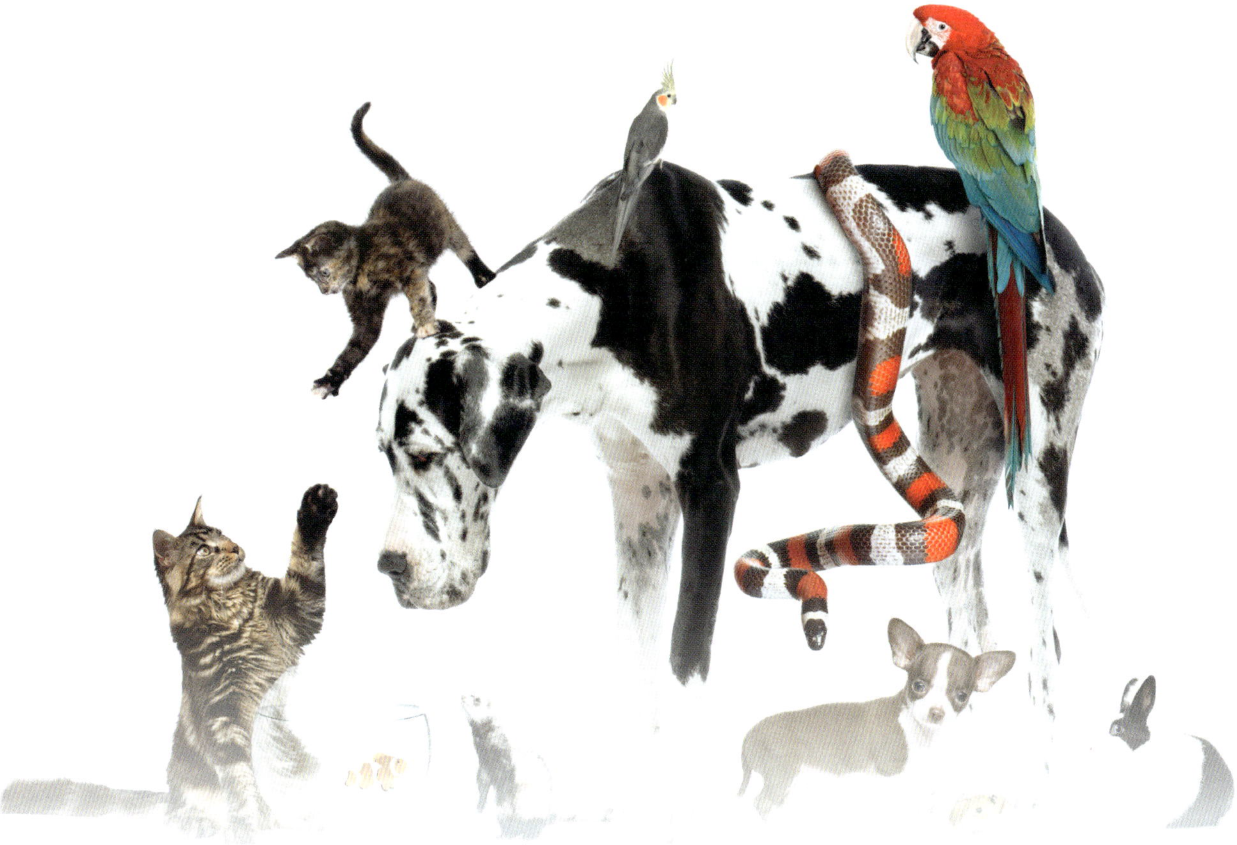

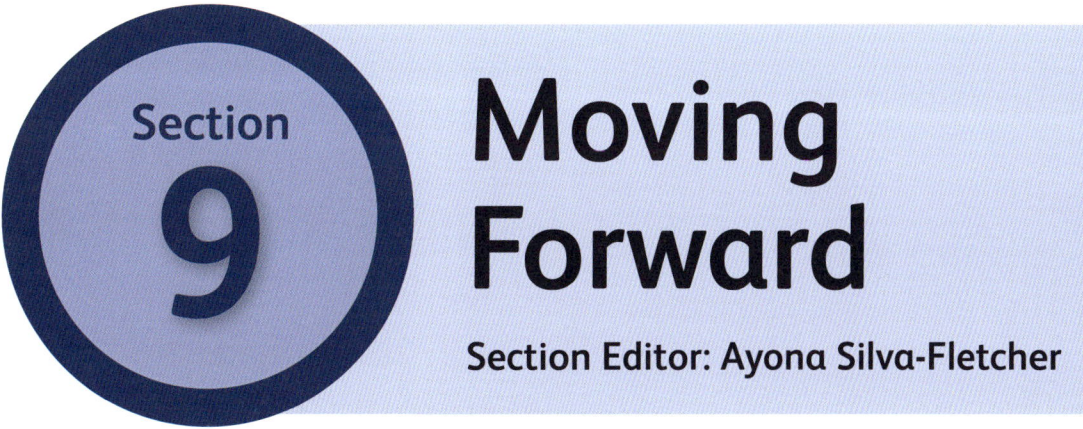

Introduction

Since the opening of the first veterinary clinical skills centre (CSC) in 2004, many new developments have taken place around the world to promote awareness and to improve the performance of these innovative teaching facilities. These developments include the introduction of novel clinical skills stations, innovative objectively structured clinical examination (OSCE) practices, efficient management structures, training for clinical tutors, conferences, websites, videos and supporting materials to share and disseminate good practice and the growth of dedicated educators. The development of new and expensive simulators has been balanced by simple, inexpensive innovations that have sometimes been introduced and driven by students. One important factor that has contributed more than any other to the progress of CSCs is the willingness to use feedback from students, OSCE assessors, clinical tutors and fledgling graduates. In this section we look to the future and we look for opportunities to further improve the performance of CSCs by considering the reflections of new graduates.

We explore the way forward by learning from the experiences and reflections of a new veterinary graduate who had been taught in a CSC.

Within this section there are three chapters as outlined below.

Chapter 23: 'Mind the Gap' – the Development, Validation and Evaluation of a Veterinary Clinical Skills Model

Chapter 24: Simulators in Veterinary Clinical Skills Education: Background and Examples

Chapter 25: The Transition between the Clinical Skills Lab and the Real World – Perspectives from a New Graduate 2 Years after Qualifying

Chapter 23 is a valuable example of how a gap was identified in veterinary clinical skills teaching and how a new resource was developed to fill this gap. In this chapter the author takes us through the steps of identification of a skills gap, the development of a new clinical skills resource and then the validation and evaluation by students who were taught using the new resource. As society demands new services and skills from the veterinary sector, this chapter illustrates how new teaching materials and methods can be rapidly and efficiently developed and deployed in the environment of CSCs. It is an ideal example of seeing what is needed

as society demands new services from the veterinary sector. The example described is based on the relative lack of suitable teaching in current education for veterinary dentistry. The description in Chapter 23 of how a dental simulator was designed, piloted and evaluated will be very useful for educators planning their future curricula. This chapter also shows how student feedback was pivotal in this development. The author goes on to consider how the introduction of more sophisticated technologies may lead to further advances in teaching this area of veterinary skills.

Chapter 24 offers an excellent background to simulators and why these are considered as the best tools for an introduction to clinical skills and to the learning of more advanced skills. The author offers evidence from educational literature to support the pedagogical underpinning of skills development, both from general and health professional-related literature. Challenges offered at different stages of design, validation and evaluation are outlined. Examples of manikins and computer hybrids that are related to small and large animals as well as generic skills are explored, leading to a discussion on the usage today. The haptic technologies are a growing area and offer a more realistic experience to the students and, despite the cost, are the fastest-growing area of simulators. The use of computer-only 3D-based technologies may offer more developments as rapid advances in these technologies will lead to more cost-effective and practical methods that can be used by the growing student numbers and larger student cohorts.

Chapter 25 describes the reflections of a recently qualified graduate about what has been learnt from a CSC and its relevance in the clinical workplace. New graduates may face the challenges of dealing with their anxiety and low confidence level and in addition the overwhelming sense of responsibility to clients, patients and other colleagues. How helpful are the skills learnt in the skills lab to reduce anxiety and increase confidence? Having knowledge of the basic practical skills such as suturing and the feel of materials and equipment gained in a CSC helps to provide the confidence required to carry out a practical procedure. Some clinical skills learnt in the skills lab are used daily, some rarely, but having the exposure to a wide array of skills may possibly reduce anxiety. A surprising discovery for this new graduate was the realization that they not only have to perform but also teach other staff at the workplace (often para-veterinary and technical helpers) how and what to do. Reflections on how they were taught in the skills centre were useful here.

23 'Mind the Gap' – the Development, Validation and Evaluation of a Veterinary Clinical Skills Model

Rachel H. Lumbis
The Royal Veterinary College, London

Introduction: Building a Skills Base – the Journey from Novice to Competent

Practical clinical skills lie at the heart of the professional practice of veterinarians and veterinary nurses, with the mastery of fundamental skills proving to be an important component of both professions. When considering the acquisition of requisite skills, it is essential to contemplate education as a process that moves the student through a series of stages from novice to competence. Miller's (1990) framework for clinical competence (Fig. 23.1) suggests that, in order for an individual to be deemed competent, a practical application of knowledge gained following the transition from 'knowing to doing' is essential. This framework implies that students will begin at the cognition stage of knowing and work their way up to the behavioural stage of doing; however, anecdotal opinion can be contradictory.

Many students can complete a practical task, yet may not fully understand the methodology, whereas others acquire the necessary knowledge, yet may require a significant amount of tuition and supervision in order to master the skill independently. It is therefore crucial to ensure that knowledge and skills are integrated at all stages of the learning process in the hope that students will ultimately become competent practitioners. This view is mirrored by Schön (1983) who argued that 'technical rationality' (the application of theory) and its conception of practice does not adequately describe the form of professional knowledge that distinguishes between the adequate and the excellent practitioner; it does not account for 'professional artistry' (intuitive knowledge).

Another issue is that a novice and an expert are fundamentally different, working and learning in different ways. For example, in terms of higher-order thinking, novices are associated with the acquisition of knowledge whereas experts utilize thoughts such as application,

analysis, synthesis and evaluation – the basis of planning and problem solving. As highlighted by Bleakley (2006, p. 152), 'there is a lack of tacit knowledge upon which to engage synthetic or holistic learning through pattern recognition'. Therefore, to assist in the transition from novice to expert, analytical principles-based 'building block' learning should be encouraged.

23.1 Identifying a Gap in Practical Teaching

One of the most common diseases in small animal patients is periodontal disease (Robinson *et al.*, 2015; Goldstein *et al.*, 2016), thus dental work is identified as a large part of modern-day practice and is one of the most common sources of revenue in general practice (Chamblee and Reiboldt, 2010). As highlighted by Goldstein *et al.* (2016), whilst clients are becoming more aware of periodontal disease in dogs and cats, a lack of visual detection until its advanced stages leaves many owners typically unaware of its presence and significance. A subsequent reliance is placed on the veterinary team to be proactive in educating owners about its detrimental impact on health and the importance of prevention, early identification and treatment. The cornerstone of periodontal therapy in small animals is considered to be dental prophylaxis, of which professional scaling and polishing is regarded as an essential element (Johnston, 2011).

Despite the high incidence rate, dental procedures can be lengthy, intricate and arduous and do not carry the same eminent image as other surgical procedures. According to Putter (2011), the delegation of this task to qualified veterinary nurses (VNs) and new veterinary graduates is associated with an accepted apathy and lack of understanding of dentistry by the majority of veterinary surgeons, often with unsatisfactory results. Whilst

© CAB International 2018. *Veterinary Clinical Skills Manual* (eds N. Coombes and A. Silva-Fletcher)

Fig. 23.1. Miller's (1990) framework for clinical competence.

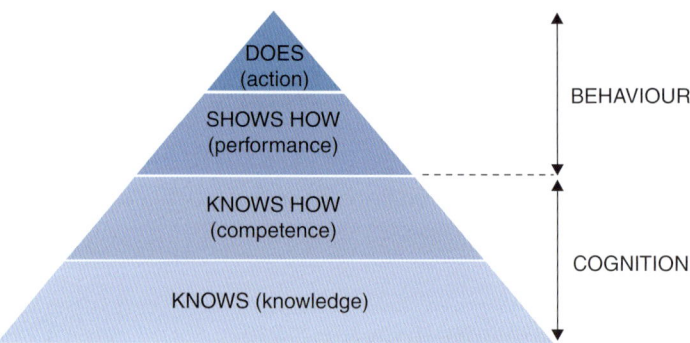

Registered Veterinary Nurses (RVNs) are prohibited from carrying out non-digital tooth extractions, they may still undertake routine dental hygiene work under veterinary direction (RCVS, 2017), a system identified by Colmery (2005) as being effective, provided that proper training has been given. However, the amount of training in veterinary dentistry received by student VNs has traditionally been viewed as minimal and on par with their veterinary colleagues, leaving them undertrained and ill equipped (Cleland, 2001).

The Royal College of Veterinary Surgeons (RCVS) is responsible for regulating the UK degrees and courses that allow veterinary surgeons and veterinary nurses to practise in the UK. Setting and monitoring the standards of veterinary and VN education is a key responsibility of the RCVS, in addition to defining the competences that need to be met by newly qualified veterinary surgeons and veterinary nurses. Courses must facilitate the acquisition of essential competences generically defined by the RCVS and Quality Assurance Agency (QAA) by the time of graduation/qualification. This is a key benchmark affecting the RCVS approval of veterinarian and VN training courses in the UK.

At the Royal Veterinary College (RVC, 2017), the *BVetMed Day One Skills Handbook* identifies the behaviour, attitudes and skills that are expected of every RVC veterinary student by the time of graduation. Those pertaining to small animal dentistry involve the preparation and operation of dental machinery, patient preparation for dental treatment and the ability to scale and polish teeth. Under Chapter 18 of the supporting guidance relating to the RCVS Code of Conduct for Veterinary Nurses and Veterinary Surgeons (RCVS, 2017), veterinary nurses, and student veterinary nurses working under the direction of a veterinary surgeon, may carry out routine dental hygiene work, excluding exodontia.

At the RVC, traditionally there was a heavy focus on knowledge acquisition by veterinary and veterinary nursing students. Core dentistry-related knowledge and low-level cognition was delivered using didactic teaching methods, such as lectures and computer-aided learning (CAL) programmes. Reaching the behaviour, action-based, domain requires attainment of physical and nimble skills, yet limited consideration was given to students' practical ability or performance. This is comparable to the attitude of dental schools nearly two decades ago when it was reported by Bartlett *et al.* (2001) that academia considered dental students' confidence in completing practical skills to be more effectively developed in general practice. Thus, dental schools focused on providing students with an understanding of the fundamental principles only. As LeBlanc *et al.* (2004, p. 378) identified, 'development of clinical skills requires mastery of two components: knowledge of the concepts of the procedure and the dexterity to perform it'.

It has often been assumed that veterinary and veterinary nursing students receive basic practical tuition on subjects such as types, care, maintenance and use of dental instrumentation whilst on extramural studies (EMS)/placement. However, student feedback does not support this assumption (BVA, 2012) and student experience is variable and dependent upon clinical case load. In addition, this arrangement has a number of associated limitations. As Schönwetter *et al.* (2006) recognized, the possession of expert knowledge and technical skills by professionals fails to ensure effective teaching. Not all clinicians possess formal training in clinical teaching, thus presenting a challenge for expert practitioners to explain complex skills to novice students. Issenberg and McGaghie (2002) emphasized that instructors require appropriate training in skills tuition as well as an understanding of the desired learning outcomes in order to facilitate students' acquisition of clinical skills. Whilst demonstration is identified as a significant factor in learning a psychomotor skill, Fugill (2005) highlighted the need for contextual teaching in the integration of knowledge and skill. This was echoed by Macluskey and Hanson (2011) who, in addition to observation, identified assistance and kinaesthetic learning as effective means of instruction in dental education. However, the potential risk to patients often impedes such student interaction, necessitating alternative, safer means of acquiring the skills that students will be expected to master prior to graduation (Fugill, 2005).

23.2 Creating a Dental Model

Simulators are increasingly being used in veterinary education. Advantages include supporting experiential learning of clinical procedural skills in a safe environment without risk of jeopardizing patient safety – factors identified as important for learning (Kneebone and Baillie, 2008). In order to address the acknowledged gap in RVC's provision of practical veterinary dentistry teaching, a prototype dental model was constructed using ceramic tiles, silicone sealant and grout to emulate teeth, gingiva and calculus, respectively (Fig. 23.2). Ceramic tiles were chosen due to being inexpensive, readily available and capable of providing a suitable substitute for real teeth. A study by Brine *et al.* (2000) to evaluate the effect of different ultrasonic scalers on canine and ceramic teeth found that, regardless of tip force, there was minimal damage to either the ceramic or the enamel surfaces, suggesting that a

ceramic surface has similar properties to tooth enamel. Despite this, ceramic teeth appeared a little softer and more easily altered by power scalers at higher tip forces.

In a pilot evaluation of the veterinary model, feedback received from two veterinarians and three veterinary nurses indicated that the model had a realistic feel and it was possible to cause damage through incorrect use of dental instrumentation (Fig. 23.3). A subsequent small-scale study was conducted to validate this simple, low-cost dental model as a tool for teaching and learning the fundamental dental skills needed to perform a professional dental cleaning technique. In addition to determining the efficacy of the model as a training tool, an objective of the study was to capture the students' attitudes regarding the use of a dental model in learning new dentistry-related skills. Ethical approval was granted by the RVC Ethics Committee.

23.3 Evaluating the Model

The sampling frame for this study consisted of third-year veterinary students studying at the RVC, all of whom had received tuition on periodontal disease (PD). This consisted of one 45 min didactic lecture on PD, with minimal coverage of the scale and polish technique, and access to a CAL programme. The CAL was developed for veterinary students by a veterinary dental specialist, Norman Johnston, and covered the fundamental principles of veterinary dentistry. Students volunteered to participate in the study and those with zero or minimal practical experience of dental scaling and polishing on small animals were selected. Purposive

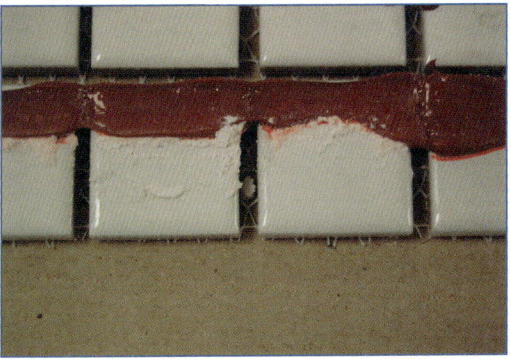

Fig. 23.2. A prototype veterinary dental model constructed using ceramic tiles, silicon sealant and grout to emulate teeth, gingiva and calculus, respectively.

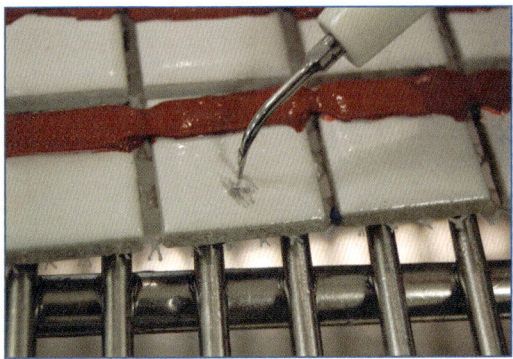

Fig. 23.3. Damage caused to the dental model through incorrect use of dental instrumentation.

sampling, a non-probability sampling technique, was an essential approach as some students had previously assisted with, or participated in, performing a dental procedure, providing a significant variable.

Using a computer-generated randomization list, the 25 student participants were assigned to two groups: group A (study) and group B (control). Within a 2-week study period, all participants in groups A and B were given access to skills sheets. These sheets consisted of text supplemented where necessary with still photographs or images and provided participants with step-by-step instructions on how to complete a scale and polish procedure. In addition, members of group A attended a skills training session incorporating use of the simulator model and members of group B had access to a video recording of how to prepare and use a dental machine and perform a scale and polish.

In subgroups of four to five students, group A participants spent up to 90 min in a laboratory training session, during which students were shown how to set up and identify the parts of a dental machine. A demonstration of how to correctly use an ultrasonic scaler and mechanical polisher was also conducted. Students were then allowed to practise these skills. Students were encouraged to trial different settings on the machine to appreciate the inefficiency of a low speed setting and the potential damage to tooth enamel that can result using a high speed setting. They were also instructed to apply excessive pressure to gain a better understanding of the appropriate force that should be applied to a patient. The model and dental machine were not available other than during the designated laboratory sessions.

Three short video clips were made available to group B participants. One detailed how to set up, correctly use and care for a dental machine as well as providing an overview of safety considerations. The other two provided a demonstration of how to scale and polish teeth on the simulator model using an ultrasonic scaler and mechanical polisher. Each clip also provided a verbal explanation of the procedure. These techniques were demonstrated and described by the author. The videos were uploaded to VetConnect, an online environment developed for RVC students and staff to share learning resources and experiences and to discuss clinical cases. Access to this site was restricted to students in group B and granted via a video link, which was distributed via an email.

All students were assessed using an objective structured clinical examination (OSCE), which provided an objective measure of technical skill. This assessment tool has been used to evaluate the clinical competence of medical students for over four decades and has proven validity at assessing technical skills of veterinary students (May and Head, 2010). The OSCE was constructed in accordance with guidelines developed by Davis *et al.* (2006). To ensure uniformity in the assessment of all students, a pre-agreed checklist format of objective steps was generated. To increase reliability and validity, the station was pilot tested and global rating scales were incorporated; good pass (GP), just pass (JP), just fail (JF) and bad fail (BF). These reflected the assessor's global opinion of each candidate's performance and were used, together with checklist scores, to calculate the pass mark.

A member of staff independent of the research team, with experience in veterinary dentistry and OSCE examining, assessed all students, thus removing inter-rater variation. Each student was assigned a number and the tutor was blinded to the group to which the student belonged. A commercially produced canine jaw model sourced from Veterinary Instrumentation was used, instead of the simulation model, to avoid advantaging group A and to provide a more realistic anatomical representation of an animal (Fig. 23.4). Yet, as with the simulator model, poor operator technique and incorrect use of dental instrumentation still resulted in visible damage being revealed (Fig. 23.5).

The results of the OSCE indicated that the model was an effective way to train students to perform a dental scale and polishing procedure and to operate a dental machine. The opportunity to acquire basic knowledge, understanding and skills in a safe environment was also recognized by students as being beneficial, which has important implications, not just for student learning but also for animal welfare. The training model also helped to boost students' confidence which may, in turn, increase their involvement with dental procedures while on clinical placements. The significantly improved performance of the model-trained students highlights the advantages of practical experience, a finding that is consistent with other studies that have evaluated the impact of simulators on veterinary training (Smeak *et al.*, 1991; Griffon *et al.*, 2000). In addition, these students achieved a higher number of key steps in relation to operator technique, use of instrumentation and safe practice.

The comparatively poor performance of video-trained students emphasizes the difficulty in

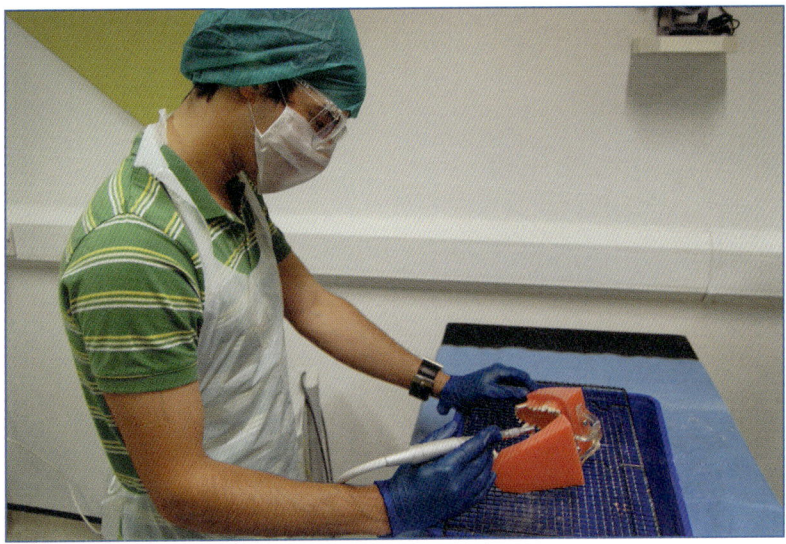

Fig. 23.4. The canine jaw model used by students in the objective structured clinical examination.

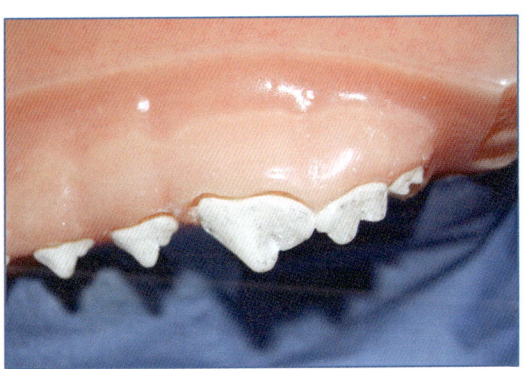

Fig. 23.5. Visible damage to the canine jaw model as a result of poor operator technique and incorrect use of dental instrumentation.

mastering a seemingly simple skill such as a professional dental cleaning procedure without the inclusion of a practical instruction method. Despite their perceived inability to offer practical experience and build confidence, videos were identified as a helpful tool for learning how to perform a professional dental cleaning procedure.

The model successfully facilitated tuition of the fundamental principles behind performing a professional dental cleaning procedure. It further enabled development of the necessary psychomotor skills required by veterinary students and future veterinarians to perform this technique safely and correctly in practice. All students identified positive themes, including those relating to practical and interactive instruction and the acquisition of skills in a safe learning environment. The simple design, tactile features and ease of use featured heavily, as did the opportunity to prepare and use dental equipment and machinery. Student comments included the following:

- 'Allowed me to see the "boundary" of where damage can be caused but in a "safe" environment, i.e. *not* a live animal!'

- 'Practical way to learn, better than trying to understand a lecture.'

- 'Being able to practise on something that didn't matter if you made mistakes.'

- 'You can see straight away how well you have done or if your technique could be improved.'

- 'Being able to use the tools and actually set up the equipment yourself.'

23.4 Meeting Student Expectations

When evaluating the type of educational resource most suited to facilitating the acquisition of veterinary dental skills, consideration has to be given to the 'visual acuity and sensory motor skills' that were considered by Steinberg *et al.* (2007, p. 1574) to be 'critical requirements for success in dentistry'. There is also an ultimate desire to create a smooth transition from preclinical laboratory to clinical environment. Whilst all students recognized the value of the dental model in facilitating the acquisition of skills for scaling and polishing teeth, the majority identified a need for tutor-assisted training in order to gain full benefit. The need for an instructor presents additional challenges in time and cost and could potentially limit access to, and use of, the model. An alternative, which has since been implemented, includes student observation of the videos as a preparatory tool, prior to a tutor-facilitated practical class involving use of the models. This has been introduced into the curriculum as part of a voluntary sign-up session for BVetMed and VN students in years one and three, respectively, and as a mandatory session for BVetMed students in year three.

Technology involving the use of simulation is adaptable to flexible scheduling, facilitates repetition of the skill to be learned in a safe environment and enables students to learn how to deal with the outcomes of their action without risk of morbidity. When questioned about the benefits of using a simulator model to learn a veterinary dental scale and polish technique, students identified similar themes including increasing confidence and learning via a practical method in a safe and stress-free environment with no risk to live patients. Student comments included the following:

- 'Amazing idea; a lot less stressful and less pressure doing it in small groups versus in practice on EMS.'

- 'A chance to practise an essential skill that is required of you upon starting a new job as a graduate. It would make me feel a lot more confident in terms of skills.'

- 'Much easier to remember how to do something if you do it practically; watching videos is helpful but can't teach you forces you need to apply and motions, etc.'

Not all study participants were able to identify aspects of the simulator model that they disliked or found ineffective, yet one of the limitations identified by several students was that it lacked certain aspects of realism, mainly in relation to the shape of the tiles. Some students commented that the model's simplicity made the task easier than on a real animal; others perceived difficulty in

applying the skills learned on broad, flat tiles to the small multi-dimensional teeth of real animals.

Other limitations included the inability to assess the effectiveness of polishing and not being able to 'crack' off heavy accumulation of calculus using tartar forceps. In addition, it did not enable students to learn sub-gingival cleaning, an important step in dental prophylaxis and one identified by Niemiec (2008) as a more complex skill to master. Other models, commercially produced, have since been purchased for teaching this and other advanced dentistry-related skills, including exodontia. These learning tools have promoted student interaction and enabled students to use the required resource repeatedly until they have mastered a skill. Yet a common limitation remains their limited ability to provide tactile and pressure-related feedback on performance. As identified by Bakr *et al.* (2015), the most obvious differences in dental instrument usage between novices and experts relate to the extent of instrument movement and the force used during the procedure. Students need to develop a fine sense of touch and pressure early in their learning cycle, warranting use of virtual reality (VR) simulation and haptic technology.

In spite of these valid limitations, the model successfully facilitated tuition of the fundamental principles behind performing a professional dental cleaning procedure and development of the necessary psychomotor skills that are required to perform this technique safely and correctly in practice, either while being observed during clinical placements or once qualified. In addition, in comparison with commercially produced models, materials were easy to source, relatively low in cost, robust and reusable, rendering the model a cost-effective teaching tool.

23.5 Future Aspirations

23.5.1 The use of more sophisticated technologies

Dental education has evolved through the years and various technologies are being incorporated into the curriculum to improve fine motor skills and hand–eye coordination in preclinical settings to allow for smooth transition to the clinical setting. Due to the nature of veterinary dentistry and the skills that are subject to assessment, the ethical and welfare issues surrounding the use of living or deceased animals are too great. The wide use of VR, simulation and haptic technologies in the instruction of competences that are considered to be dangerous, painful or rare reflects the realization that the clinical setting is not an ideal environment for skills training in healthcare professions. These types of technologies can provide an effective training method for the development of operative dental skills and offers the provision to practise in a realistic, yet safe, environment, filled with objective and rapid feedback. VR has also been acknowledged as enabling students to progress from the acquisition to the application of knowledge at a faster rate. Such a notion is important for student users of the RVC Clinical Skills Centre who have traditionally commented on a perceived limited amount of time to master their practical skills. Jasinevicius *et al.* (2004) further identified the ability of VR to highlight students who may require additional instruction – an issue that may go undetected, particularly when teaching large student numbers, and therefore an important consideration for educators.

23.5.2 Summative assessment of veterinary dentistry

Biggs's (1999) notion of constructive alignment optimized the conditions for quality learning and promoted the successful integration of teaching and learning methods. By this, an inference is made that desirable higher-order and deeper learning processes can be elicited by reviewing the teaching and assessment systems together as one, ensuring that they are most appropriate to the course curriculum and requisite learning outcomes.

Currently, RVC veterinary and VN students' knowledge of veterinary dentistry is assessed through the completion of multiple-choice and short-answer questions, yet as Hodges (2006) proclaimed, knowledge tests alone are unlikely to be adequate in examining skills or attitudes. Therefore additional assessment methods that consider the students' ability to perform basic prophylactic dental skills are also required. The addition of a small animal veterinary dental simulator and haptic component at the RVC would enable greater sophistication in creating simulations of various veterinary dental examination techniques and periodontal procedures, facilitating a smoother transition to the clinical environment. When combined with modification of

learning objectives, this could also assist in the development of higher-level thinking aptitudes such as tactile, critical analysis, decision making and problem-solving skills. Since such tools are computer driven, there is the feasibility to monitor students' progress, frequency of use and assessment of performance (Steinberg *et al.*, 2007), thus helping to produce a unified system of teaching, learning and assessment.

23.5.3 Inter-professional education

Another aspiration is to promote peer-assisted learning and to further develop undergraduate inter-professional collaboration through the use of the dental model and associated teaching station. Attitudes of RVC students towards inter-professional education (IPE) for the acquisition of elementary veterinary dental skills prior to and after use of the dental model have been sought. Unpublished findings concurred with comparable research in identifying the delivery of IPE during the pre-qualification stage of training as facilitating future collaborative approaches to clinical practice and enhancing future working relations. IPE using the veterinary dental model positively influenced attitudes towards veterinary dental education with students identifying the need for and advantages associated with inter-professional learning of this subject.

The study also raised student awareness of the requirement for students to learn similar skills and knowledge associated with routine dental hygiene work, in addition to highlighting the differences between professional roles in relation to the provision of veterinary dental care and treatment. More consistent inter-professional use of the model is predicted to positively influence attitudes towards collaborative veterinary dental practice. In turn, this is expected to improve awareness of professional roles, dental skills and clinical experience, promote positive working relationships and advance the quality of dental healthcare to veterinary patients.

23.6 The Outcome of the Development of this Model

Although small scale, this study has emphasized that a simple, inexpensive model has proven effectiveness in facilitating the acquisition of basic veterinary dental skills and students recognized its value as a training tool. Whilst there remains a need for traditional instruction methods, a dental model is a useful adjunct for the acquisition of foundation-level veterinary dental skills including scaling and polishing, use of dental instrumentation and manual dexterity. Integration of the use of this model into the curriculum can better prepare students to assist with the technique on live animals, leading to enhanced student confidence and more rapid skills acquisition.

The results of this study have been written up, presented and defended as part of a successful RVC MSc in Veterinary Education project. In addition, a manuscript by Lumbis *et al.* (2012) has been published in the *Journal of Veterinary Medical Education*. The skills sheets, tutor's teaching notes and instructions for making the model are available to others online, enabling students around the world to benefit from a validated training tool for learning the important skills necessary for performing a dental scale and polish.

References: Bakr, M.M., Massey, W.L. and Alexander, H. (2015) Can virtual simulators replace traditional preclinical teaching methods: a students' perspective? *International Journal of Dentistry and Oral Health* 2(1). http://dx.doi.org/10.16966/2378-7090.149.

Bartlett, D.W., Coward, P.Y., Wilson, R., Goodsman, D. and Darby, J. (2001) Experiences and perceptions of vocational training reported by the 1999 cohort of vocational dental practitioners and their trainers in England and Wales. *British Dental Journal* 191(5), 265–270.

Biggs, J. (1999) What the student does: teaching for enhanced learning. *Higher Education Research & Development* 18(1), 57–75.

Bleakley, A. (2006) Broadening conceptions of learning in medical education: the message from teamworking. *Medical Education* 40, 150–157.

Brine, E.J., Manfra Marretta, S., Pijanowski, G.J. and Siegel, A.M. (2000) Comparison of the effects of four different power scalers on enamel tooth surface in the dog. *Journal of Veterinary Dentistry* 17(1), 17–21.

BVA (2012) British Veterinary Association and the Association of Veterinary Students Survey results 2012. Available at: https://www.bva.co.uk/uploadedFiles/BVA % 20AVS % 20 Survey % 20results % 202012.pdf (accessed 7 May 2017).

Chamblee, J. and Reiboldt, M. (2010) *Financial Management of the Veterinary Practice.* American Animal Hospital Association Press, Lakewood, Colorado, USA.

Cleland, W.P. (2001) Opportunities and obstacles in veterinary dental drug delivery. *Advanced Drug Delivery Reviews* 50, 261–275.

Colmery, B. (2005) The gold standard of veterinary oral health care. *Veterinary Clinics of North America: Small Animal Practice* 35, 781–787.

Davis, M.H., Ponnamperuma, G.G., McAleer, S. and Dale, V.H.M. (2006) The objective structured clinical examination (OSCE) as a determinant of veterinary clinical skills. *Journal of Veterinary Medical Education* 33(4), 578–587.

Fugill, M. (2005) Teaching and learning in dental student clinical practice. *European Journal of Dental Education* 9, 131–136.

Goldstein, G., Chapman, A., Herzog, L. and McClure, G.D. (2016) Routine use of a thiol-detection test in every wellness examination increased practice dental revenues and enhanced client compliance with dental recommendations in veterinary general practice clinics. *Journal of Veterinary Science & Technology* 7(2). doi:10.4172/2157-7579.1000312.

Griffon, D.J., Cronin, P., Kirby, B. and Cottrell, D.F. (2000) Evaluation of a hemostasis model for teaching ovariohysterectomy in veterinary surgery. *Veterinary Surgery* 29, 309–316.

Hodges, B. (2006) Medical education and the maintenance of incompetence. *Medical Teacher* 28(8), 690–696.

Issenberg, S.B. and McGaghie, W.C. (2002) Clinical skills training – practice makes perfect. *Medical Education* 36, 210–211.

Jasinevicius, T.R., Landers, M., Nelson, S. and Urbankova, A. (2004) An evaluation of two dental simulation systems: virtual reality versus contemporary non-computer-assisted. *Journal of Dental Education* 68(11), 1151–1162.

Johnston, N. (2011) Periodontal disease: systemic consequences in wider focus. *Veterinary Times* 41(22), 10–12.

Kneebone, R. and Baillie, S. (2008) Contextualised simulation and procedural skills: a view from medical education. *Journal of Veterinary Medical Education* 35(4), 595–598.

LeBlanc, V.R., Urbankova, A., Hadavi, F. and Lichtenthal, R.M. (2004) A preliminary study in using virtual reality to train dental students. *Journal of Dental Education* 68(3), 378–383.

Lumbis, R., Gregory, S. and Baillie, S. (2012) Evaluation of a dental model for training veterinary students. *Journal of Veterinary Medical Education* 39(2), 128–135.

Macluskey, M. and Hanson, C. (2011) The retention of suturing skills in dental undergraduates. *European Journal of Dental Education* 15(1), 42–46.

May, S.A. and Head, S.D. (2010) Assessment of technical skills: best practices. *Journal of Veterinary Medical Education* 37(3), 258–265.

Miller, G.E. (1990) The assessment of clinical skills/competence/performance. *Academic Medicine* 65(9) S63–S67.

Niemiec, B.A. (2008) Periodontal therapy. *Topics in Companion Animal Medicine* 23(2), 81–90.

Putter, G. (2011) Pet dentistry: are we still only scratching the surface? *Veterinary Business Journal* 102, 8–10.

RCVS (2017) *Delegation to Veterinary Nurses.* Available at: http://www.rcvs.org.uk/advice-and-guidance/code-of-professional-conduct-for-veterinary-surgeons/supporting-guidance/delegation-to-veterinary-nurses/ (accessed 7 May 2017).

Robinson, N.J., Dean, R.S., Cobb, M. and Brennan, M.L. (2015) Investigating common clinical presentations in first opinion small animal consultations using direct observation. *Veterinary Record* 176(18), 1–7. doi:10.1136/vr.102751.

RVC (2017) *Bachelor of Veterinary Medicine Day One Skills Handbook*. Available at: http://www.live.ac.uk/Media/LIVE/PDFs/day_one_handbook.pdf (accessed 3 October 2017).

Schön, D. (1983) *The Reflective Practitioner: How Professionals Think in Action*. Temple Smith, London.

Schönwetter, D.J., Lavigne, S., Mazurat, R. and Nazarko, O. (2006) Students' perceptions of effective classroom and clinical teaching in dental and dental hygiene education. *Journal of Dental Education* 70(6), 624–635.

Smeak, D.D. Beck, M.L. Schaffer, C.A. and Gregg, C.G. (1991) Evaluation of video tape and a simulator for instruction of basic surgical skills. *Veterinary Surgery* 20(1), 30–36.

Steinberg, A.D., Bashook, P.G., Drummond, J., Ashrafi, S. and Zefran, M. (2007) Assessment of faculty perception of content validity of PerioSim©, a haptic-3D virtual reality dental training simulator. *Journal of Dental Education* 71(12), 1574–1582.

Simulators in Veterinary Clinical Skills Education: Background and Examples

24

Tierney Kinnison
The Royal Veterinary College, London

Introduction

The terms simulator, simulation and models can be confusing in the context of clinical skills training. The *Oxford English Dictionary*'s definition of a 'simulator' is 'a machine that imitates the controls and conditions of a real vehicle, process, etc., used for training or testing' (OED, 2012). An obvious example of such a machine would be a flight simulator. A flight simulator requires the trainee pilots to use multiple skills and competences in carrying out a whole task, flying an aeroplane, as if for real. It is more than practising a skill in isolation. This chapter does not aim to discredit the value of bench-top models and fully acknowledges the importance of mastering individual skills in such an effective manner. However, it is also imperative that trainees building up these skills are able to use them within their future context and within the context of their current education.

The beginning of this chapter will draw frequently on the work of Roger Kneebone and his teams, due to his significant contribution and influence in the world of medical simulation. Kneebone (2003) supported the above statements in his outline of the importance of locating simulators within education and clinical practice. His team also identified that contextualized 'distributed simulation' provides an ideal stage between bench-top models and real surgery (Kassab *et al.*, 2012).

In their article about simulators for veterinary professional and clinical skills, Scalese and Issenberg (2005, p. 461) defined simulators as 'a device or set of conditions that aims to imitate real patients, anatomic regions, or clinical tasks, and/or to mirror the real life situations in which medical services are rendered'. Therefore, within this chapter, the focus will remain on tools that allow veterinary students to practise multiple skills or whole competences *within their real-life context* (either part of the whole animal, the whole animal, or the full real-life context). Considering the Day One

Competences by the Royal College of Veterinary Surgeons, there are a couple of competences that clearly fit with this notion of simulators: 'Perform a complete clinical examination' and 'Perform first aid' (RCVS, 2014).

24.1 Why Simulators?

Simulators can have many benefits for veterinary students, educators and animals (and therefore their owners). Chapter 1 in this volume ('Developing Veterinary Clinical Skills: The Pedagogy' by Stephen A. May) provides an excellent introduction to the benefits for student learning of tools that develop clinical skills. For example, the chapter discusses deliberate practice and active learning. For students, simulators can provide an opportunity for deliberate practice that is a significant factor in explaining the development of expertise (Kulasegaram *et al.*, 2013). In addition to the opportunity for ongoing practice, students from veterinary schools have been suggested to prefer learning by physical activity (active) and prefer hands-on learning (sensing), as opposed to being reflective and intuitive (Neel and Grindem, 2010). Kolb's learning cycle also outlines the importance for learning of a concrete experience, within a cycle of reflective observation, abstract conceptualization and active experimentation (Kolb, 1984). Simulators are ideal for providing hands-on concrete experiences. Mirroring the suggestions of May in Chapter 1 regarding clinical skills centres in general, Kneebone (2003) considered advantages of simulators to include a 'safe' learning environment, where the learning can be student-centred with effective feedback. Simulator experiences are safe for the students, in that they can make a mistake with no fear of causing actual harm, and can then learn from the mistake. Subsequently this is likely to make patients safer too. Other factors of simulators leading to effective learning include

© CAB International 2018. *Veterinary Clinical Skills Manual* (eds N. Coombes and A. Silva-Fletcher)

incorporating a range of difficulty levels, multiple learning strategies and capturing clinical variation (Issenberg *et al.*, 2005). The complementary nature of simulators and Vygotsky's Zone of Proximal Development (ZPD) has also recently been identified (Clapper, 2015). The ZPD is the area between which a student is in their comfort zone in terms of learning, and where learning is out of their reach. It is an area where scaffolding of a student's understanding using simulators is an ideal way to assimilate new knowledge and skills into the student's own practice.

Teaching unsighted examinations is a challenge for educators. In an article called 'Hidden practice revealed', Low-Beer *et al.* (2011) evaluated the teaching of digital rectal examination for humans by a group of medical experts, and identified that if you are only able to listen to the expert, and not see what they are doing, you will miss many steps in the procedure. Simulators assist clinical experts in becoming expert teachers, as they often allow the student to see what they are required to do, or allow the expert to see what the student is doing and provide feedback. Simulators also offer educators the chance to provide learning opportunities that would not ordinarily arise at all, or as often, in the university's real life caseload.

It is perhaps easy to see the benefits for animals of introducing simulators into veterinary curricula. Veterinary students can be more confident and competent prior to ever practising on a real animal, and in theory will subsequently require less practice to reach proficiency. Simulators allow veterinary students to maintain the regard and respect for animals that is at the heart of the veterinary profession's ethos (Martinsen and Jukes, 2005). As such, global veterinary curricula have reacted to the views of their students, staff and regulatory governors and have reduced the use of animals where appropriate, which provides an example for other areas where animal use is still occurring (for example, in secondary schools) (Hart *et al.*, 2005). The correlation between safer animal patients and happier clients is obvious.

24.2   Challenges of Simulators

Although many students are conscious of the ethical issue of using animals within their education, a study in 2002 identified that students at that time preferred live animal use over models due to the ability to learn certain aspects of the task, including tissue handling, dissection, haemostasis and anaesthesia (Hedlund *et al.*, 2002). The realism of some methods of using computer-based simulations has also been questioned and limits the opportunity of replicating some tasks; for example, those requiring a whole hand, or two hands (Baillie *et al.*, 2003; Baillie *et al.*, 2005b). However, it is not suggested that simulators can totally replace all practice on live, or dead, animals. Nevertheless, this chapter argues that they can often provide an appropriate and effective adjunct to traditional teaching.

An obvious challenge in the use of simulators is that many of the high-tech simulators, and indeed models, are costly to purchase and require space to be housed and used. However, in addition to cost, the ultimate cost–benefit ratio should be considered. In one medical study, the authors considered multiple bench models to be better value than training in operating rooms (Scott *et al.*, 2000) when they factored in the estimation that 'the annual cost of training residents in the operating room is $53 million' in the USA (Bridges and Diamond, 1999; p. 31).

24.3   Types of Simulator

Simulators can be of varying fidelity (meaning how well they replicate reality). Fidelity does not necessarily correlate with learning potential, but does often correlate with cost. Models, such as bench-top models, will sometimes be called simulators (often low fidelity). However, as identified earlier, the term tends to relate more to the ability to practise multiple skills within their real-life context (to a degree). Typically, therefore, they can allow a more complete understanding of a whole procedure. A hybrid simulation combines a physical model with a computer (Kneebone, 2003), thus benefiting from the advantages of each: a realistic experience but with the flexibility of a computer's potential for creating different simulations. In medicine, such hybrid simulations can replace the physical model with a real simulated patient, and an example with a simulated client (farmer) in the veterinary field will be explored later. It should be noted that this chapter does not seek to discuss simulated patients in isolation, as that relates more to communication skills and is, therefore, outside the current scope of the chapter.

The examples of simulators within this chapter will include both manikin-based simulators and computer-hybrid simulations. In addition, a brief discussion of computer-only simulators, which involve less practical hands-on learning, will be provided.

The hybrid simulators use haptic technology, a type of virtual reality. The word 'haptic' pertains to the sense of touch. A haptic simulator facilitates a human–computer interaction that allows the user (student) to feel the images they are seeing on the screen, via the use of a robotic device. The types of haptic device used in the simulators identified below are 'grounded', meaning that the device can provide actual force feedback. This feedback pushes back against the student's hand as they hold on to the device. In this way, the student assumes they are touching something, or the device can even move the student's hand. Haptic devices are able to simulate size, shape, texture and softness. A challenge of creating haptic virtual reality simulators is the requirement of computing language-coding skills. However, even this is not insurmountable, as an interactive proto-typing tool exists (Forrest and Wall, 2006). The benefits of haptic technology include being able to transfer between simulations easily and its validation for use.

Validity of educational strategies and assessments is just as important with regard to simulations as with regard to any other type of learning. The same types of validity considerations occur with simulators (Carter *et al.*, 2005):

- Face validity – a group (usually experts) judges how well the simulator resembles the real-life activity.

- Content validity – the degree to which the simulator covers all of the aspects of the real-life activity.

- Construct validity – the ability of the simulator to differentiate between those with different abilities or experience.

- Predictive validity – a comparison of performance of the simulator with performance on established assessment methods for the same skills.

The veterinary haptic simulators presented in this chapter are quite unusual in their published record of predictive validity, which enables us to identify that the simulators are improving the competence of students, and not only their confidence (or nothing at all) (Baillie *et al.*, 2005a; Baillie and Rendle, 2008).

Another way to consider the evaluation of these pedagogical tools is to apply Kirkpatrick's four levels (Kirkpatrick, 1998). These relate to an evaluation of a training programme's effects on student reaction, learning, behaviour and results. In the field of medical inter-professional education, Hammick *et al.* (2007) adapted these levels to consider the following: (1) reaction; (2a) perceptions and attitudes; (2b) knowledge and skills; (3) behaviour; (4a) service delivery; and (4b) patient/client care. These levels are not increasing in worth; all levels are worthy of research. However, they typically increase in difficulty of evaluation and hence more publications focus on student opinions than future behaviour or effects upon patient care.

There are some challenges related to evaluating any educational initiative. For example, students trained on 'anything plus traditional methods' are likely to outperform students trained with 'traditional methods alone', simply because they spend more time on learning. In addition, students trained on a simulator are likely to perform better than those trained with traditional methods (for however long), if their ability is tested on a simulator.

24.4 Designing a Simulator

In order to increase the simulator's validity and positive evaluation, it is imperative that it is designed appropriately. Firstly, simulators should be designed to address a gap in the teaching, and educators are best placed to identify these gaps. Once the idea has been formulated for a worthwhile simulator, it may be tempting to jump straight into making the simulator resemble the real-life activity as closely as possible and then to test it with students. However, it has been observed that a teaching protocol in conjunction with the simulator provides the best teaching opportunity (Baillie *et al.*, 2005a; Read and Baillie, 2013). One way to create a teaching protocol is to use cognitive task analysis (CTA). CTA typically involves observing experts conducting a task as normal, while 'thinking aloud', and/or as if teaching a novice. The researcher records and analyses the tasks and breaks them down into parts, including where decisions are made. This method circumvents the problems of tacit knowledge, where experts are unable to describe exactly how they do a task, because it has become almost automatic, such as the intricacies of driving a car. A prime example is Read and Baillie's CTA for creating a teaching protocol for bovine dystocia (Read and Baillie, 2013).

24.5 Pedagogy with Simulators

As far as possible, it is beneficial for simulators to be integrated into the curriculum and to be timetabled. This integration demonstrates the importance of the learning to the students. Baillie *et al.* (2005b) gave an example of how a simulator, the Haptic Cow, was integrated into a veterinary curriculum.

Simulators can be freely available for students to use; however, with the large costs of some simulators this may not be advisable. More importantly, the learning potential may be limited due to the absence of a taught protocol. Students could be taught on a one-to-one basis with the simulator but this is very resource intensive. Two alternative solutions were proposed by Baillie and colleagues for the Haptic Cow: an automated version and peer-assisted learning. The automated version has been validated for use, through demonstrating the improved ability of those students who had undergone the training (Baillie *et al.*, 2010a). Peer-assisted learning (where students are trained and then teach their own year group) was also very successful, improving the tutors' confidence, providing them with teaching skills and providing the trainees with a teacher who was less intimidating (Baillie *et al.*, 2009).

As previously discussed in this chapter, simulators aim to include an element of context for a competence or series of skills. A narrow focus on just the technical aspects of this can provide the student with a distorted view of reality, by excluding the other aspects of every task, namely communication and professionalism skills. Examples of simulators that include these typically termed 'non-technical skills' are rare but do exist and may increase in the future through developments in client-focused simulation.

24.6 Examples of Veterinary Clinical Skills Simulators: Manikins and Computer Hybrids

Within this section, examples of simulators designed to teach veterinary clinical skills are explored. The examples primarily come from a search of the *Journal of Veterinary Medical Education* (*JVME*) for the term 'simulation' and are enhanced through awareness of other simulators, which may not have been written

about in the educational literature. The author does not suggest that this list is exhaustive. The examples are split into categories of species, as many simulators are species specific, mirroring the importance of context for simulators. However, some simulators focus on one general skill that is appropriate within different contexts, and we shall start with these.

24.6.1 General

Levi *et al.* (2016) compared two simulators for teaching veterinary students basic laparoscopic surgery skills. They found that both competence and confidence increased after using both simulators. One simulator (tablet trainer) was significantly cheaper than the other simulator (box trainer) and therefore may be preferred.

Read *et al.* (2016) compared two simulators for teaching ovariohysterectomy. The term simulator for one of the tools is perhaps misleading, as it is low-fidelity and low-cost, and focuses on the single task without certain lifelike features, such as a thick enough dermis. It is therefore more akin to a model. An evaluation of live animal ovariohysterectomy allowed comparison of the effectiveness of the simulator, model and traditional teaching (lab manual and video only). Students who used either the simulator or the model outperformed the other students. Odds ratio analysis identified a benefit of the simulator on six of 46 checklist items and of the model on one item. However, recent advances to the model were outlined, which makes this an equally useful teaching method.

In addition to these examples, a human simulator has been used within veterinary education (Modell *et al.*, 2002). The simulator appeared to improve students' confidence with real patients; and students trained on the simulator scored significantly higher in an examination when dealing with concepts reviewed by simulation, but not when dealing with more general concepts reviewed by methods other than simulation.

24.6.2 Small animal

Williamson (2014) validated a previously developed small animal thoracocentesis simulator, which included a chest, silicone skin, fur, ribs, intercostal spaces and reusable reservoirs. The evaluation included face and content validity through survey results and construct validity via assessing novice (student) and expert (veterinarian) performance. The survey provided favourable results and students scored significantly lower on global rating scores and took significantly longer than veterinarians take to complete the procedure, suggesting that the simulator is valid.

The vast majority of small animal simulators that have been written about in the *JVME* are canine simulations. The remainder of this section, therefore, relates to dogs.

Gopinath *et al.* (2012) described the development of an ovariohysterectomy simulator model (OSM). The simulator is silicon based and is of a medium to large breed dog in dorsal recumbency. The simulator is just part of a new initiative at the University of Sydney's Faculty of Veterinary Science, which has adapted its soft tissue surgical skills training to be in line with Day One competences and has incorporated new lectures, tutorials, clinics and an e-portfolio for tracking learning.

A simulator for cardiopulmonary resuscitation has been created via an adapted part of a human patient simulator with a dog manikin (Fletcher *et al.*, 2012). The level of evaluation of the simulator was on student reaction, perception and attitude. Students were engaged with the teaching method, wanted more opportunities to use simulators and appreciated the additional skills they were practising, such as communication and teamwork.

Usón-Gargallo *et al.* (2014a) described the development of the Canine Laparoscopic Simulator (CLS). The simulator was considered important to give student and graduated veterinarians practice with minimally invasive surgery. Tapia-Araya *et al.* (2016) validated the use of the CLS. Face validity was identified via veterinarians' perceptions of usefulness. Construct validity was identified through experienced individuals performing tasks better and faster than a control group; and in addition, a 'training' group performed better on their second attempt. Content validity was defined differently to the current chapter, namely as the appropriateness of the simulator as a teaching method, which was considered to have been valid due to the construct validity results.

Members of the same research and development team also validated a simulator, Simuldog, for gastrointestinal endoscopy training in dogs (Usón-Gargallo *et al.*, 2014b). The simulator was evaluated in having face, content and construct validity. Simuldog can be used within an operating room, where various monitors display endoscopic images. In addition, an assistant can be incorporated, which allows for communication practice at the same time as clinical skills practice.

A canine prostate palpation simulation was developed by a group in Brazil (Capile *et al.*, 2015). The group assessed student opinions and identified that students largely felt better prepared having used the simulator, and were especially pleased to be learning in a way that did not negatively affect dog welfare.

24.6.3 Large animal: bovine

'Breed'n Betsy' is probably one of the most well known bovine simulators based on a model. It is a whole package, which allows training for artificial breeding, pregnancy diagnosis and embryo transfer (Pickford, 2017). In an evaluation of Breed'n Betsy, it was demonstrated that students trained with live cows were significantly better at finding the uterus, and finding and evaluating the ovaries, than students trained on the simulator (Bossaert *et al.*, 2009). This study also identified that rectal palpation of 200 live cows was insufficient for students to demonstrate a consistent level of expertise. It was concluded that although the simulator cannot replace live animal training, it is a useful addition to traditional teaching methods.

The Haptic Cow (or Bovine Rectal Palpation Simulator) is another well known bovine simulator. In comparison with Breed'n Betsy, it is a computer hybrid, which has several advantages over model-based simulators, though also some drawbacks. Advantages include the ease of changing between simulations, while drawbacks may include a more artificial experience, with the requirement of teachers to explain aspects not involved in the simulation (Baillie and Rendle, 2008). Professor Sarah Baillie, the inventor of the Haptic Cow, has been previously mentioned in this chapter for her extensive contribution to the field of veterinary simulators. The range of publications regarding the Haptic Cow are able to demonstrate its biggest advantages: its validation for transferable skills to the real-life situation (predictive validity) and its range of effective teaching modalities. Baillie *et al.* (2003) described the development and preliminary evaluation of the Haptic Cow. Within this study, expert veterinarians assessed the haptic properties (as well as the teaching protocol and other aspects of the simulator). The haptic properties were rated as either good, or adequate for teaching, or inadequate, and any inadequate aspects were amended based on feedback. In 2005, Baillie and colleagues described the integration of the Haptic Cow into a veterinary curriculum (Baillie *et al.*, 2005b) and the validation of the simulator (Baillie *et al.*, 2005a). This validation study demonstrated that students trained with the Haptic Cow were significantly better at finding and identifying the uterus in a real cow than were students trained traditionally. Then, as outlined earlier, Baillie and colleagues successfully evaluated the use of peer teaching with the Haptic Cow (Baillie *et al.*, 2009) and the use of an automated Haptic Cow (Baillie *et al.*, 2010a) to combat challenges with teaching requirements. In addition, the Haptic Cow has been used as part of a contextualized simulation, where the simulator provides one part of the task, which also includes taking a history from a 'farmer' (who is a simulated client), making a diagnosis and deciding on treatment (Baillie *et al.*, 2010b). This Simulated Fertility Visit allows the students to behave as if they are real veterinarians and bring in several different skills, such as scientific knowledge, communication with clients, decision making in real time and professionalism. As it is a haptic simulator, it is easy to move forward in time and skip to a follow-up visit where the students can feel the results of their diagnosis and treatment from the preceding visit. Through evaluating students' perceptions, the article suggested that the Simulated Fertility Visit provides a safe opportunity to make mistakes and learn from them.

Veterinary Simulator Industries (VSI) (VSI, 2017) has a selection of bovine simulators, such as a Hereford dystocia simulator, compact dystocia model, calf dystocia, Holstein dystocia simulator, bovine theriogenology and a bovine captive-bolt gun training model. VSI is a Canadian company and works in collaboration with Emma Read, who has been cited already several times in this chapter for her contribution towards veterinary simulators.

24.6.4 Equine

Fox *et al.* (2013) designed and evaluated an equine joint injection simulator. The simulator provides an excellent example of instant feedback for students without the need for a facilitator, through the use of a buzzer that buzzes when the needle is placed into the joint correctly. Students who had learned via a textbook were significantly less likely to perform one type of injection correctly (though not another) than students who had learned on the simulator. A group who had learned on a cadaver performed even better, but due to the unavailability of cadavers, the simulator provides an effective and easy-to-access alternative.

In addition to the Haptic Cow there is a Haptic Horse, designed for training veterinary students in

diagnosing colic via rectal palpation. The Haptic Horse was evaluated as a training tool and it has been demonstrated that students trained on the simulator were more systematic in their technique of palpating the horse and were better able to differentiate normal structures from abnormal structures (Baillie and Rendle, 2008).

VSI also has a selection of equine models and simulators, which include equine theriogenology, equine neck venepuncture injection and an equine colic simulator (VSI, 2017).

24.7 Examples of Veterinary Clinical Skills Simulators: Computer-only

There are simulators that do not have a physical model, but are purely computer based. Examples include:

- DairySim dairy herd health simulator (Allore *et al.*, 2001).
- Virtual ventilator computer simulation to teach mechanical ventilation (Keegan *et al.*, 2009).
- Virtual slaughterhouse simulator (Seguino *et al.*, 2014).
- Virtual exam room (Balogh, 2014) (this is a great example of a whole examination room using high-fidelity 3D simulation to allow case-based learning).
- Interactive computerized dog's head to teach cranial nerve knowledge (Bogert *et al.*, 2015).

These simulators have similar advantages and disadvantages to simulators with a model or hybrid aspect. However, they also aid the ability for students to practise cognitive skills related to clinical skills at any time or place.

24.8 The Future

Due to continuing advances in computer technology, it is possible that the range and benefits of simulators will continue to grow exponentially. In addition, with the ever-increasing awareness of the importance of communication skills (both between veterinarian and client and between veterinary inter-professional colleagues), it is possible that patient-focused and team-focused hybrid simulators will grow in demand.

There is, it could be suggested, no point in reinventing the wheel. If these simulators are of interest to you as a veterinary educator, you could consider contacting the authors or the companies and purchasing a version for your own veterinary school. In addition, there is a group of very active developers who are continuously creating homemade simulators and who are always willing to offer their advice. This group can be found on www.noviceproject.eu. NOVICE was an EU-funded Lifelong Learning Programme project which still has as an active website designed for the 'network of veterinarians in continuing education'. It is free to join if you are a veterinary student, veterinary surgeon or an educator within a veterinary school. The 'Veterinary Clinical Skills & Simulation' group was started by Sarah Baillie and includes other authors on veterinary simulators, such as Emma Read. Please register with NOVICE and join this group if you would like to become more active in developing and disseminating veterinary clinical skills models and simulators.

References: Allore, H.G, Haferkamp-Wise, C., Gröhn, Y. and Warnick, L.D. (2001) Teaching dairy herd health dynamics using a web-based program. *Journal of Veterinary Medical Education* 28(3), 140–144.

Baillie, S. and Rendle, D. (2008) A virtual reality simulator for training veterinary students to perform rectal palpation of equine colic cases. In: *International Meeting for Simulation in Healthcare*, San Diego, Vol. 2(4).

Baillie, S., Crossan, A., Reid, S. and Brewster, S. (2003) Preliminary development and evaluation of a bovine rectal palpation simulator for training veterinary students. *Cattle Practice* 11, 101–106.

Baillie, S., Crossan, A., Brewster, S., Mellor, D. and Reid, S. (2005a) Validation of a bovine rectal palpation simulator for training veterinary students. *Studies in Health Technology and Informatics* 111, 33–36.

Baillie, S., Mellor, D., Brewster, S.A. and Reid, S.W. (2005b) Integrating a bovine rectal palpation simulator into an undergraduate veterinary curriculum. *Journal of Veterinary Medical Education* 32(1), 79–85.

Baillie, S., Shore, H., Gill, D. and May, S.A. (2009) Introducing peer-assisted learning into a veterinary curriculum: a trial with a simulator. *Journal of Veterinary Medical Education* 36(2), 174–179.

Baillie, S., Crossan, A., Brewster, S.A., May, S.A. and Mellor, D.J. (2010a) Evaluating an automated haptic simulator designed for veterinary students to learn bovine rectal palpation. *Simulation in Healthcare: The Journal of the Society for Simulation in Healthcare* 5(5), 261–266.

Baillie, S., Pierce, S.E. and May, S.A. (2010b) Fostering integrated learning and clinical professionalism using contextualized simulation in a small-group role-play. *Journal of Veterinary Medical Education* 37(3), 248–253.

Balogh, M. (2014) Applying games technology to veterinary teaching. *Veterinary Record* 174(3), 63–64.

Bogert, K., Platt, S., Haley, A., Kent, M., Edwards, G., *et al.* (2015) Development and use of an interactive computerized dog model to evaluate cranial nerve knowledge in veterinary students. *Journal of Veterinary Medical Education* 43(1), 1–7.

Bossaert, P., Leterme, L., Caluwaerts, T., Cools, S., Hostens, M. *et al.* (2009) Teaching transrectal palpation of the internal genital organs in cattle. *Journal of Veterinary Medical Education* 36(4), 451–460.

Bridges, M. and Diamond, D.L. (1999) The financial impact of teaching surgical residents in the operating room. *American Journal of Surgery* 177(1), 28–32.

Capile, K.V., Gabriela, C., Campos, G.M.B., Stedile, R. and Oliveira, S.T. (2015) Canine prostate palpation simulator as a teaching tool in veterinary education. *Journal of Veterinary Medical Education* 42(2), 146–150.

Carter, F.J., Schijven, M.P., Aggarwal, R., Grantcharov, T., Francis, N.K. *et al.* (2005) Consensus guidelines for validation of virtual reality surgical simulators. *Surgical Endoscopy and Other Interventional Techniques* 19(12), 1523–1532.

Clapper, T.C. (2015) Cooperative-based learning and the zone of proximal development. *Simulation & Gaming* 46(2), 148–158.

Fletcher, D.J., Militello, R., Schoeffler, G.L. and Rogers, C.L. (2012) Development and evaluation of a high-fidelity canine patient simulator for veterinary clinical training. *Journal of Veterinary Medical Education*, 39(1), 7–12.

Forrest, N. and Wall, S. (2006) ProtoHaptic: Facilitating rapid interactive prototyping of haptic environments. In: McGookin, D. and Brewster, S. (eds) *Haptic and Audio Interaction Design (HAID): First International Workshop*. Springer, Heidelberg, Germany, pp. 21–25.

Fox, V., Sinclair, C., Bolt, D.M., Lowe, J. and Weller, R. (2013) Design and validation of a simulator for equine joint injections. *Journal of Veterinary Medical Education* 40(2), 152–157.

Gopinath, D., McGreevy, P.D., Zuber, R.M., Klupiec, C., Baguley, J. and Barrs, V.R. (2012) Developments in undergraduate teaching of small-animal soft-tissue surgical skills at the University of Sydney. *Journal of Veterinary Medical Education*, 39(1), 21–29.

Hammick, M., Freeth, D., Koppel, I., Reeves, S. and Barr, H. (2007) A best evidence systematic review of interprofessional education: BEME Guide no. 9. *Medical Teacher* 29(8), 735–751.

Hart, L.A., Wood, M.W. and Weng, H.-Y. (2005) Mainstreaming alternatives in veterinary medical education: resource development and curricular reform. *Journal of Veterinary Medical Education* 32(4), 473–480.

Hedlund, C.S., Hosgood, G. and Naugler, S. (2002) Surgical education: attitudes toward animal use in teaching surgery at Louisiana State University. *Journal of Veterinary Medical Education* 29(1), 50–55.

Issenberg, S.B., McGaghie, W.C., Petrusa, E.R., Lee Gordon, D. and Scalese, R.J. (2005) Features and uses of high-fidelity medical simulations that lead to effective learning: a BEME systematic review. *Medical Teacher* 27(1), 10–28.

Kassab, E., Kyaw Tun, J. and Kneebone, R.L. (2012) A novel approach to contextualized surgical simulation training. *Simulation in Healthcare: Journal of the Society for Simulation in Healthcare* 7(3), 155–161.

Keegan, R., Henderson, T. and Brown, G. (2009) Use of the Virtual Ventilator, a screen-based computer simulation, to teach the principles of mechanical ventilation. *Journal of Veterinary Medical Education* 36(4), 436–443.

Kirkpatrick, D. (1998) *Evaluating Training Programs: The Four Levels*, 2nd edn. Berrett-Koehler, San Francisco, USA.

Kneebone, R. (2003) Simulation in surgical training: educational issues and practical implications. *Medical Education* 37(3), 267–277.

Kolb, D.A. (1984) *Experiential Learning: Experience as the Source of Learning and Development*. Prentice Hall, Englewood Cliffs, New Jersey, USA.

Kulasegaram, K.M., Grierson, L.E.M. and Norman, G.R. (2013) The roles of deliberate practice and innate ability in developing expertise: evidence and implications. *Medical Education* 47(10), 979–989.

Levi, O., Michelotti, K., Schmidt, P., Lagman, M., Fahie, M. and Griffon, D. (2016) Comparison between training models to teach veterinary medical students basic laparoscopic surgery skills. *Journal of Veterinary Medical Education* 43(1), 1–8.

Low-Beer, N., Kinnison, T., Baillie, S., Bello, F., Kneebone, R. and Higham, J. (2011) Hidden practice revealed: using task analysis and novel simulator design to evaluate the teaching of digital rectal examination. *American Journal of Surgery* 201(1), 46–53.

Martinsen, S. and Jukes, N. (2005) Towards a humane veterinary education. *Journal of Veterinary Medical Education* 32(4), 454–460.

Modell, J.H., Cantwell, S., Hardcastle, J., Robertson, S. and Pablo, L. (2002) Using the human patient simulator to educate students of veterinary medicine. *Journal of Veterinary Medical Education* 29(2), 111–116.

Neel, J. A. and Grindem, C.B. (2010) Learning-style profiles of 150 veterinary medical students. *Journal of Veterinary Medical Education* 37(4), 347–352.

OED (2012) *Oxford English Dictionary*. Oxford University Press, Oxford, UK.

Pickford, B. (2017) *Complete Bovine & Equine Training Simulation Packages*. Available at: http://www.breednbetsy.com.au/ (accessed 7 February 2017).

RCVS (2014) *Day One Competences*. Available at: http://www.rcvs.org.uk/document-library/day-one-competences/ (accessed 26 June 2015).

Read, E.K. and Baillie, S. (2013) Using cognitive task analysis to create a teaching protocol for bovine dystocia. *Journal of Veterinary Medical Education* 40(4), 397–402.

Read, E.K., Vallevand, A. and Farrell, R.M. (2016) Evaluation of veterinary student surgical skills preparation for ovariohysterectomy using simulators: a pilot study. *Journal of Veterinary Medical Education*, 43(2), 1–24.

Scalese, R.J. and Issenberg, S.B. (2005) Effective use of simulations for the teaching and acquisition of veterinary professional and clinical skills. *Journal of Veterinary Medical Education* 32, 461–467.

Scott, D.J., Bergen, P.C., Rege, R.V., Laycock, R., Tesfay, S.T. *et al.* (2000) Laparoscopic training on bench models: better and more cost effective than operating room experience? *Journal of the American College of Surgeons* 191(3), 272–283.

Seguino, A., Seguino, F., Eleuteri, A. and Rhind, S.M. (2014) Development and evaluation of a virtual slaughterhouse simulator for training and educating veterinary students. *Journal of Veterinary Medical Education* 41(3), 233–42.

Tapia-Araya, A.E., Usón-Gargallo, J., Enciso, S., Pérez-Duarte, F.J., Díaz-Güemes Martin-Portugués, I. *et al.* (2016) Assessment of laparoscopic skills in veterinarians using a canine laparoscopic simulator. *Journal of Veterinary Medical Education* 43(1), 71–79.

Usón-Gargallo, J., Tapia-Araya, A.E., Díaz-Güemes Martin-Portugués, I. and Sánchez-Margallo, F.M. (2014a) Development and evaluation of a canine laparoscopic simulator for veterinary clinical training. *Journal of Veterinary Medical Education* 41(3), 218–224.

Usón-Gargallo, J., Usón-Casaús, J.M., Pérez-Merino, E.M., Soria-Gálvez, F., Morcillo, E. *et al.* (2014b) Validation of a realistic simulator for veterinary gastrointestinal endoscopy training. *Journal of Veterinary Medical Education* 41(3), 209–217.

VSI (2017) VSI Home. Available at: http://vetsimulators.net/ (accessed 6 February 2017).

Williamson, J.A. (2014) Construct validation of a small-animal thoracocentesis simulator. *Journal of Veterinary Medical Education* 41(4), 384–389.

25 The Transition between the Clinical Skills Lab and the Real World – Perspectives from a New Graduate 2 Years After Qualifying

Desiree Janine Herrick

Vets4Pets, Basildon, UK

Introduction

As a new graduate, the transition from veterinary school into the 'real' world can hit you with shock and an overwhelming sense of responsibility. The safe environment that you have stayed in for the past 4 or 5 years is gone, and a wealth of responsibility has been thrust upon you. You are left with feelings of incompetence and intimidation of expectations in the work place. Suddenly, you go from asking questions to the one who is having questions asked of you. This steep learning curve is frightening, exciting and full of challenges not yet experienced, as one takes the next step from university to general practice.

I have been qualified just over 2 years now and nobody tells you just how much of being in practice meets your expectations and falters at the same time. No amount of studying and practice at university can quite prepare you for the sudden reality and the absolute amount of responsibility that falls upon you when you start. It does not matter whether you are a newly qualified veterinary student or veterinary nurse; it is an overwhelming rush the moment you step through that practice door where you might be expected to perform immediately. This transition period is where our critical learning and practice make an intersection.

The more confident a new graduate can feel in their capabilities, with regards to both their knowledge and practical skills, the more likely it is that this will have a positive impact on the start of their career, and on the practice that they are joining. Universities are always changing their structure and format to help to acclimate students in better preparation for their chosen career. For veterinary students, this means the importance of not only a wealth of knowledge, but also a handful of critical practical skills with which they are expected to hit the ground running.

25.1 Clinical Skills Centre (CSC) as a Student

As a student, the CSC allows you to observe a demonstration of a skill, understand the theoretical application of it and then try it hands on. Additionally, it provides you with resources to complement learning. For me, this was always the best way to learn. I had to learn by doing in order to remember anything worthwhile. This was often reflected in my rotation scores, which consistently graded my practical skills higher than my knowledge. These essential skills are integrated into our student placements and ultimately your chosen career path. Unique to the CSC are its teaching methods. A variety of skills sets are taught and practised with the underlying aim of acquainting students with the practical aspect of their skills. Its hands-on approach focuses on perfecting methods commonly used in practice, where you ultimately learn by doing. As a student, you commonly focus on how to do these methods step by step. It is not until you venture into placements or graduate and start practice that you begin to realize that the methods taught in the CSC are simply a guide; other methods do exist as well. Often co-workers or mentors on placement suggest other ways to do a skill set. These other ways sometimes offer students a better way to adapt to a skill they were previously struggling with. Not everyone learns through the same method: some grasp a concept better from reading, others from doing. The CSC provides a good mix of resources for its students. Having spoken with friends and classmates who have gone through the CSC, all agreed that the teaching methods done at the skills centre were far more consistent than experienced in lectures or on rotations. Educational knowledge in the veterinary field can be tricky, as often even experts have more than one argument and answer for the same question. The CSC

© CAB International 2018. *Veterinary Clinical Skills Manual* (eds N. Coombes and A. Silva-Fletcher)

focuses on an underlying tone of teaching solid practical methods and often the answers are far more direct. Consistency and a hands-on approach helps students to learn, but also helps those concepts to stick.

Students are given the clinical freedom to come and go as they please within the CSC. There are resounding resources within the skill centre, true to the motto that 'you get out what you put in'. Opportunities vary from completely independent learning, to smaller group sessions. Often this is a nice method as students can tie it directly to what is being covered in lectures, while others can focus on areas which they would like to strengthen. In my experience, final-year students use the CSC more than most other years. The expectations on rotations are high and the build-up to the exams at the CSC – the objectively structured clinical examinations (OSCEs) – means that students flood in and out throughout the final year. Rotation students find themselves utilizing the space to freshen up skills such as gowning and gloving or hand ties for surgical rotations. The suturing station is also quite commonly accessed to perfect techniques that might be assessed on lucky dip. Other students need to familiarize themselves with ultrasound equipment or setting up for radiographs. It was not uncommon for our rotation group to practise in the centre before starting a new rotation.

Prior to graduation, students often have limited ability to practise Day One skills and a lot depends on your placements as a student. Each placement varies; some provide students with plenty of hands-on opportunities while others do not, which makes access to the lab even more important. I was fortunate, as many of my placements allowed me to practise anything from surgery to dentals. Many of them allowed me to pick areas that I wanted practise in, and let me delve in hands on. Unfortunately, not all of my friends were as fortunate with their placements. Having the CSC helps to level the field and presents students with an opportunity to familiarize themselves with a certain skill set before it really matters.

25.2 Early Skill Development in Practice

Once immersed in a clinical setting, the discrepancies between education and work become apparent. Clinical settings sometimes, but not always, push away from the idealism seen in education. This can be frustrating when freshly qualified and when ideal practice has been what you are most familiar with.

There is a great deal of information that employers know will come with years on the job – those more complicated surgical procedures such as exploratory operations, diagnosing the occasional rare medical case such as myasthenia gravis, etc. But there is a great amount of pressure on new graduate students to hold a set of basic practical skills. These are skills that you are expected not only to know but also to feel competent in. The Day One skills identified by the Royal College of Veterinary Surgeons (RCVS) list the application of certain principal skills as well. Senior staff members at the practice are aware that new graduates will need some looking after and reassurance when it comes to getting things right. They do not, however, want to have to oversee need-to-know skills such as gowning, gloving or how to place a catheter. Day One skills are made clear to students prior to graduation, but it is not until that point when you go to perform a task that you realize why lecturers had insisted you should practise it a hundred times. There is nothing more intimidating than when you go to scrub and glove for your first surgical procedure in practice, with all eyes on you, wondering if you know what you are doing. A safety net no longer exists if it all goes wrong.

It is near impossible to make a direct translation from examples in the CSC to real life, but the more realistic the examples can be, the smoother can be the transition into practice. Speaking with fellow classmates, techniques that were more hands on and similar to what we have each experienced are the ones we struggle less with in practice. Take, for example, our dental practical. We were each given a tile with paint on it. We were taught how to use the dental equipment and then shown how to apply that equipment to the tile as if we were performing a dental. The feel of the scaler when it flicked off the paint from the tile was similar to the feel of removing tartar from a tooth. That stuck with me. The feel of the equipment and the response of the equipment within that setting simulated what I should see and feel during a dental. That direct application of technique is one of the best ways for me to understand what I am expecting during a real-life dental. It is easier to translate how and what, when you have had a near-similar experience before.

This applies not only to technique, but materials and equipment as well. It can be as simple as using the same brand of vet wrap or radiology equipment. Even now in general practice, I have nurses who are disgruntled when we order a different brand of cannula, as one gets used to using a particular type. The same applies to students when having to make the translation from lab to life. We become comfortable handling certain materials and brands within the lab and we are lucky when those same ones appear in practice: it is one less aspect from our teachings that has to be applied differently. When things are different, it is not the end of the world; it is just a matter of adjusting the familiar.

25.3   The Employer

Graduation is a strange mix of emotions: happiness in completing the course but also an unsettling mix of anxiety and an employer's expectations that the new graduate was not expecting. Some students are lucky enough to have been offered jobs through previous extramural studies (EMS) placements. Securing a job prior to graduation helps students to plan ahead but also allows them to start practice in a familiar space.

Unlike several of my friends, I refused even to look at jobs until I could confirm that I had passed exams. I did not want or need additional pressure on myself, while I was already overwhelmed with finals. This was both a blessing and a curse. While I eliminated pressure from the exam room, I gained it once I qualified. Friends from the classroom and rotations had now also become my competitors in the job hunt. There are few things that newly qualified veterinary students can do to make them stand out from other newly qualified vets. This alone can feel like enormous pressure when searching for employment prospects.

Expectation levels of new graduates will vary from practice to practice and from employer to employer. While going through the interview process soon after graduation, I noticed how desirable practical skills were to potential employers – not just surgical experience but handling techniques, familiarity with equipment, ability to get blood samples or place intravenous lines. Most interviewers wanted theoretical evidence of how well studied a potential candidate was, but many were also keen on the practical application of skills.

Apart from formal interviews, members of my class (myself included) commonly experienced working interviews. This unique approach to watching a candidate in the working environment can give an employer a thorough indication of whether or not your skills match your CV. As a student who has prided herself on practical application, working interviews to me were my chance to stand out. A combination of previous experience, hours in the CSC and time on placements had made me comfortable in a working setting. They gave me a chance to highlight my talent and initiative and show how I could make a strong contribution to the team. These day-to-day skills are an asset to any new graduate's CV. As a recent graduate, it also means you are more likely to bring up-to-date skills with you alongside a modern research initiative. General practices constantly aim to maintain the newest standards and to modernize the way they work, and the clients love it. The ability of a student to bring in new techniques can help a clinic to grow firmly and stabilize its place in modern veterinary practice.

25.4   Adapting to Clinical Practice

The CSC acts as a guideline, a testing ground for students to trial new skills, refresh old ones and ask questions in a safe environment before venturing out in general practice. Once transitioning into practice, students will note the theory versus practical incongruities. The CSC gives you the ability to learn the concept but it is up to you to apply it in the clinical context. There is a structure behind everything we are taught at university but it is very grey. With practical application in particular, there is no right way. In the end, you learn that there are a dozen different ways to accomplish the same outcome. Working in a team means working with people of different backgrounds and education levels, often collaborating together to form multiple perspectives.

From time to time, I end up not necessarily needing certain skills in practice, or at least, not using them extensively. Some skills I use almost daily, others weekly and some monthly. While we are taught a variety of skills, sometimes a role ends up being expected of others, rather than myself. At my particular practice, radiography is often given to the nurses to complete. If there is a staff shortage, or if I am available, I am then expected to step in and know what to do. Likewise, a nursing friend of mine recently told me that she rarely uses skills such as intubation or suturing, as the vets are the ones who most often perform those tasks. However, in a given situation she would be expected to know how to carry out these skills if requested. Real life is all about adaptability; whether we use the skills or not, we need to have at least a basic structure of what to do should it be necessary. There are other skill sets that can be disregarded depending on the type of practice one goes into. Companion animal practice will not necessarily use the skills taught for equine or farm practice, and vice versa. These are vital to learn and be competent in for educational purposes, but do not necessarily apply, depending on the practice you seek.

Soon after qualifying, I remember being asked by one of the nurses to assist with a set of limb radiographs, but to my amazement I could barely remember a thing about positioning. Fear, perhaps, held back my initial ability, as it was the first time I had to apply what I had learned at university in a clinical context. My lack of consistency in doing such tasks had made me wary of jumping straight in for fear of doing it wrong. Unfortunately, this is only one example of what often happens to new graduates. We think things in practice are black and white like we see at university. This is simply not the case in reality and yet it takes us time to reconcile with it. We forget that, within the teaching setting, we are given examples but nothing is 'cookie cutter' in life. Those hesitations eventually fade and practical application often becomes second nature.

University can only prepare students so much, but ultimately many skills are developed and honed in practice. Students can be prepared, but not wholly ready, for the transition state that follows shortly after graduation. No class can fully prepare you for what you will encounter in the workplace. A lot, too, comes down to timing. In the lab or classroom, it is easy to take your time with each step and process it as you complete it. However, timing is everything in practice. It is easy to place a cannula on a non-moving object, but entirely different when your patient is trying to bite you at the same time. It is far harder to maintain an idealistic way to perform a task when you are dealing with live animals and have consultations waiting. Proficiency does eventually come, with time, practice and patience. If anything, I like to think my practical and theoretical skills have improved with the time pressures sometimes placed upon me in practice.

25.5 Co-workers

Since starting in practice, my co-workers have easily become my biggest mentors. You teach one another, you learn from one another and seek to improve the working environment together. This collaboration benefits not only the patients that we work with, but also the practice as a whole. A lot of what I have learned outside of university and since starting in practice, I have learned from my co-workers – shared techniques, tips for surgery and advice on what might interest me. I have found that the ability to ask them questions and observe skills has made a huge difference to my professional and personal growth. This alone helps to make the connection from everything I had learned at university and allows me to see its application in the real world. The ability to connect those dots has helped me become a more rounded veterinary surgeon. What I may lack in one area, a colleague can assist me with and vice versa. We each have areas of strengths, or even interests, and we aim to help one another achieve the most we can in these areas. This is both good and bad, as my skills in one area may flourish but may lack in another. One of my interests lies in cardiology, which has allowed me to gain a lot of confidence in using the ultrasound equipment and trying out echoes. However, I have fallen behind on my ability to perform tasks such as dentals, as I tend to hand them over to colleagues who enjoy them. If I am ever feeling less than satisfied in one area of my skills, I am confident that I can ask a colleague to allow me to attempt the procedure and also get their guidance when doing so. Together, we often address the areas of weakness of what is not textbook perfect. It is important to look out for one another and to help each other to better ourselves.

Mentoring within the practice happens on a daily basis. In the past few years, I have become more confident with spays and felt eager to expand my skills by learning how to perform them with keyhole surgery. Several members of staff at my practice have attended various courses on this and have routinely been practising this technique at the clinic for years. I approached them about my desire to start learning keyhole techniques and they were more than happy to guide me. The process started with me simply watching keyhole procedures, to get a generalized picture of what was going on and how. After a few times, I began to scrub in to the procedures themselves. This allowed me to take what I had previously processed through observation and let me come to terms with the hands-on effect of the procedure. During these events, my colleagues explained the equipment, the process and the steps necessary to achieve the desired outcome. Soon, I was able to take what they had shown and taught me and I was able to do small parts of the procedure with their guidance. With some additional practice, I should be able to perform these on my own. Similarly, some newer colleagues have shown an interest in learning about echocardiography (echoes). While not a specialist, I had done further Continuous Professional Development (CPD) training in this and they began to watch me when we had cases in-house for work-up. As I had done for the keyhole procedures, my colleagues started by watching only. Once they felt comfortable enough, they began trying them hands on. I stayed to help, reassuring them when images looked good or making suggestions when needed, based on what my course had taught me. Additionally, I gave them notes from the CPDs I had attended to supplement their learning. Now, not only are my colleagues more confident in performing a basic echocardiography, but it also proves beneficial to the practice if I am away or unable to do one on a certain day.

Sometimes in practice my colleagues and I support one another in new surgical procedures at the same time. Recently, my colleague and I performed a liver mass removal on a cat. Neither of us had done this exact procedure before but we scrubbed in together and assisted one another. Before the surgery, we had read up on the necessary literature in *Small Animal Surgery* (Fossum, 2013). We then planned out our drugs together, making suggestions based on knowledge and experience in similar cases we had dealt with. Once in surgery, the two of us bounced suggestions back and forth, or provided words of encouragement when the other was unsure. Our senior staff member was able to come in from time to time to offer words of support and was contactable if needed. Both of us were able to mentor and support each other in that surgery, while never having done that exact procedure before. We were able to use our cumulative knowledge from other surgeries we had done, each of us having an area of strength, and we were able to progress in our surgical skills. Now, having done this procedure once with a colleague, I feel more confident to perform it again, especially if I am in a situation where I might be by myself. I may not be perfect in performing the surgery, but I would certainly be in a better position to handle similar cases if I were to come across them in the future.

Small acts of mentoring are also common, perhaps even more so on a daily basis. It is not uncommon for several members of staff to meet around the blood machine for a chat about results and possible outcomes. Together, we share ideas or facts from different but similar cases. At other times, we seek out the opinion of someone who has more experience in dealing with a specific diagnosis. For example, I often seek out the opinion of a colleague who has a lot of experience and interest in internal medicine: I present her with the case and the work-up I have done so far, then state my thoughts about where I want to take the case and see if I am on a reasonable track. Often, her extensive knowledge of the subject matter allows her to recommend further testing that I did not know would be helpful, or to present a diagnosis I had not considered. Now, thanks to her guidance, when faced with similar cases I feel that I have more options and can better treat patients. Again, these small acts help to improve the practice further, as we become more rounded individuals with a more extensive array of skills.

As previously mentioned, a common aspect of being in practice is developing other methods for similarly taught objectives. Both nursing and veterinary friends have mentioned this, citing what they have picked up from co-workers. As a novice within the field, you learn from peers. The working environment is not at a standstill when it comes to learning. Commonly, co-workers share what they have learned from attending CPD events with a plethora of new knowledge or techniques. These traits get passed around and developed within the practice. Different protocols get brought in and old techniques are modernized to adapt to the ever-changing field of medicine. When I initially started performing bitch spays, our practice used only catgut for ligatures and had done for years. I struggled placing my ligatures to an adequate tightness, as I had only ever used vicryl during my student placements. A colleague saw me struggling and suggested switching to polydioxanone (PDS) suture, as he was trying to adapt our older methods to be more in parallel with the gold standard recommendations he had recently heard from a CPD event. This simple recommendation made the absolute difference for my surgeries. Additionally, this adjustment allowed us to upgrade all of our surgical material and ditch the catgut for good.

25.6   Self-assessment

In reality, we actually begin self-assessment of these skills before we even leave campus. On rotations, clinicians frequently asked students to attend the CSC and try to familiarize themselves with specifics to the core modules prior to starting a specific course. One in particular that stands out is the surgical rotation. Before even starting this rotation, many students went to the CSC to study surgical materials, instruments and surgical technique. It allowed students to perfect gowning and gloving before our superiors could assess us officially. During these sessions, we were often on our own, left to decide whether our examples were sufficient or not. We would often comment to one another, 'Yes, that suture looks too tight,' or 'No, you did not break sterility.' We practised suturing on the imitation skin in preparation for our final at the end of the rotation.

This peer-to-peer evaluation also affected how we studied for finals. During OSCE preparation, peers helped to reflect on the good and bad techniques. Together, we worked through the sheets, refreshing the exact skill set in our memories and then trying it out. In these situations, one person attempted the skill, while the other observed like an examiner. This method of teaching helps you to learn a skill, demonstrates your ability to perform the task asked and teaches both of you self-critique. Prior to finals, it was not uncommon for us to get to together and create mock exam situations. The underlying result was to test your ability to perform the task but also to recognize flaws and think analytically. Together, we could discuss concerns about whether we were doing what was expected or not. Being able to recognize a flaw is characteristic when you go on to general practice. Repetitions of skills prior to examination also helped them to stick.

In a busy practice especially, there is often no one there to stop you when you are doing something wrong. It comes down to you, the individual, to assess yourself. It is an odd pressure that you put upon yourself, to decide whether or not you stick by what you have been taught. During OSCEs, students are asked whether or not they have maintained sterility during surgical procedures. This mental awareness is not just to tick a box on an exam sheet, but rather to get the student thinking about what is correct and incorrect. At the end of the day, if you break sterility in practice and nobody sees it, will you know that you have done wrong and will you take the steps to correct it? Ultimately it comes down to responsibility of performing tasks in an appropriate and safe manner. Self-assessment is important in practice, especially as we all develop bad habits as time goes on. Skills I used to know and perform with complete care and diligence, I now perform more quickly and as I have become more competent I do not need to think how I do them. It is easy to cut corners if you know you

can or will get away with it, however it breaks from the traditional teaching methods.

It is a scary, almost shocking, moment when you realize you have gained the responsibility of teaching, especially when it seemed as though you were just the one learning the skills. This moment hit me quite suddenly in practice when one of our nursing students asked for my help while studying for his OSCEs. Suddenly, I was the one who was meant to know things – not just know them, but also know them properly. No cutting corners, or cheating. Small details that I had not even thought about since my OSCE finals suddenly had to be dredged up and thought about. It is sometimes a harsh reality admitting to yourself that maybe you have not been keeping up with information as well as you should have or applying that knowledge sufficiently in practice. I and many of my friends have kept our skills sheets so that we can refer to procedures we may not have carried out for quite some time. Those sheets, like textbooks, hold valuable information that allows us to refer back and keep things fresh in our mind.

Self-assessment also comes through employers who are proactively involved in your teaching. The importance of sitting down and objectively looking at your progress and checking that it is up to date is critical. Frequent feedback forces you to pause and assess your strengths and weakness from your first few months to years in practice. It also aids in feeling effective in your role within the working environment and the progress that you make. Professional assessment is also available to some, depending on the practice. We often have an orthopaedics specialist visiting every 2 weeks, who evaluates the quality of our radiographs. Prior to working with him, my limbs radiographs were less than desirable. After collaborating with him and discussing the pros and cons of the images taken, the quality of those radiographs improved dramatically. Every pointer was learned from shared techniques and small details from his career, which ultimately helped me improve myself as a clinician.

Communication is a skill that is undervalued by students and it is difficult for universities to teach it well. However, the importance of such skills becomes apparent when you start in practice. During these past 2 years, I have learned and adapted better ways of communicating and handling these challenges; however, it has taken me a lot of practice, patience and stress to get to a point where I feel reasonably competent in addressing the issues. Providing students at university with more opportunities to address these issues, in realistic settings, can hopefully build competent communication skills and allow students to come to terms with the harsh reality they are likely to face.

25.7 Conclusion

Education, both at university and in practice, will take place in a manner where you need to build one level before the next, adding one skill at a time. It is important to remember that what happens in the skills centre does not necessarily always happen in life. The CSC is a model, an adaptation from real life to help to structure learning. In practice, the dog or cat will not always stand still while its leg is being bandaged, or stand perfectly still when you are trying to perform a fundic examination. Sometimes, you have to adapt your skills to fit your situation and it is often more difficult than you would think. At the same time, this is ultimately why the CSC is so important. If you can get a framework skills set and understand how and why things need to be done in a certain way, you will be far better off. Your employer and co-workers will help you to fill in the blank spaces of what you may not know, but you will at least have a clear step up compared with the majority of freshly graduated students.

References: Fossum, T.W. (2013) Part 1: General Surgical Principles. In: *Small Animal Surgery*, 4th edn. Elsevier Mosby, St Louis, Missouri, USA.

Glossary

Abscess – an enclosed collection of liquefied tissue, otherwise known as pus, somewhere within the body.

Adhesions – the formation of scar tissue as a response to inflammation, resulting in two surfaces adhering to each other.

Anaemia – a medical condition characterized by an abnormally low concentration of red blood cells.

Analgesia – insensibility or inability to feel pain without loss of consciousness, often created using drugs or medicines.

Anthelmintic – a group of anti-parasitic drugs used to expel parasitic worms and other internal parasites from the body.

APL valve – adjustable pressure-limiting valve, used during manual ventilation in anaesthesia.

Apnoea – the cessation of breathing.

Asepsis – the absence of bacteria, viruses and other micro-organisms.

Aspirate – to draw material in using a sucking motion. When performed on tissues, a needle and syringe is used.

Arytenoid lateralization – corrective surgery for laryngeal paralysis.

Atelectasis – the collapse of part of a lung.

Autoclave – a pressure chamber used to sterilize surgical equipment.

Bilirubin – a yellow pigment which is formed by the liver and excreted in bile.

Biochemistry – a branch of science that explores the chemical processes that occur within living organisms. It links the biology and chemistry of living cells.

Biosecurity – the set of measures taken to limit or counter the spread of disease or biological contamination.

Box joint – joint between the bones in a finger or a digit.

Bradycardia – a slower than normal heart rate.

Bronchoalveolar lavage – a diagnostic procedure in which a bronchoscope is passed into the lungs, saline infused and then aspirated for the examination of cells (cytological examination).

Canthus – either corner of the eye where the upper and lower eyelids meet. There are medial and lateral canthi: the medial one is closer to the mid-point of the face (closer to the nose) and the lateral away from the midpoint of the face.

Capillary action – the ascension of a liquid through a thin tube due to adhesive and cohesive forces interacting between the liquid and the surface.

Capnography – the monitoring of the partial pressure of carbon dioxide in the exhaled respiratory gases, usually presented as a graph.

Catheterization – the passage of a catheter into a body channel or cavity.

Caudal – towards the tail.

Coagulation – the process by which platelets are activated, adhere and aggregate to form a blood clot.

Cognition – the mental action or process of acquiring knowledge and understanding through thought, experience and the senses.

Collimation – a process that narrows a beam of particles or waves to be more aligned in a specific direction.

Contamination – the presence of an infectious agent.

COSHH – Control Of Substances Hazardous to Health.

Corticosteroids – a group of steroid hormones produced by the adrenal gland or manufactured synthetically. There are two kinds: glucocorticoids and mineralocorticoids.

CPR – cardiopulmonary resuscitation.

Cranial – towards the head.

Cytotoxic – toxic to living cells.

Decubitus ulcer – an ulcer or an open wound caused by pressure, also called bed sore on the skin.

Dehiscence – a surgical complication in which the wound ruptures along the incision site.

Dental calculus – a hard concretion that forms on the teeth through calcification of dental plaque, otherwise known as tartar.

Diff-quik stain – a commercial Romanowsky stain variant, commonly used in histological staining to rapidly stain and differentiate a variety of smears such as blood smears.

Disbudding – a common procedure to remove the horn buds from a young animal.

Distal – situated away from a certain point.

Dorsal – relating to the upper surface of an animal.

Dystocia – difficult birth/labour due to size or position of the fetus or abnormality or size of the mother's birth canal.

Echocardiography – a diagnostic procedure using ultrasound waves to create an image of the heart.

Echogenicity – the ability of a tissue or object to return a signal during an ultrasound examination (echogenicity is higher when more sound waves are reflected).

EDTA - ethylenediaminetetraacetic acid, an anti-coagulant.

Efficacy – the capacity or ability to achieve the desired effect.

Endoscopy – a non-surgical visual examination of interior structures of the body, using a flexible tube with a light and camera attached to it which is called the endoscope.

End-tidal – relating to the end of normal expiration during breathing.

Eppendorfs – small tubes used in laboratory work (especially for centrifuges) made of polypropylene, which is a relatively inert plastic characterized by low 'wettability' and high dimensional and mechanical stability across a wide temperature range.

Exodontia – the extraction of teeth.

Fenestrated – having one or more openings or pores

Flexnerian – in 1910 Abraham Flexner wrote a report called 'Medical Education in the United States and Canada' in which he suggested that clinical teaching should be underpinned by basic scientific knowledge and this gave birth to the preclinical–clinical divide in the curriculum; this is called the Flexnerian curriculum.

Fluoride oxalate – an anticoagulant that is used when taking blood for analysis. It also prevents glucose breakdown in blood and is therefore used when it is necessary to measure glucose in blood.

Grid (in relation to radiography) – a grid, made of lead, which is placed between the patient and X-ray film to reduce the scattered radiation.

Haematology – branch of medicine/veterinary medicine concerning the study of blood, the blood-forming organs and blood diseases.

Haematoma – a localized swelling that is filled with blood due to a break in the wall of a blood vessel.

Haemolysis – the rupturing of red blood cells.

Haemorrhage – the escape of blood from a ruptured blood vessel.

Haemostasis – a process by which bleeding stops.

Heparin – an anticoagulant.

Horner's syndrome – a syndrome resulting from interruption of the sympathetic nerve supply to the face and eye.

Hypoventilation – breathing at an abnormally low rate, resulting in an increased amount of carbon dioxide in the blood.

Hypovolaemia – a state of decreased blood volume.

Hypoxia – diminished availability of oxygen to the body tissues.

Iatrogenic – relating to illness caused by medical examination or treatment.

Intensifying screen (in relation to radiography) – screen used in the cassette to intensify the effect of the X-ray. The X-ray energy is absorbed by the intensifying screen material and a portion of it is converted into light. The light, in turn, exposes the film.

Isotonic crystalloid – a solution that is designed to match most closely to blood plasma so that it can be injected directly to blood (intravenously).

Jaundice/icterus – a yellowish discoloration of the skin, mucous membranes and sclera caused by elevated bilirubin levels in the blood.

Ketones – chemically known as ketone bodies, these are by-products of the breakdown of fat in the body.

kVp – kilovoltage peak, the maximum or peak voltage applied to the X-ray tube.

Laparoscopy – is a surgical procedure that uses a thin, lighted tube (endoscope) put through a cut (incision) in the belly to look at the abdominal organs.

mAs – milliamperage-seconds, a measure of radiation produced (milliamperage) over a set amount of time (seconds) via an X-ray tube.

Mastitis – inflammation of the mammary gland.

Minute volume – the volume of gas inhaled into the lungs per minute.

Myasthenia gravis – an autoimmune disease affecting the neuromuscular junction. Affected animals may show signs of weakness, difficulty in swallowing and drinking, and regurgitation.

Myoglobin – an iron- and oxygen-binding protein found in muscle tissue.

Necrotic – a form of cell death, resulting in death of cells and tissues in living tissue by autolysis.

Nerve block – a procedure performed to prevent the passage of impulses through a nerve. Often used as a component of analgesia.

Obtunded – an abnormal mental state, with reduced alertness and decreased sensitivity to pain.

Oedema – an abnormal excess accumulation of serous fluid in a tissue that can cause swelling.

Oesophagostomy tube – a feeding tube which is surgically placed into the oesophagus to provide nutrition when an animal cannot or will not eat.

Orthopnoea – the sensation of breathlessness when lying in a recumbent position.

Osmotic pressure – when pure liquid water is separated by a membrane, permeable to water but not to anything dissolved in water (called solute), then water will pass from the pure water side to the other side until both sides have equal solute. The pressure needed to stop this water movement is the osmotic pressure.

Ossifying – the process of formation of or conversion to bone.

Palmar – relating to the palm of the fore paw.

Plantar – relating to the sole of the hind paw.

Pedagogy – the method and practice of teaching.

Periodontal disease – disease affecting the tissues that support and anchor the teeth.

Peritoneal tap (also known as abdominocentesis) – the act of inserting a needle into the peritoneal space in the abdomen (which is the space unoccupied by organs) to aspirate peritoneal fluid.

Photodiodes (in relation to radiography) – a semiconductor device used to convert light into an electrical current.

Pluck (in terms of post-mortem examination) – the heart, trachea, lungs and liver of an animal.

Pneumothorax – an abnormal accumulation of air in the pleural (chest) space.

Portosystemic shunt – an abnormal vascular connection between the portal vein and another vein, resulting in blood bypassing the liver. It may be congenital or acquired.

Proximal – situated towards a certain point.

Retractors – a surgical device for retracting or opening of two surfaces, for example holding open the abdomen during surgery.

Septic thrombophlebitis – a condition characterized by blood clot formation within a vein (venous thrombosis), inflammation and bacteraemia.

Sinus arrhythmia – the normal increase in heart rate that occurs during inspiration phase of breathing.

Sphygmomanometer – a device used to measure blood pressure.

Sterility – the absence of all biological contaminants.

Stipple – the creation of a pattern by using small dots.

Somatic cell count – the number of somatic cells found in a millilitre of milk.

Stuporous - an abnormal mental state in which the animal can only be aroused by a vigorous or unpleasant stimulus.

Surgical dead space – a space remaining in the tissues as a result of failure to properly close surgical wounds, permitting the accumulation of blood or serum.

Surgical scrubs – surgical attire or suit, protective clothing worn by operating room personnel.

Sustentaculum tali – an anatomical term to describe a horizontal shelf that arises from the anteromedial portion of the heel bone or the calcaneus.

Tachycardia – a faster than normal heart rate.

Tetracyclines – a class of antibiotics which inhibit protein synthesis.

Theriogenology – the discipline of animal reproduction.

Thoracocentesis – surgical puncture and drainage of the thoracic cavity; it can be both diagnostic and therapeutic.

Thrombus – a blood clot within a blood vessel.

Tracheostomy tube – a surgical procedure in which a tube is placed into the trachea on the ventral aspect of the neck to maintain a patent airway.

Urobilinogen – a colourless by-product of bilirubin reduction which is formed in the intestine and excreted in the urine.

Venepuncture – the puncture of a vein as part of a procedure; typically to withdraw blood or give an intravenous injection.

Ventral – relating to the lower surface of an animal.

Volatile anaesthetic – anaesthetic agents which are liquid at room temperature but evaporate for inhalation.

WHO – World Health Organization.

Zoonotic disease – an infectious disease that can be transmitted between humans and animals.

Index

Note: bold page numbers indicate figures and tables.

abdominal drain 173
abdominal palpation 172
Aberdeen knot 63, 70, 71
abscess 10, 311, 319, 383
abscesses, draining 10
active learning 2, 3–4, 9
adhesions 46, 383
adrenals **260**, **262**
alfaxalone 113
alginate dressing **192**
Alleveyn (dressing material) 197
alpacas 224, 225
ammonium urate **166**
ampicillin 209
anaesthesia **13**, 17, 27, 93–128
    and apnoea 106, 113
    and blood pressure 112–113
    breathing systems *see* breathing systems
    checking depth of 110–111
    concentration administered 100
    and crystalline fluid therapy 175
    further reading on 101, 113
    and heart/respiratory rates 111, 113
    intubation *see* intubation
    monitoring 110–113, **111**, **112**
    and pain in patient 113
    and pulse oximeter 112
    questions to ask before administering 108–109
    ventilating patient 113
    and volatile anaesthetic 96, 97, 99–100, 105, 106, 385
anaesthetic machines 94, 95–104
    anatomy of **96**
    anti-hypoxic devices 97
    back bar 96
    Bodok seals 99
    changing oxygen cylinder 100–101, 104
    checking oxygen cylinder 98, **98**, **100**
    circuit check for leaks 104
    emergency oxygen flush **96**, 99, **102**
    filling keys 100, **100**
    flowmeters/rotameters 99, **103**
    further reading on 101
    health and safety issues with 95

    nitrous oxide supply 97
    and OSCE assessment 333, 335, **336**, 337, 339, **339**
    oxygen alarm 99
    oxygen supply 96–97, **96**, 333
    pin index 97, **98**
    pipeline connectors **96**, 97
    pressure gauges **96**, 99
    pressure relief valve **96**, 99
    pressure-reducing valves 99
    scavenging systems, passive/active 99
    setting up 102–104, **102**, **103**, **104**
    stand/wall bracket 96
    vacuum-insulated evaporator (VIE) 97
    vaporizer **96**, 99–100, **103**
analgesia/analgesics 97, 113, **206**, 383
anatomy 27
Animal Health Project (AHP) 20
animal welfare 203, 225–228, 331, 350, 362
antimicrobial silver dressing **192**
antiseptics 33
APL valve 105, 110, 383
apnoea 106, 113, 383
artery forceps **57**
arytenoid lateralization 66, 383
aseptic procedures 10, 30, 31, 32, 383
    and abdominal drains 174
    and breaches in sterility 33, 34, 185, 189
    for instrument pouches 50–51
    and opening of equipment packaging 33
    see also scrubbing techniques
assessment of clinical skills *see* OSCE
atelectasis 249, 383
attitude, professional 3, 20, 21
auditory stations 227–228
autoclave **52**, 53, 383
Ayres T-piece breathing system 94, 106, 107, **123–124**, 125, **125**, 126

Baillie, S. 370, 371, 372–373, 374
Bain breathing system 106, 107, 108, 120, **120–121**, 122, **122**, 126
Bakr, M.M. 364

bandages/dressings 17, 27, **186**, 190–202
    advanced 192
    canine forelimb, applying 194–196, **194**, **195**, **196**
    chest drain 193, 197–199, **197**, **198**
    ear, applying 190, 193, 200–202, **200**, **201**, **202**
    further reading on 193
    homemade 'doughnuts' 191, **193**
    and iatrogenic injuries 191
    impregnated dressings **192**
    layers of 190, 191, **192**
    lower limb (for horses) 241–245, **241**, **242**, **243**, **244**, **245**
    practising application of 192
    purpose of dressings 191
    stable (for horses) 237–240, **237**, **238**, **239**
    and sterility 192
    tail (for horses) 234–236, **234**, **235**, **236**
    tension of 190, 191, 195, **198**, 199
Bartlett, D.W. 360
behaviourism 4
Biggs, J. 365
bilirubin **160**, **161**, 383
biopsy 27, 133
    see also FNAB
biosecurity 10, 383
    see also aseptic procedures
birds 133, 220, 222
bits (horses' tack) 223
'Blacksmith Buddy' 319, **320**
Bleakley, A. 359
blood collection tubes **132**, 133, **143**
    Vacutainer 129, 135–138, **135**
blood pressure 112–113
blood samples 6, 128, 132–133, 292
    collection by syringe/needle 137–139, **137**, **138**, **139**
    collection by Vacutainer 129, 135–138, **135**
    equine 298, 299–300
    from coccygeal vein 227, **227**
    from facial venous sinus 300
    from jugular vein 299–300
    and OSCE assessment 339
    sites for 299
    tube selection **132**, 133
    Vacutainer system 129, 135–138, **135**, 300
blood smears/stains 27, 148, 152–154, **152**, **153**, **154**
blood withdrawal 27
bovine dystocia simulator **23**, 370, 373
bovine sterile milk sampling method 293, 296
bradycardia 113, 383
breathing systems 105–109
    APL valve 105, 110, 383
    Ayres T-piece 94, 106, 107, **123–124**, 125, **125**, 126
    Bain 106, 107, 108, 120, **120–121**, 122, **122**, 126
    calculating flow rates 99, 107, 108, 116, 117, 119, 122, 123, 125, 126
    and capnography 108, 110
    checking 107–108
    circle 107, 117, **117–119**, 119, 126
    clinical skills sheets for 105, 108
    and controlled ventilation 105, 106
    further reading on 113
    Lack 106, 107, 114, **114–116**, 126
    Magill 106, 107, 126
    Mapleson classification of 107
    mini-Lack 107, 126
    non-rebreathing 106, 107, 126
    rebreathing 106–107, 126
    types of, choosing 106, **106**
Breed'n Betsy 372
bronchoalveolar lavage 133, 383
bulls 223
buprenorphine 208
business management 21, 27
buster collar 174
BVetMed Day One Skills Handbook (RVC) 360

cadaver legs 319, **320**
CAL (computer-aided learning) 360, 361
calcium oxalate **166**
California Milk Test (CMT) 292, 293, 294–295, **294**
camelids 225
Canine Laparoscopic Simulator (CLS) 372
cannula placement 17
canthus 179, 250, 299, 303, 383
capillary tubes **152**, **156**
    disposal of **131**, 334
capnography 108, 110, 383
cardiopulmonary cerebral resuscitation (CPR) **13**, 372, 383
cardiovascular system 172, **172**
carotid artery 300
castration 226–227, **226**
catheterization 6, 27, 383
    see also intravenous catheter
cats **175**, 220
    handling 219, 221, 350
cattle *see* cows
cattle crush 224, **224**
cefuroxime 208
Centres for Excellence in Teaching and Learning 5, 17
cephalic vein **175**, 183–184, **183**, **184**, 299
chest drain bandage 193, 197–199, **197**, **198**
Chifney bit 223
Chinese finger-trap suture 71
chlorohexidine gluconate 33
circle breathing system 107, 117, **117–119**, 119, 126
Clinical Learning Improvement Program (CLIP, Sri Lanka) 22
clinical practice 376–382
    and communication skills 381–382
    and CPD 380
    and employer 378
    and experience gained in CSC 376–377, 380–381, 382
    and mentoring 379–380
    and self-assessment 380–382
    and skill sets 378–379

clinical skills 169–211, 358
    building competence in 359
    log books/lists 28
    model *see* veterinary clinical skills model
    pharmacy *see* pharmacy
    physical examination *see* physical examination
    tube/drain management *see* tube/drain management
clinical skills centres (CSCs) 2, 5–6, 9, 16–28, 32
    and access 2, 16, 23
    animal specimens/bone specimens in 27
    assessments at 330, 350–351
    at Lincoln Memorial University (USA) 18–20, **19**
    at Royal Veterinary College (UK) 16–18, **17**
    Cambridge Vet School 22–25, **24**
    and clinical skills log books/lists 28
    and curriculum integration 12–14
    and deliberate practice *see* deliberate practice
    development of 12–14
    and equine hoof removal 319
    and feedback 5, 12, 19
    field training 20, 21
    and handling skills 218
    in Jordan 26–29
    and learning theories/teaching skills 11
    and model creation/research 19–20
    in Mongolia 20, **21**
    portable/field-based 227–228
    reductionist approach of 6
    and simulation-based training 6, 9, 12
    and skills assessment 16, 20
    in Sri Lanka 21–22, **23**
    in Sweden 25–26, **26**
    and transition to work 376–378, 380–381, 382
    and veterinary nurses/technicians 6
Clinquest (software) 334, 339–340
CLIP (Clinical Learning Improvement Program, Sri Lanka) 22
CLS (Canine Laparoscopic Simulator) 372
CMT (California Milk Test) 292, 293, 294–295, **294**
coccygeal vein 227, **227**
cognitive task analysis (CTA) 370
colic 302, 313, 314, 373
collagen dressing **192**
Colmery, B. 360
combination dipstick **161**
communication skills 5, 6, **10**, 17, 18, 27, 381–382
    and OSCE 351, 353, 354
    and simulators 369, 371, 372, 373
computer-aided learning (CAL) 360, 361
conjunctiva 179
continuing professional development (CPD) 380
Control of Substances Hazardous to Health (COSHH, 2002) 204, 383
controlled ventilation 105, 106
coplin jar **153**, **154**
core knowledge 3
cornea/corneal reflex 178, 179
corticosteroids 168, 383

cows
    with calf 223
    coccygeal vein 227, **227**
    pain markers of 226
    placement of IV catheter for **175**
    and pregnancy assessments 6
    and sterile milk samples *see* milk samples, sterile
    and udder health *see* udder health
cows, handling 23, 219, 220, 224–225, **224**
    putting halter on 246–248, **246**, **247**, **248**
CPD (continuing professional development) 380
cranial nerve examination 173, 177–178
crystalloid fluid therapy *see* fluid therapy
CSCs *see* clinical skills centres
CTA (cognitive task analysis) 370
curriculum, outcome-based 2, 3, 9–14, 18–19
    and Day-One competency/skills 9, 10
    and development of CSC 12–14
    development of 9, 20–21
    and domains of clinical skills 10–11, **10**
    integration in 4, 12–14
    and learning theories/teaching skills 11, **11**
    and safe learning environment 14
    and simulators *see* simulation-based training
cystine **166**
cytology collection 133
cytotoxic drugs 204

DairySim (simulator) 373
Day-One competency/skills (D1C/D1S) 9, 10, 20, 23, 30, 148, 372, 377
    and large animals 292
    and OSCEs 331–332, 350
    patient handling/diagnostics 214
dazzle reflex 179
Debakey forceps 65
decubitus ulcers **94**, 383
deer 225
Defra (Department for Environment, Food and Rural Affairs) 203
dehiscence 70, **70**, 191, 383
deliberate practice 4, 9, 12
dentistry 113, 377, 384
    building competency in 359
    and CAL programmes 360, 361
    gap in teaching 359–361
    and OSCE in 362
    and periodontal disease/procedures 359, 361, 365, 385
dentistry simulator 359–366
    canine jaw model 362, **363**
    creating 361, **361**
    evaluating 361–363, **361**
    future prospects for 364–365
    and inter-professional education 365
    outcome of development of 365–366
    and role of instructors 364
    and student expectations 363–364

dentistry simulator (*continued*)
    and video-trained students 362–363, 364
    and visual acuity/sensory motor skills 363–364
    VR 364–365
Department for Environment, Food and Rural Affairs
    (Defra) 203
diagnostic imaging 249–271
    further reading on 259
    radiography *see* radiography
    ultrasound *see* ultrasound
diagnostics 10, **10**, 20, 27, 213–290
Diastix (urine dipstick) **161**
dioptic lens 179, 180, 218
disbudding 224, 384
disease control *see* aseptic procedures
disinfectants 33
dogs
    applying forelimb bandage to 194–196, **194**, **195**, **196**
    caudo-cranial stifle in **252**, **257**, 266–268, **266**, **267**, **268**
    in CSCs 23
    drug calculations for 208–209
    eye examination on 179–180
    handling 219, 220, 221
    hip dysplasia in 264–265
    imaging BVA/KC hips of 263–265, **263**, **264**, **265**
    intravenous catheter placement for **175**, 183–185, **183**, **184**
    intravenous catheter set-up for 186–189, **186**, **187**, **188**, **189**
    olfactory sense of 220–221
    sheep-224–225
    simulations 372, 373
Doppler 112
'doughnuts' (homemade bandages) 191, **193**
drains 71, 173
    see also tube/drain management
draping 30, 35
    four-quadrant technique for 47–48, **47**, **48**
ducks 222
Dundee (UK) 5
duodenum **260**, **262**
dystocia 384
    simulator **23**, 370, 373

ear bandages/dressings 190, 193, 200–202, **200**, **201**, **202**
Easifix (bandage) 197
echo-cardiography 379, 380
echocardiography 380, 384
echogenicity of organs 259, **260**, **261**, **262**, 384
Edinburgh (UK) 5
EDTA (ethylenediaminetetraacetic acid) 133, **143**, 144,
    152, 384
education–work transition 5, 376–382
Elastoplast 198, 242
elastration 225–226, **225**
electrolytes 175, 189
emotions in learning 4–5, 6, 9
EMS (extramural studies) placements 31, 32, 360, 364, 378

endoscopy 27, 384
endotracheal (ET) tube 109, **109**, **110**
enrofloxacin 208
eOSCE (software) 339
equine procedures 292, 298–317
    fluid therapy 304–308, **304**, **305**, **306**, **307**, **308**
    giving intramuscular injection 14, 301–302, 309, **310**, **311**
    giving intravenous injection 298–299
    passing nasogastric tube 302–303, 313–317
    placing intravenous catheter 300–301
    taking blood sample 298, 299–300
equine shoe removal 292, 318–328
    equipment for **321**
    from forelimb 318–319, **322**
    from hindlimb **322**
    and hoof anatomy 318, **319**, **321**
    method 322–324, **322**, **323**, **324**
    models for 319, **320**
    opportunities for practising 319
    and paring sole/trimming hoof wall 325–328, **325**, **326**,
        327, **328**
equine simulators 19, 27, **27**, 373
equine tarsus, radiography of 272–290
    and desensitizing horse's leg 273
    dorsolateral-palmaromedial oblique (DLPMO) view
        272, 276, **286**, 289, **289**
    dorsomedial-palmaromedial oblique (DMPLO) view
        272, 276
    dorsopalmar (DP) view 272, **273**, **275**, **277**, 279–280,
        279, **280**, **286**
    dorsoplantar view 288, **288**
    dorsoproximal-palmarodistal oblique views 281–283, **281**,
        282, **283**
    lateromedial (LM) view **273**, **275**, **277**, 278–279, **278**,
        279, 286–287, **287**
    opportunities for practising 274
    overview **277**
    palmaro-45°-proximal palmarodistal oblique view 283–285,
        284, **285**
    plantaro-45°-lateral dorsomedial (PLDMO) view 290, **290**
    and tarsus anatomy 273
    views/positions, help sheet for 275–276, **275**, **276**
ethylene oxide **52**, 53
ethylenediaminetetraacetic acid (EDTA) 133, **143**, 144,
    152, 384
euthanasia 299
evidence-based approach 2
Excel Pivot Table (software) 340
extramural studies (EMS) placements 31, 32, 360, 364, 378
eye examination *see* ophthalmic examination
eyelids 179
eyes
    canthus 179, 250, 299, 303, 383
    and depth of anaesthesia 110, **111**
    medications for **211**
    see also ophthalmic examination
eyesight 219–220

facial sensation 178
facial venous sinus 299, 300
faecal analysis 27, 128
    McMaster technique 159, 162, **162**, 167–168
farm visits 6
farriers 318, 319, 351
feedback, students' 5, 12, 19, 21, 22, 26, 334, 353, 358, 360, 368
Fibregee (bandage) 237
field teaching stations 20, 21
fine-needle aspirate biopsy (FNAB) 133, 140–141, **140**, **141**
Flamazine (dressing) **192**
flehmen response 220
Flexnerian curriculum 3, 384
fluid therapy 17, 175, 186–189, **188**, **189**
    equine 304–308, **304**, **305**, **306**, **307**, **308**
    equipment for 186–187, **186**, **187**, 304, **304**
fluoride oxalate **142**, 144, 384
fluoroscein dye 173
foot/hoof trimming
    goats 225
    horses 325–328, **325**, **326**, **327**, **328**
    sheep 338, **342**, 353
forceps
    artery **57**
    Debakey/haemostatic 65
    holding **57**, 58, **59**, **64**
    rat-tooth 65, **87**
    thumb *see* thumb forceps
formalin 133, 134
Fox, V. 373
fracture repair 27
fundic exam 180

gallbladder 134, **260**, **262**
Gamgee (bandage) 237, 242, 244
gastrointestinal tract (GIT) 302
General Medical Council (GMC) 3, 9
Giemsa–Wright stain 148
gloving techniques 27, 30, 43–46
    closed 35, 43–44, **43**, **44**
    open 35, 45–46, **45**, **46**
glucose 142, **161**
gluteal muscles 301, 302, 309, 311, **311**, 312
goats 225
good practice 30, 49, 91, 94, 128
    and Code of Conduct/SOPs 129–130
    see also health and safety; laboratory skills
Gopinath, D. 372
gowning techniques 27, 30, 41–42, **41**, **42**
    and colour coding 34
granny knot 60, 62
guinea pigs 222
gynaecology 20

haematology 133, 143, 144, 384
haematoma 299, 384
haemolysis 133, 137, **153**, 384
haemostatic forceps 65
haemostatic pressure bandage 192
Halstead's principles 63
halters/haltering 246–248, **246**, **247**, **248**
Hammick, M. 370
hamsters 219
hamstrings 309, 311, **311**
hand drying 34, 39–40, **39**, **40**
hand washing 34, 130
    OSCE assessment 351, 355
handling/restraint 10, 17, 20, 24, 27, 171, 217–248
    and animal behaviour 218–219
    and animals' sensory perception 219–221
    and flight distance 219, 222
    further reading on 228
    future ideas for 227–228
    and handler behaviour 219, 223
    and human facial expressions 219
    and human voice 219, 223
    of large animals *see* large animal handling skills
    and pain 218, 219, 225–226
    PAWS system for 218
    practising with manikins 218, 226–227, **226**, **227**
    of small animals *see* small animals handling skills
    and stress 218, 219, 221, 222
    TREAT policy for 219
    welfare issues with 225–228
Hanson, C. 361
Haptic Cow 6, 371
Haptic Horse 373
Harden, R.M. 331
Hartmann's solution 113, **187**
health and safety 49, 65, 95, 129–130, 204
    and personal protective equipment (PPE) 130, 162, 221, 225
Health and Safety at Work Act (1974) 204
hearing, animals' sense of 220
heart
    monitoring 111, 113, 172, 259
    post mortem examination of 134
    and stress 218
    and ultrasound 259, **260**, **261**
Hebridean sheep 225
heifers 223
hep-saline 183, 184, **187**, 189
heparin 133, 384
Hodges, B. 365
horses
    colic in 302, 313, 314, 373
    and human voice 219, 223, 234
    intramuscular (IM) injection in 292
    models/simulators 19, 27, **27**, **316**
    pain markers/facial expressions of 226
    paring soles/trimming hoof walls of 325–328, **325**, **326**, **327**, **328**

horses (*continued*)
    and placement of IV catheter **175**
    and radiography **13**, 275–276, **275**, **276**
    radiography of foot *see* equine tarsus, radiography of
    removing shoes from *see* equine shoe removal
    taking blood sample from 292
    see also equine procedures
horses, handling 23, 219, 220, 223–224
    applying lower limb bandage 241–245, **241**, **242**, **243**,
        244, **245**
    applying stable bandage 237–240, **237**, **238**, **239**
    applying tail bandage **13**, 234–236, **234**, **235**, **236**
    and OSCE assessment 336–337, **337**
    rugging up 229–231, **229**, **230**, **231**
    tying up **232–233**
Humphrey breathing system 106, 107
hydration status 148, 175, 182
hydrocolloid dressing **182**
hydrogel dressing **192**
hydrogen peroxide **52**, 53
hypodermic syringes/needles 27, **131**, 137–139, **137**, **138**, 292
    safe use of 204
    see also intramuscular (IM) injection; intravenous (IV) injection
hypovolaemia 175, 384
hypoxia 97, 384

iatrogenic injuries 191
ileum **250**, **260**
injections, giving *see* hypodermic syringes/needles
inter-professional education (IPE) 365
intermittent positive pressure ventilation (IPPV) 106
internal medicine 20, 380
intramuscular (IM) injection 292, 298, 301–302
    equipment required for 301
    for gluteals 302, 311, **311**, 312
    for hamstrings 311, **311**
    for neck 302, 310, **310**, 312
    for pectorals 301, 309, 310, **310**
    sites for 301, 309–312
intravenous catheter (IVC) 298, 300–301
    equipment required for placing 300
    and euthanasia 299
    fluid set-up 175, 186–189, **186**, **187**, **188**, **189**
    method of placing 301
    placement **13**, 27, 175, **175**, 183–185, **183**, **184**
    preparation for placing 300
intravenous (IV) injection 292, 298–299
    avoiding carotid artery in 300
    equipment for 299
    sites for 299
intubation 105, 109–110, **109**, 378–379
    alternatives options to 110
    choosing size of tube 109, **110**
IPPV (intermittent positive pressure ventilation) 106
iris 179
iris diaphragm 146, **146**, **151**

isoflurane 100, 113
isothenuria **160**
isotonic crystalloid solutions 175, 384
Issenberg, S.B. 360, 368
IVC *see* intravenous catheter

Jasinevicius, T.R. 365
jaw tone test 178
Jordan University of Science and Technology (JUST) 26–29
Journal of Veterinary Medical Education (JVME) 371, 372
jugular vein 299

Keto-diastix (urine dipstick) **161**
ketones **161**, 384
Ketostix (urine dipstick) **161**
kidneys **260**, **262**
Kirkpatrick's four levels of evaluation 370
Kneebone, Roger 368
Knitfix (bandage) 194, 197, 200, **242**
knots 5, 27, 30, 60–63
    Aberdeen 63, 70, 71
    granny 60, 62
    instrument tie 61
    modified miller's/strangle 61–62
    number of throws 60–61
    one-handed tie 61, 73, **73–77**, 77
    practising with ultrasound gel 85
    quick-release **232–233**
    security 65, 85
    slip (half-hitch) 60, 62, 63
    square 60, 61, 62, 85, **89–91**
    surgeon's 60, 61, 71
    and suture material 61
    two-handed tie 61, 78, **78–84**, 85
Kolb, D.A. 368
KY jelly 303

laboratory skills 17, 129–132
    and appropriate attire 130
    and appropriate conduct 130
    and disposal of consumables *see* waste disposal
    and personal protective equipment (PPE) 130
    sample collection *see* sample collection
Lack breathing system 106, 107, 114, **114–116**, 126
lambing 218, 219
lambs 225
    manikin, for elastration practice 225–226, **225**
laparoscopy 371, 384
    simulator for 372
large animal handling skills 23, 222–225, 292
    and bottle-fed species 223
    camelids 225
    cattle *see* cows, handling
    deer 225

goats 225
and group characteristics 219, 220, 222
horses *see* horses, handling
pigs 225
protective equipment for 223
safety tips for 223
sheep 219, 220, 222–223, 224–225
large animal skills 291–328
laryngoscope 109–110
larynx 66, **314**
learning theories/principles 2, 3
Lifelong Independent Veterinary Education (LIVE) Centre 5
Lincoln Memorial University (USA) 18–20, **19**
lithium heparin 133
liver 68, **260**, **262**
mass removal operation on 380
llamas 225
local anaesthetic 298
Low-Beer, N. 369
Lumbis, R. 36
lymph nodes 133, 133–134, 260, **262**

Macluskey, M. 361
McMaster technique 159, 162, **162**, 167–168
Magill breathing system 106, 107, 126
Management of Health & Safety at Work Regulations (1999) 204
manikins *see* simulators
manuka honey dressing 192
mastitis 292, 293, 384
May–Grunwald–Giemsa (stain) 148
meatus anatomy 314, **314**
medetomidine 112
Medicines (Labelling) Regulations (1976) 206
Melolin **241**
menace response 179
mentoring 379–380
mice 221
microhaematocrit tubes *see* capillary tubes
microscopes 128, 145–158
care of 147
components of **146**
further reading on 148
and oil immersion 146–147
and PCV measurement 133, 148, 156–158, **156**, **157**
procedure following use of 147
setting up 149–151, **149**, **150**, **151**
and stain use 27, 148, 152–154, **152**, **153**, **154**
techniques for viewing slides 145–146, **147**
and urinalysis 162, 165–166, **165**, **166**
and Vernier scale 147, **147**
milk samples, sterile **13**, 293–296
bovine sterile milk sampling method 293, 296
and California Milk Test (CMT) 292, 293, 294–295, **294**
key points for 293
and somatic cell count (SCC) 294
Miller's assessment pyramid 332, **332**

Miller's pyramid of competency 11, 359, **360**
mini-Lack breathing system 107, 126
minimum alveolar concentration (MAC) 100
Misuse of Drugs Act/Regulations (1971) 203, 205
modified miller's knot 61–62
Mongolian Veterinary School 20, **21**
mosquito haemostats 71
myasthenia gravis 377, 384–385
myoglobin **160**, **161**, 385

nasogastric tube 292, 298, 302–303, 313–317
anatomical considerations with 302
common problems with 314
equipment for passing 302, 315, **315**
and meatus anatomy 314, **314**
other uses for 314
simulator for 313–316, **315**, **316**
nasopharynx 303
needle holders 62, 63–64, 67, 70
grips for 63–64, **64**
handling **57**, 58, 63–64, **64**, **86**
suturing with 87–90
nerve blocks 113, 385
neurological system **172**
New Methylene Blue (stain) 148
nictitating membrane/third eyelid 179
Niemiec, B.A. 364
nitrous oxide 97
no-touch method 204
NOVICE project 374
'Novice to Master' model 11, **11**
nystagmus 178

OBE (Outcome-Based Education) 9
obstetrics 20
ocular reflexes 177, 179
oesophagostomy tube 71, 385
oesophagus 303, 317
off-label medication 205
olfaction 177, 220–221
olfactory stations 227
ophthalmic examination **13**, 173, 177, 178, 179–180
direct/indirect 180
ophthalmoscope **13**, 173, 179, 180, 218
Orthoband (bandage) 183, 194, **194**, 197, 200, 242
orthopnea **172**, 385
OSCE (objectively structured clinical examination) 16, 27, 330, 331–356, 377
and alternative methods 334, 335
and analysis of marks 339–341, **340**, **341**, **342**
authors of/expertise in 350
and bias, overcoming 343
and blueprinting assessment 332–333, **332**, 350
and checklists 333–337, 338, 339–340, 342–343, 362
and checklists, errors in 338, **338**

OSCE (*continued*)
    and chunking of items 333, 334, 336
    circuit of stations 346–347, **347**, **348**, **356**
    and Day One skills 331–332, 333, 350
    in dentistry 362
    dilemmas in assessment 339
    equipment/consumables for 351
    and exam infrastructure 350–351
    and maps/layouts of sites 351, 352
    and Optical Mark Reading (OMR) process 334, 339, 340
    and order of performing actions 334–336, **336**
    percentage of students performing each item 336–337
    planning/setting up 351–352
    and precise terminology 336
    and red line actions 337–338
    role of 349
    selection of stations for 347–348
    selection/training of assessors for 348–349
    siting of 249–250
    and standard setting 341–343, **343**
    station grading sheet, example of 332, 333, **345**
    subjective judgement in 332, 338, 339, 341–342, 343
    timeline for 352–354
    timing of, in students' career 349
    training of students for 349
    use of simulators in 333
    and weighting of items 333–334, 336–337, 338, 339
OSCEOnline 339
osmolality **160**
ovaries **260**, **262**, 372
ovariohysterectomy 371, 372

packed cell volume (PCV) testing 133, 148, 156–158,
    156, **157**
pain 113, 218, 219, 225–226
palpebral reflex 178, 179
pancreas **260**, **262**
parasites, detecting *see* faecal analysis
PAWS (pause/assess/welfare/seek assistance) system 218
pectoral muscles 301, 309, 310, **310**
pedagogy 3–6, 385
    and active learning 2, 3–4, 9
    and clinical skills centres *see* clinical skills centres
    and curriculum *see* curriculum, veterinary
    and deliberate practice 4, 9
    and feedback 5
    and integrated skills 4, 6
    and simulators/models *see* simulation-based training
    and student anxiety 4–5, 6
peer-assisted learning 371
Penrose drain 71
periodontal disease/procedures 359, 361, 365, 385
peritoneal tap 133, 385
personal protective equipment (PPE) 130, 162, 221, 225
Peyton's four-stage model 11, **11**
pharmacy 170, 203–211

and '5 rights' 207–208
    cytotoxic drugs 204
    dispensing/labelling 205–206, **207**
    drug calculations 208, **210**
    further reading on 211
    and health and safety 204
    and legislation 203
    off-label medication 205
    online resources for 209
    prescribing/dispensing categories 205, **205**
    prescriptions 206–207, **207**
    record keeping/stock control/storage 204
    and regulation of premises 203
    and routes of administration 209, **210**, **211**
    and schedules of controlled drugs 205, **206**
    and waste disposal 204–205
pharynx 178, **316**
pheromones 220
physical examination 170, 171–173
    cranial nerve 173, 177–178
    further reading on 176
    ophthalmic 173, 177, 178, 179–180
    and safe handling/patient welfare 171
    triage 172, **172**
pigs 225
pneumothorax 97, 133, 253, 385
polydioxanone (PDS) suture 61, 67, **67**, **68**, 380
portosystemic shunt **68**, 385
post-mortem 134
povidone–iodine 33
PPE (personal protective equipment) 130, 162, 221, 225
preclinical–clinical divide 3, 6
pregnancy assessments 6
prescriptions 206–207, **207**
propofol 113
prostate **260**, **262**
    palpation simulation 372
pulse, feeling for 111, **111**
pulse oximeter 112
pupillary light reflex (PLR)/pupil size 177, 179
Putter, G. 359

QMHA (Queen Mother Hospital for Animals) 218
Queen's Veterinary School Hospital Pauline Brown Clinical Skills
    Centre (Cambridge) 22–25, **24**

rabbits **175**, 220, 222
racehorses 20
radiography 10, **13**, 17, 27, 249–256, 378
    and animal movement 250–251
    BVA/KC hips imaging 263–265, **263**, **264**, **265**
    caudo-cranial stifle imaging **252**, **257**, 266–268, **266**,
        267, **268**
    and collimation 265, 383
    and contrast 251, **251**, **252**

and digital artefacts 253–254, **254**, **255**, **256**, **257**, **258**

of equine foot *see* equine tarsus, radiography of

and exposure 251, **253**

and film faults 250–251, **250**, **251**

and film marks 254–255, **256**

further reading on 259

positioning, terminology/guidelines for 249–250, 272, 275–276, **275**, **276**

PPE for 130, 272

safety points for 272

rams 220, 225

rat-tooth forceps 65, **87**

rats 220, 221

RCVS (Royal College of Veterinary Surgeons) 9, 203, 205, 211, 360

Read, E.K. 370, 371, 373, 374

rectal palpation models 19, 27, 373

reflux 314

refractometer 160–161, **160**, 163, **163**

reindeer 225

reptiles 133

respiratory system **172**, 174–175

Robert Jones bandage 192

rodents, handling 220, 221, 222

Romanowsky stain 148

Rondopad (dressing material) 194, 197

Royal Pharmaceutical Society 205

Royal Veterinary College (RVC) 5, 6, 12–14, **13**, 16, 219, 227

CSC at 16–18, **17**, 32, 298

and dentistry 360, 365

Ethics Committee 361

MSc in Veterinary Education 366

OSCEs at 330, 346, 347, **348**

QMHA at 218

RVNs (Registered Veterinary Nurses) *see* veterinary nurses/technicians

sample collection 132–144

blood *see* blood samples

cytology 133

FNAB 133, 140–141, **140**, **141**

packing/posting 134, 142–144, **142**, **143**, **144**

post-mortem 134

sample collection tubes **142–143**

see also blood collection tubes

Scalese, R.J. 368

scalpels/scalpel blades 51, **131**

handling **58**, **59**, 65, **66**

SCC (somatic cell count) 294, 385

Schirmer tear test strips 173

Schön, D. 359

Schönwetter, D.J. 360

scissors, handling **58**, 65

scrubbed personnel 32, 52

scrubbing techniques 27, 30, 33–34, 37–38, **37**, **38**

and disinfectants/antiseptics 33

and drying hands 34, 39–40, **39**, **40**

variety of applications for 34

scrubs, surgical (attire) 33, 385

SDC (Swiss Agency for Development and Cooperation) 20

self-directed learning 2

sensory perception of animals 219–221

septic thrombophlebitis 301, 385

sevoflurane 100, 113

sharps 49, 51, 130, **131**, 204

sheep

foot trim 338, **342**, 353

lambing 218, 219

rams 220, 225

see also lambs

sheep, handling 219, 220, 222–223, 224–225

and OSCE assessment 339

sheepdogs 224–225

Sheffield (UK) 5

silver antimicrobial dressings **192**

Simulated Fertility Visit 373

simulators 5–6, 9, 12, 18, **19**, **27**, 358, 368–374

benefits of 16, 368–369

and blood withdrawal 27, 227, **227**

bovine 372–373

bovine dystocia **23**, 370, 373

Breed'n Betsy 372

Canine Laparoscopic Simulator 372

challenges of 369

computer-hybrid 369, 370

computer-only 37

contextualized 373

and Day One Competences 368

defined 368

and dentistry *see* dentistry simulator

designing 370

for different levels of training **13**, 14

for elastration practice 226–227, **226**

equine 19, 27, **27**, 373

future prospects for 373–374

Haptic Cow 6, 371, 372–373

haptic devices in 370

human 371

for laparoscopic surgery skills 371

online developers/groups 374

for ovariohysterectomy 371, 372

pedagogy with 371

and peer-assisted learning 371

prostate palpation 37

research/creation of new models 19–20

small animal 371–372

types of 369–370

and validity/evaluation 370, 372

and Zone of Proximal Development 369

Simuldog 372

skills assessment 16, 20

see also OSCE

slaughterhouse simulator 373
slip knot 60, 62, 63
small animal handling skills 221–222
    and cages/vivaria 221
    and OSCE assessment 339
    protective equipment for 221
Soffban (bandage) 186, 194, 195, 201
somatic cell count (SCC) 294, 385
spaying 50, 62, 379, 380
sphygmomanometer 112, 385
spleen **260**, **262**
Sri Lanka 21–22, **23**
Standard Operating Procedures (SOPs) 130
Steinberg, A.D. 364
sterilizing surgical instruments 51–53
    expiration dates 53
    manual cleaning 51
    methods for, advantages/disadvantages of **52**
    monitoring 52–53
    packing for 52
    ultrasonic baths 51–52
    washer/disinfectors 52
steroids *see* corticosteroids
stethoscope, oesophageal 111, **112**
stomach **260**, **262**, 303, 317
    suturing 69–70
strabismus 177
strangle/modified miller's knot 61–62
stress 14, 16, 172, 218
struvite (triple phosphate) **166**
supravital stains 148
surgeon's knot 60, 61, 71
surgical instruments 30, 49–59
    care/maintenance of 49, 52
    further reading on 53
    handling/selection 57–59, **57–59**, 63–65
    health and safety issues with 49, 65
    materials in manufacture of 50
    opening pouch 50–51, 54–56, **54–55**
    practising handling of 49
    sets of, familiarity with 50
    sharps 49, 51, 130
    sterilization procedure *see* sterilizing surgical instruments
    for suturing *see under* suturing
    trolley, placing/removing from 51
surgical rotations 377, 381
surgical scrubs (attire) 33, 385
surgical scrubs (washing) *see* scrubbing techniques
surgical theatre skills 6, 10, 17, 18, 29–91
    aseptic procedures *see* aseptic procedures
    attire for 33
    and breach in sterility 33
    and circulating staff 32
    draping patient/surgical area *see* draping
    drying hands 34, 39–40, **39**, **40**
    further reading on 36
    gloving *see* gloving techniques

gowning *see* gowning techniques
    models for 20, 25
    opportunities for students to practice 31, 32
    and roles in theatre 32–33
    and scrubbed personnel 32, 52
    scrubbing up *see* scrubbing techniques
    teamwork in 32–33
    see also suturing
suture materials 61, 66–67, **86**, 380
    choosing, practical tips for 66, 67
    classification systems for 66
    qualities of **66**, **67**
    and tissue type **68**
suture needles 51, 67–69, **69**, **131**
    care with 67
    round-bodied/cutting 68–69
    swaged-on/eyed 67–68
suture patterns 69–71
    appositional/inverting/everting 69
    continuous/interrupted 69, 70, **70**
    one-layer/two-layer closure 69–70
    starting/finishing 70
    tension-relieving 70
suturing 27, 30, 60–91, 378–379
    absorbable/non-absorbable 65
    Chinese finger-trap 71
    choosing patterns *see* suture patterns
    coming up through incision **87**, 91
    and dehiscence 70, **70**, 191, 383
    in drains 71
    and haemostatic forceps 65
    and Halstead's principles 63
    instrument 86, **86–91**, 91
    and instrument handling 63–65
    knot techniques *see* knots
    and needle holders *see* needle holders
    and surgical dead space 63, 385
    and thumb forceps *see* thumb forceps
swallowing gag reflex 178
Sweden 25–26, **26**

T-piece breathing system *see* Ayres T-piece
    breathing system
tablet counters 204
tail docking 226–227, **226**
tail vein 227, **227**, 299
Tapia-Araya, A.E. 372
temporal muscle mass 178
tetracyclines **160**, 385
theriogenology 27
thoracic cavity 133, 134
thoracic vein, lateral 299, 300
thoracocentesis 385
    simulator 371–372
thoracostomy tube 174
3Rs (Replacement/Reduction/Refinement) 19

thumb forceps 64–65
    handling **57**, **59**, **64**
Tomorrow's Doctors (GMC) 3, 9
tongue 178
touch, animals' sense of 219
trachea 303, 317
tracheostomy tube 174–175, 385
TREAT (time/restraint/equipment/assistance/training) policy 219
triage examination 172, **172**
tube/drain management 170, 173–175
    abdominal drain 173
    fluid set-up 175
    IV catheters *see* intravenous (IV) catheter
    thoracostomy tube 174
    tracheostomy tube 174–175, 385
    urethral catheter 173–174
turkeys 222
twitches 302

udder health 293–296
    and mastitis 292, 293, 384
    and milk samples *see* milk samples, sterile
ulcers 66, **94**, 383
ultrasound 27, 256–259, 379
    echogenicity/echotexture of organs on 259, **260**, **261**, **262**
    further reading on 259
    knobs/buttons on 258, **262**
    organs examined using 259
    physics of 256–257
    set-up 269–271, **269**, **270**, **271**
    transducer movements 258, **261**
United States (USA) 3, 9, 18–20, **19**
upper respiratory tract 174
urethral catheter 173–174
    and assessment of urinary output 181–182, **181**, **182**
urinalysis 27, 128, 159–162
    and appearance/odour of sample 159, **160**
    dipstick analysis 159, 161, **161**, 163–164, **164**
    further reading on 162
    key terms in **160**
    microscope analysis 162, 165–166, **165**, **166**
    preparation/equipment for 161
    and refractive index (RI) 159
    and refractometer 160–161, **160**, 163, **163**
    and specific gravity (SG) 159, **160**, 163, **163**
    and urine crystals **160**, 162, 165, **166**
urinary bladder 134, **260**, **262**
urine scalding 173, 174

Uristix (urine dipstick) **161**
urobilinogen **161**, 385
Usón-Gargallo, J. 372
uterus **260**, **262**, 372, 373

Vacutainer system 129, 135–138, **135**, 300
vacuum-insulated evaporator (VIE) 97
venepuncture 385
    see also blood samples; catheterization; hypodermic
        syringes/needles
Vernier scale 147, **147**
veterinary clinical skills model 358, 359–366
    and dental procedures 359–361
    and framework of competency 359, **360**
    and gap in practical teaching 359–361
'Veterinary Clinical Skills and Simulation' group 374
Veterinary Medicines Directorate (VMD) 203, 205, 207, 211
Veterinary Medicines Regulation (VMR) 203
veterinary nurses/technicians 6, 31, 32, 129, 359–360, 378
veterinary school graduate, reflections of 358, 376–382
Veterinary Simulator Industries (VSI) 373
veterinary surgeons/surgery 32, 359, 380
Vetrap (bandage) 186, 194, 197, 198, 199, 200,
    242, 245
volatile anaesthetic 96, 97, 99–100, 105, 106, 385
vomeronasal organ 220
Vygotsky's Zone of Proximal Development (ZPD) 369

waste disposal 130–132, 204–205
    clinical waste 130–131
    cytotoxics 131, 204
    general waste 131–132
    pharmaceuticals 130
    sharps 130, **131**, 204
Williamson, J.A. 371–372
World Organization for Animal Health 9
wound management 191, 192–193, **192**
    see also bandages/dressings
Wrights–Giemsa stain 148

X-rays *see* radiography

Zone of Proximal Development (ZPD) 369
zoonotic diseases/hazards 129, 134, 385
Zorbopad (dressing material) 194